# Breast Cancer

*Editor*

LISA A. NEWMAN

# SURGICAL ONCOLOGY CLINICS OF NORTH AMERICA

www.surgonc.theclinics.com

*Consulting Editor*
NICHOLAS J. PETRELLI

July 2014 • Volume 23 • Number 3

**ELSEVIER**

1600 John F. Kennedy Boulevard ● Suite 1800 ● Philadelphia, Pennsylvania, 19103-2899

http://www.theclinics.com

**SURGICAL ONCOLOGY CLINICS OF NORTH AMERICA Volume 23, Number 3
July 2014 ISSN 1055-3207, ISBN-13: 978-0-323-31173-1**

Editor: Jessica McCool
Developmental Editor: Stephanie Carter

*Surgical Oncology Clinics of North America* (ISSN 1055-3207) is published quarterly by Elsevier Inc., 360 Park Avenue South, New York, NY 10010-1710. Months of publication are January, April, July, and October. Business and Editorial Offices: 1600 John F. Kennedy Blvd., Ste. 1800, Philadelphia, PA 19103-2899. Customer Service Office: 3251 Riverport Lane, Maryland Heights, MO 63043. Periodicals postage paid at New York, NY and additional mailing offices. Subscription prices are $290.00 per year (US individuals), $421.00 (US institutions) $140.00 (US student/resident), $330.00 (Canadian individuals), $533.00 (Canadian institutions), $205.00 (Canadian student/resident), $410.00 (foreign individuals), $533.00 (foreign institutions), and $205.00 (foreign student/resident). Foreign air speed delivery is included in all *Clinics* subscription prices. All prices are subject to change without notice. **POSTMASTER**: Send address changes to *Surgical Oncology Clinics of North America,* Elsevier Health Science Division, Subscription Customer Service, 3251 Riverport Lane, Maryland Heights, MO 63043. **Customer Service: 1-800-654-2452 (US and Canada). 314-447-8871 (outside US and Canada). Fax: 314-447-8029. E-mail:** journalscustomerservice-usa@elsevier.com (for print support); journalsonline support-usa@elsevier.com (for online support).

*Reprints.* For copies of 100 or more, of articles in this publication, please contact the Commercial Reprints Department, Elsevier Inc., 360 Park Avenue South, New York, New York 10010-1710. Tel. 212-633-3874; Fax: 212-633-3820; E-mail: reprints@elsevier.com.

*Surgical Oncology Clinics of North America* is covered in *MEDLINE/PubMed (Index Medicus)* and *EMBASE/ Excerpta Medica, Current Contents/Clinical Medicine, and ISI/BIOMED.*

# Contributors

## CONSULTING EDITOR

### NICHOLAS J. PETRELLI, MD, FACS
Bank of America Endowed Medical Director, Helen F. Graham Cancer Center at Christiana Care, Newark, Delaware; Professor of Surgery, Thomas Jefferson University, Philadelphia, Pennsylvania

## EDITOR

### LISA A. NEWMAN, MD, MPH, FACS, FASCO
Professor of Surgery; Director, Breast Care Center, University of Michigan Comprehensive Cancer Center, Ann Arbor, Michigan

## AUTHORS

### PRASANNA ALLURI, MD, PhD
Research Fellow, Department of Radiation Oncology, University of Michigan, Ann Arbor, Michigan

### TIFFANY NICOLE S. BALLARD, MD
Section of Plastic Surgery, Department of General Surgery, University of Michigan Health System, Ann Arbor, Michigan

### KRISTEN A. BAN, MD
Department of Surgery, Loyola University, Maywood, Illinois

### JESSICA BENSENHAVER, MD
Assistant Professor, Department of Surgery, University of Michigan Health System, Ann Arbor, Michigan

### ABIGAIL S. CAUDLE, MD, MS
Department of Surgical Oncology, The University of Texas MD Anderson Cancer Center, Houston, Texas

### ANEES B. CHAGPAR, MD, MSc, MPH, MA, FRCS(C), FACS
Director, The Breast Center – Smilow Cancer Hospital at Yale-New Haven; Associate Professor, Department of Surgery, Yale University School of Medicine, New Haven, Connecticut

### JULIE A. CUPP, MD
Department of Surgical Oncology, The University of Texas MD Anderson Cancer Center, Houston, Texas

### AMY E. CYR, MD, FACS
Assistant Professor, Department of Surgery, Washington University School of Medicine, St Louis, Missouri

**CONSTANTINE V. GODELLAS, MD, FACS**
Department of Surgery, Loyola University, Maywood, Illinois

**KELLY K. HUNT, MD, FACS**
Hamill Foundation Distinguished Professor of Surgery in Honor of Dr. Richard G. Martin, Sr.; Chief, Surgical Breast Oncology, Department of Surgical Oncology, The University of Texas MD Anderson Cancer Center, Houston, Texas

**ISMAIL JATOI, MD, PhD**
Division Chief, Division of Surgical Oncology & Endocrine Surgery, Department of Surgery, University of Texas Health Science Center San Antonio, San Antonio, Texas

**TARI A. KING, MD**
Associate Attending Surgeon, Breast Service, Department of Surgery; Jeanne A. Petrek Junior Faculty Chair, Memorial Sloan-Kettering Cancer Center; Associate Professor of Surgery, Weill Medical College of Cornell University, New York, New York

**HENRY M. KUERER, MD, PhD**
Department of Surgical Oncology, The University of Texas MD Anderson Cancer Center, Houston, Texas

**CHRISTINE LARONGA, MD, FACS**
Comprehensive Breast Program, Department of Women's Oncology, Moffitt Cancer Center; Department of Surgery, University of South Florida, Tampa, Florida

**MEEGHAN A. LAUTNER, MD**
Resident, Department of Surgery, University of Texas Health Science Center San Antonio, San Antonio, Texas

**JULIE A. MARGENTHALER, MD, FACS**
Associate Professor, Department of Surgery, Washington University School of Medicine, St Louis, Missouri

**ASHLEY C. MCGINITY, MD**
Resident, Department of Surgery, University of Texas Health Science Center San Antonio, San Antonio, Texas

**ADEYIZA O. MOMOH, MD**
Section of Plastic Surgery, Department of General Surgery, University of Michigan Health System, Ann Arbor, Michigan

**MONICA MORROW, MD**
Chief, Breast Service, Department of Surgery, Evelyn H. Lauder Breast Center, Anne Burnett Windfohr Chair of Clinical Oncology, Memorial Sloan-Kettering Cancer Center; Professor of Surgery, Weill Medical College of Cornell University, New York, New York

**LISA A. NEWMAN, MD, MPH, FACS, FASCO**
Professor of Surgery; Director, Breast Care Center, University of Michigan Comprehensive Cancer Center, Ann Arbor, Michigan

**MELISSA PILEWSKIE, MD**
Assistant Attending Surgeon, Breast Service, Department of Surgery, Evelyn H. Lauder Breast Center, Memorial Sloan-Kettering Cancer Center, New York, New York

**JORGE S. REIS-FILHO, MD, PhD, FRCPath**
Member and Attending Pathologist; Affiliate Member, Human Oncology and Pathogenesis Program; Department of Pathology, Memorial Sloan-Kettering Cancer Center, New York, New York

**MICHAEL S. SABEL, MD, FACS**
Associate Professor, Department of Surgery, University of Michigan, Ann Arbor, Michigan

**PAUL SMITH, MD**
Department of Surgery, University of South Florida, Tampa, Florida

**MEDIGET TESHOME, MD**
Department of Surgical Oncology, The University of Texas MD Anderson Cancer Center, Houston, Texas

**DAVID P. WINCHESTER, MD**
Medical Director, Cancer Programs, American College of Surgeons, Chicago, Illinois; Department of Surgery, NorthShore University HealthSystem, Evanston Hospital, Evanston, Illinois

# Contents

This article outlines the current incidence, prevalence, and mortality of breast cancer and reviews the epidemiology of the disease. Major risk factors for the development of breast cancer are covered, including reproductive, genetic, and environmental variables. Understanding the epidemiology of breast cancer will help clinicians identify high-risk patients for appropriate screening and informed disease management decisions.

With increasing public awareness of the risk for breast cancer and modern techniques of reconstruction, the option of surgical prophylaxis for risk reduction is becoming increasingly popular. Bilateral prophylactic mastectomy for women at increased risk of developing breast cancer and contralateral prophylactic mastectomy for those with unilateral breast cancer seeking symmetry, risk reduction, and ease of follow-up are acceptable options for many women. However, prophylactic surgery is not an inconsequential decision, and careful consideration should be given to the risks and benefits of such procedures.

This article reviews the relevant data on breast magnetic resonance imaging (MRI) use in screening, the short-term surgical outcomes and long-term cancer outcomes associated with the use of MRI in breast cancer staging, the use of MRI in occult primary breast cancer, as well as MRI to assess eligibility for accelerated partial breast irradiation and to evaluate tumor response after neoadjuvant chemotherapy. MRI for screening is supported in specific high-risk populations, namely, women with BRCA1 or BRCA2 mutations, a family history suggesting a hereditary breast cancer syndrome, or a history of chest wall radiation.

Breast cancer is now considered a heterogeneous and phenotypically diverse disease. Molecular profiling is used in clinical practice in 2 broad categories: (1) characterization of breast cancers beyond the standard histopathologic features such as tumor grade, histologic subtype, and biomarker profile for prognostic information; and (2) prediction of response to therapy and clinical outcome. This article addresses the importance and application of molecular subtype analysis, and provides an in-depth analysis of the clinical application of the molecular prognostic indices for ductal carcinoma in situ, node-negative invasive breast cancer, and node-positive invasive breast cancer.

For patients with primary breast cancer, nodal status remains a key determinant for overall prognosis. Sentinel lymph node biopsy (SLNB) has become standard care for staging patients who have clinically node-negative disease. However, a new dilemma has arisen: how to manage the clinically negative axilla in patients with ipsilateral breast tumor recurrences (IBTRs). Are outcomes in these patients improved with repeat SLNB? Although observational studies suggest SLNB is feasible in patients with IBTR and a clinically node-negative axilla, the overall impact on morality and local recurrence is not yet known as no randomized trials have addressed this issue.

The presence of nodal metastases is the most important prognostic indicator in breast cancer, making accurate assessment of the axillary nodal basin critical to delivering optimal therapy in breast cancer. Clinically node-negative women can be reliably staged in a minimally invasive manner using sentinel lymph node dissection (SLND). In node-negative patients receiving neoadjuvant chemotherapy, SLND can be performed after chemotherapy, allowing for a single surgical procedure and a decreased probability of requiring axillary lymph node dissection (ALND). Clinically node-positive patients are currently recommended to undergo ALND, although these recommendations may change with emerging trial data.

Lobular neoplasia (LN) is characterized by a dysfunctional E-cadherin-catenin axis, and loss of E-cadherin plays a causative role in the typical morphology of LN cells. LN is both a nonobligate precursor and a risk indicator of invasive breast cancer, and in particular, of invasive lobular carcinoma. Despite the evidence supporting the precursor role of LN, its impact on clinical management has been a matter of controversy, and conservative management remains the mainstay of treatment. In this article, an update is provided on the pathology and genetics of LN, and the management of these lesions in surgical practice is discussed.

Neoadjuvant systemic therapy in breast cancer treatment was initially utilized for inoperable disease. However, several randomized prospective studies have demonstrated comparable survival with adjuvant chemotherapy in early-stage, operable breast cancer while also decreasing tumor size facilitating breast conservation without significant increases in local recurrence. Response to therapy can predict outcome, with improved survival associated with pathologic complete response (pCR). Triple negative and HER2-positive subtypes show increased pCR rates. A multidisciplinary approach is necessary with neoadjuvant treatment. This can improve rates of breast conservation, provide insights into tumor biology and predict patient outcomes.

biologically more aggressive pattern of disease. The two terms, however, are not synonymous, and some TNBC cases are prognostically more favorable. TNBC differs from non-TNBC in risk-factor profile, pattern, and rate of metastatic spread.

African American women have a lower lifetime incidence of breast cancer than white/Caucasian Americans yet have a higher risk of breast cancer mortality. African American women are also more likely to be diagnosed with breast cancer at young ages, and they have higher risk for the biologically more aggressive triple-negative breast cancers. These features are also more common among women from western, sub-Saharan Africa who share ancestry with African Americans, and this prompts questions regarding an association between African ancestry and inherited susceptibility for certain patterns of mammary carcinogenesis.

The surgical management of breast cancer has evolved significantly, facilitated by advancements in technology and imaging and improvements in adjuvant therapy. The changes in surgical management have been characterized by equal or improved outcomes with significantly less morbidity. The next step in this evolution is the minimally invasive or noninvasive ablation of breast cancers as an alternative to lumpectomy. In this article, the various modalities for nonsurgical breast cancer ablation and the clinical experience are reviewed, and some of the next steps necessary for their clinical implementation are outlined.

Evidence has shown that multidisciplinary specialist team evaluation and management for cancer results in better patient outcomes. For breast cancer, breast centers are where this evaluation and management occurs. The National Accreditation Program for Breast Centers has helped standardize multidisciplinary breast cancer care by defining services and standards required of accredited breast centers.

# SURGICAL ONCOLOGY
# CLINICS OF NORTH AMERICA

**RELATED INTEREST**

*Radiologic Clinics of North America,* May 2014 (Vol. 52, Issue 3)
**Breast Imaging**
Christopher E. Comstock and Cecilia L. Mercado, *Editors*
Available at: http://www.radiologic.theclinics.com/

DOWNLOAD
Free App!

*Review Articles*
THE CLINICS

**NOW AVAILABLE FOR YOUR iPhone and iPad**

# Foreword
# Breast Cancer

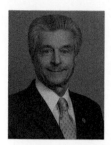

Nicholas J. Petrelli, MD, FACS
*Consulting Editor*

This issue of the *Surgical Oncology Clinics of North America* is devoted to breast cancer. The guest editor is Lisa Newman, MD, MPH, Professor of Surgery and Director of the Breast Care Center at the University of Michigan. Dr Newman has put together with her colleagues a diverse group of topics for this issue. For example, Dr Michael Sabel, Chief of Surgical Oncology at the University of Michigan, discusses the nonsurgical ablation of breast cancer. Dr Lisa Newman herself discusses breast cancer disparities with high-risk breast cancer in women of African ancestry. These are just two examples of the 14 outstanding articles in this issue.

The American Cancer Society estimates that in 2014 there will be 235,030 new cases of breast cancer in the United States and 40,430 breast cancer deaths. Although progress has been made, there is still much work to be done. Breast cancer is the most common cancer in women in the United States and the second leading cause of female cancer deaths. It is important that as the country moves toward a health care environment where high quality of care and low cost will replace fee for service and payment based on volume, that the multidisciplinary care of patients with breast cancer becomes more important now and in the future than ever before.

I want to thank Dr Newman and her colleagues for this issue of the *Surgical Oncology Clinics of North America*, where the subject matter was due for an update. Like all of the issues of the *Surgical Oncology Clinics of North America*, I encourage senior surgeons to share this information with their trainees.

Nicholas J. Petrelli, MD, FACS
Helen F. Graham Cancer Center at Christiana Care
4701 Ogletown Stanton Road, Suite 1233
Newark, DE 19713, USA

E-mail address:
npetrelli@christianacare.org

Surg Oncol Clin N Am 23 (2014) xiii
http://dx.doi.org/10.1016/j.soc.2014.03.015
1055-3207/14/$ – see front matter © 2014 Elsevier Inc. All rights reserved.

# Preface

# Breast Cancer

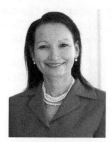

Lisa A. Newman, MD, MPH, FACS, FASCO
*Editor*

The twenty-first century has seen wonderful advances in the management of breast cancer and outcomes following treatment. Translational research has traversed the bench-to-bedside gap; we now routinely apply genetic profiling and targeted therapeutic technology in our treatment plans. These exciting improvements are not limited to the medical oncology aspect of care; locoregional treatments have also evolved dramatically, and multidisciplinary management has benefited from applications of novel imaging, minimally invasive axillary staging, breast-conserving as well as mastectomy surgery, and breast reconstruction. Our patients have expanded options regarding the extent of surgery, selection of systemic therapy, and sequence of care, but understanding the various strategies is a complex process. They rely on the oncology treatment team for guidance, and since surgeons are usually the clinicians most intimately involved with the initial diagnostic process, we are appropriately seen as the leader in the coordination of care. It is therefore incumbent on the surgical breast oncology community to be knowledgeable and comfortable with all multimodality aspects of breast cancer treatment planning.

This issue of *Surgical Oncology Clinics of North America* is therefore dedicated to reviewing many of the complicated and often controversial approaches to breast cancer management that have emerged in recent years. These discussions are presented by several internationally renowned leaders in the oncology field, as well as many rising stars in academia. As guest editor for this issue, I am grateful to all for investing their time and energy in the drafting of these outstanding articles. I also express my appreciation to Consulting Editor, Dr Nicholas Petrelli, for including this important topic in the *Surgical Oncology Clinics of North America* series, and for inviting me to oversee its production. Working with the authors, with Dr Petrelli, and with the editorial staff (especially Stephanie Carter and Jessica McCool) has been an absolute pleasure and a

Surg Oncol Clin N Am 23 (2014) xv–xvi
http://dx.doi.org/10.1016/j.soc.2014.03.016
1055-3207/14/$ – see front matter © 2014 Published by Elsevier Inc.

surgonc.theclinics.com

tremendous honor. I am confident that this issue will be an invaluable educational tool for trainees and faculty around the world.

Lisa A. Newman, MD, MPH, FACS, FASCO
Breast Care Center
University of Michigan Comprehensive Cancer Center
1500 East Medical Center Drive
Ann Arbor, MI 48167, USA

E-mail address:
lanewman@umich.edu

# Epidemiology of Breast Cancer

Kristen A. Ban, MD*, Constantine V. Godellas, MD

## KEYWORDS

- Breast cancer • Epidemiology • Risk factors

## KEY POINTS

- Breast cancer remains the most common invasive cancer in women and is the second leading cause of cancer death; in the United States, mortality continues to decline despite stable to slightly increasing incidence.
- Major risk factors for breast cancer fall under 3 major categories: reproductive (hormone exposure), genetic, and environmental.
- Relatively few risk factors are easily modifiable; therefore, epidemiology plays an important role in identifying high-risk patient populations for effective screening measures.

## INTRODUCTION

Breast cancer is the most common invasive cancer to affect women both in North America and in the world. It is the second highest cause of cancer death in women after lung cancer. Improvements in breast cancer detection methods have increased incidence, but mortality has steadily declined. An improved understanding of the epidemiology of breast cancer, including reproductive, genetic, and environmental risk factors, has led to more informed patient counseling and helped guide screening and management practices.

## INCIDENCE, PREVALENCE, AND MORTALITY

The Surveillance, Epidemiology, and End Results (SEER) program has been an invaluable tool for researchers studying the epidemiology of breast cancer in the United States and is the main source of data regarding incidence, prevalence, and mortality.[1]

In the United States, it is estimated that breast cancer claimed the lives of more than 39,000 men and women in 2012, with more than 229,000 new diagnoses the same year. Worldwide, it is estimated that 1.4 million women a year receive a diagnosis of

The authors have nothing to disclose.
Department of Surgery, Loyola University, 2160 South First Avenue, Maywood, IL 60153, USA
* Corresponding author.
E-mail address: kban@lumc.edu

Surg Oncol Clin N Am 23 (2014) 409–422
http://dx.doi.org/10.1016/j.soc.2014.03.011
1055-3207/14/$ – see front matter © 2014 Elsevier Inc. All rights reserved.

surgonc.theclinics.com

breast cancer, while 458,000 die of the disease.[2] On average, 1 in 8 women will be diagnosed with breast cancer in her lifetime. In 2010, it was estimated that 2.8 million women living in the United States had a prior diagnosis of breast cancer, including both women with active disease and women previously treated. Historically, breast cancer incidence in the United States increased slightly more than 1% per year until the 1980s, when incidence increased abruptly, likely due to increased use of screening mammography (**Fig. 1**).[3] In the 1990s, incidence remained fairly stable, and in the 2000s, incidence declined slightly; it is hypothesized that this decline was caused by decreased use of postmenopausal hormone replacement therapy (HRT).[4] Since 2004, incidence has been stable.

Since 1950, mortality from breast cancer has decreased on average 0.6% per year in the United States, with an overall decrease of more than 34% over this time period. The 5-year relative survival has increased dramatically from 60% in 1950 to 1954 to almost 92% in 2003 to 2009. Between 2004 and 2008, breast cancer mortality in the United States continued to decrease by 2.3% despite stable to slightly increased incidence.

### Race, Ethnicity, Socioeconomic Status

Notable differences exist in incidence and mortality among different races (**Fig. 2**). According to SEER data in the 2000s, in the white population, incidence (per 100,000) was 127.4. Total mortality was 12.3 (per 100,000) and 5-year survival was 90.4%. In the black population, incidence was 121.4. Total mortality was 18.2, and 5-year survival was 78.6%.

The number of SEER capture sites recently expanded to improve data on other minority groups including Hispanics. These figures suggest that Hispanics have a lower incidence and mortality compared with white and black women. Incidence

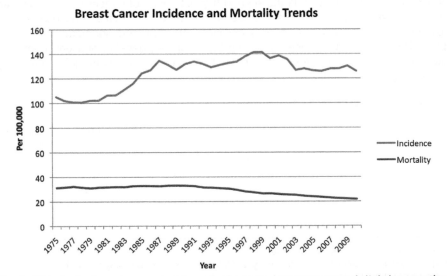

**Fig. 1.** Historically, breast cancer incidence in the United States increased slightly more than 1% per year until the 1980s; in the 1990s, incidence remained fairly stable, and in the 2000s, incidence declined slightly. Since 2004, incidence has been stable. (*Data from* Howlader N, Noone AM, Krapcho M, et al. SEER cancer statistics review, 1975-2010. Bethesda (MD): National Cancer Institute. Available at: http://seer.cancer.gov/csr/1975_2010/. Accessed March 11, 2014.)

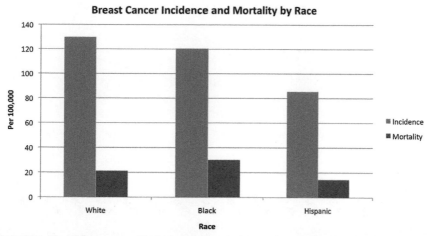

**Fig. 2.** Notable differences exist in incidence and mortality among different races. (*Data from* Howlader N, Noone AM, Krapcho M, et al. SEER cancer statistics review, 1975-2010. Bethesda (MD): National Cancer Institute. Available at: http://seer.cancer.gov/csr/1975_ 2010/. Accessed March 11, 2014.)

(per 100,000) was 90.8, and total mortality was 14.8. Despite these favorable numbers, studies suggest that Hispanic women are diagnosed at a younger age and, like black women, have a relatively higher risk of triple negative phenotype.[5]

Why is it that despite having a lower overall incidence of breast cancer, black individuals are more likely to die of the disease? Numerous studies have examined contributory factors, including socioeconomic status, access to health care, and genetics. Socioeconomic and health care access disparities in part contribute to worse outcomes,[6] but more aggressive tumor biology also plays a role. When socioeconomic factors are accounted for, African American ethnicity itself is associated with a breast cancer mortality hazard of 1.19.[7] Black women are more likely to be diagnosed with advanced stage disease, and they are disproportionately affected by triple-negative tumors.[8] Despite a lower overall incidence of breast cancer, they are more likely than white women to be diagnosed before the age of 45.[1] Taken together, these data suggest that socioeconomic factors in conjunction with different tumor biology in black women contribute to the measured survival disparity.

## RISK FACTORS
### Reproductive

#### Age
The risk of developing breast cancer increases with age, as shown in **Fig. 3**. Of note, trends exist with regard to age and the estrogen receptor (ER) status of breast cancer. ER-positive breast cancer incidence increases with age. This pattern contrasts with the incidence of ER-negative breast cancer, which increases until age 50, but then remains constant. ER-positive tumors, therefore, are more likely to occur in postmenopausal women.[9]

**Age at menarche** Early age at menarche is an important breast cancer risk factor for both premenopausal and postmenopausal women, with a 2-year delay in menarche corresponding to a 10% risk reduction.[10] Various mechanisms have been proposed to explain these effects, all related to higher lifetime exposure to endogenous

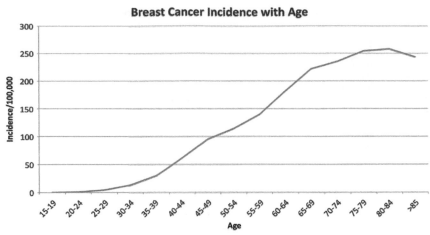

**Fig. 3.** The risk of developing breast cancer increases with age. (*Data from* Howlader N, No-one AM, Krapcho M, et al. SEER cancer statistics review, 1975-2010. Bethesda (MD): National Cancer Institute. Available at: http://seer.cancer.gov/csr/1975_2010/. Accessed March 11, 2014.)

hormones. Early onset of regular menses corresponds to longer lifetime exposure to estrogen.[11] After menarche, overall estrogen levels in the body are higher and remain so for the duration of a woman's reproductive years.[12] Interestingly, women who have early menarche (before age 12) not only have longer lifetime estrogen exposure, but are also subject to higher levels of hormone stimulation during a given cycle compared with women who have menarche later (after age 13).[12,13] Although it is well-established that early menarche increases the risk of developing breast cancer, conflicting research exists regarding the effect of early menarche on breast cancer prognosis and survival once it has been diagnosed.[14,15]

**Age at first pregnancy (full-term)** Younger age at the time of first full-term pregnancy is protective against development of breast cancer later in life.[16] The relative risk for women with older age at first pregnancy (>35 years) has been measured to be between 2.25 and 3.7 compared with women with a first pregnancy in their early to mid-20s.[17,18] This effect applies in particular to hormone receptor–positive breast cancers[19] and to women who are diagnosed after menopause.[20]

**Parity** Parous women have an overall lower risk of breast cancer compared with women who have never given birth; however, this relationship is timing-dependent. Immediately following pregnancy, a woman's risk is higher, but 10 years out from pregnancy, the effect is protective.[21] This protective effect is lasting and overall outweighs the transient risk. The short-term adverse effect is thought to result from elevated hormone levels and rapid proliferation of breast epithelial cells during preg-nancy.[22] In the long-term, breast epithelial cells undergo differentiation following a first pregnancy. Differentiated cells have longer cell cycles and are thus less sensitive to the effects of carcinogens and have more time to undergo DNA repair.[22]

The increased risk following birth is most pronounced for women over the age of 35, with an odds ratio 5 years after delivery of 1.26 (compared with nulliparous women).[21] Odds ratios decrease to as much as 0.7 by 30 years out from pregnancy for uniparous women.[21] Additional pregnancies have a less profound effect, estimated at a 7% rela-tive risk reduction for each subsequent birth.[23]

**Breast-feeding** Breast-feeding appears to have a protective effect against the development of breast cancer, with a dose-response relationship. Studies have yielded inconsistent results in Western countries where few women cumulatively breast-feed more than 1 year. In contrast, significant risk reduction has been demonstrated in non-Western countries.[24] In China, women who breast-fed for a total of 10 years or more had a risk reduction of 64%.[25] A large-scale pooled analysis showed a relative risk reduction of 4.3% for every 12 months of breast-feeding.[23]

Results regarding menopausal status have been inconsistent, but the protective effect of breast-feeding seems to apply primarily to premenopausal women.[24] The protective effect is also greater for BRCA1 mutation carriers who benefit from a 32% risk reduction after breast-feeding for at least 1 year. BRCA2 mutation carriers do not seem to benefit from this effect.[26] Interestingly, women who breast-fed and subsequently developed breast cancer are 3 times more likely to have ER-positive disease compared with women who had not breast-fed.[27]

Breast-feeding suppresses ovulation and may reduce breast cancer risk by decreasing a woman's lifetime estrogen exposure.[28] It has also been shown that estrogen levels in breast fluid are lower during breast-feeding independent of serum estrogen levels.[29] At the cell level, breast-feeding may cause terminal differentiation of breast epithelial cells, making these cells less susceptible to carcinogenic effects or mutations during cell division.[30]

**Abortion** The effect of spontaneous and induced abortion on breast cancer risk has been controversial. It was hypothesized that abortion might increase breast cancer risk by promoting proliferation of breast tissue cells without subsequent cell differentiation. Initial studies suggested an increased risk associated with induced, but not spontaneous abortion; however, results in these studies were inconsistent.[31,32] Subsequent studies demonstrated no increased risk of breast cancer associated with either spontaneous or induced abortion.[33,34] Overall, current evidence does not support a link between spontaneous or induced abortion and increased breast cancer risk.

**Age at menopause** Older age at menopause is associated with an increased risk of breast cancer. Each year delay in the onset of menopause corresponds to a 3% increase in breast cancer risk.[35] Premenopausal women have a higher risk of developing breast cancer (relative risk [RR] 1.43) than postmenopausal women of the same age, particularly for ER-positive tumors.[36]

Artificial menopause via bilateral oophorectomy decreases breast cancer risk dramatically—women who undergo bilateral oophorectomy at age 40 have a 50% lower lifetime risk of breast cancer compared with women who undergo natural menopause. It is hypothesized that the marked and sudden decline in endogenous hormone levels following oophorectomy explains this effect.[11] Simple hysterectomy does not affect breast cancer risk. This risk reduction is profound in carriers of BRCA1 or BRCA2 mutations—bilateral oophorectomy reduces breast cancer risk by more than 50%.[37]

*Exogenous hormones*
**Contraceptive hormones** The use of contraceptives containing exogenous hormones (estrogen and progestin) has been associated with a slightly increased risk of breast cancer. Current use of an oral contraceptive pill (OCP) is associated with an increased risk of 24% compared with women who have never used OCPs. The triphasic OCP formulation containing levonorgestrel may account for a disproportionate amount of the risk elevation.[38] There is no increased risk of a breast cancer diagnosis 10 years

or more after cessation of OCP use, and the duration of OCP use does not affect risk.[39] Interestingly, women with a history of OCP use have less advanced breast cancer on diagnosis compared with never-users.[40]

Despite the slightly elevated risk associated with current OCP use, it is unlikely that OCPs contribute significantly to the breast cancer disease burden—most women use OCPs in their second and third decades when the absolute risk of breast cancer is low. By the time most former OCP users are at an age of increased absolute risk, the elevated risk associated with OCP use has dissipated.

**Hormone replacement** Current or recent use of postmenopausal HRT is associated with an increased risk of breast cancer in a dose-response relationship related to duration of use.[41] This risk is higher for combination HRT (estrogen/progesterone [PR]) than for estrogen therapy alone.[42,43] Meta-analysis calculated an annual odds-ratio increase of 7.6% per year of combination HRT.[44] This increase corresponds to an increased risk of 15% at 5 years of use and 34% at 10 years of use.[45] The elevated risk dissipates by 5 years following cessation of therapy, regardless of treatment duration.[41]

HRT has a stronger effect in specific patient populations. Lean women have a higher risk from HRT compared with obese women, although obesity itself is a risk factor for breast cancer, making the absolute risk difference small.[46] Women with higher breast tissue density are also more affected.[47] Conversely, women with a BRCA1 mutation who undergo prophylactic bilateral oophorectomy are not subject to an increased risk on HRT.[48]

Specific tumor histology has been associated with HRT, including low-grade tumors and tumors that are ER/PR-positive.[49,50]

Following the publication of studies in the early 2000s suggesting a link between HRT and increased breast cancer risk, HRT use declined in many countries. Interestingly, a corresponding decline in breast cancer incidence followed, particularly among women over the age of 50. These results were demonstrated in Australia, the United States, France, and other countries.[4] Analysis of SEER data in the United States revealed an 8.6% decrease in annual age-adjusted incidence between 2001 and 2004 that applied primarily to women over 50 and to ER-positive tumors.[51]

### Genetic factors

A family history of breast cancer is a well-documented risk factor; women with an affected mother or sister are at double the risk of the general population.[52] Additional familial risk factors suggesting a genetic predisposition include early onset of disease, bilateral disease, or an affected male relative. Inheritance of high-risk genes accounts for part, but not all, of this risk.

**BRCA1/BRCA2** Mutations in the BRCA1 and BRCA2 genes represent the most well-known genetic link to breast cancer. These gene mutations are inherited in an autosomal-dominant pattern and account for approximately 5% to 10% of all breast cancer diagnoses.[53] A deletion mutation in either gene corresponds to a 10-fold increased relative risk of developing breast cancer. A prospective study of women with known BRCA gene mutations showed a cumulative risk of developing breast cancer by age 70 of 60% for BRCA1 carriers and 55% for BRCA2 carriers.[54] The prevalence of both genes in the general population varies among geographic regions and ethnicities, but is generally low (0.4%–0.7% for BRCA1, 1%–3% for BRCA2); however, penetrance of these genes is high.[55]

Both BRCA1 and BRCA2 are involved in repair of DNA double-strand breaks via homologous recombination.[56] Deficiencies in this important function contribute to tumorigenesis.[57] A recent study suggests there may be a component of anticipation (earlier age at diagnosis in subsequent generations due to increased DNA instability) with BRCA1/2 breast cancers as in diseases like Fragile X syndrome or Huntington disease.[58]

BRCA1 breast cancers often have a basal-like phenotype that is ER/PR/human epidermal growth factor receptor 2 (HER2)-negative. BRCA2 cancers are also usually HER2-negative, but tend to be ER/PR-positive.[59]

**P53/Li-Fraumeni syndrome** P53 is another high-penetrance gene with a proven link to breast cancer. Mutations in P53 are associated with Li-Fraumeni syndrome (LFS), which carries an increased risk of breast cancer as well as leukemia and malignancies of the lung and brain.[60] Women with LFS have a 50% risk of breast cancer by age 60.[61] LFS and P53-associated malignancies may account for up to 7% of all breast cancers diagnosed in women under the age of 40.[62] Breast tumors in women with LFS are predominantly ER/PR/HER2-positive.[63]

**PTEN/Cowden syndrome** Mutations in the PTEN gene result in PTEN hamartoma-tumor syndrome/Cowden syndrome, characterized by the growth of numerous hamartomas and an increased risk of thyroid, endometrial, and breast cancer.[60] PTEN is a tumor suppressor gene in the MAPK/mTOR pathways that is inherited in an autosomal-dominant manner.[64] Although the prevalence of PTEN mutation is low, individuals with germline PTEN mutations have an estimated lifetime risk of breast cancer of 85%.[65]

**Low-penetrance genes** Numerous other genes have been linked to an increased risk of breast cancer. These genes tend to be low-penetrance and contribute less to the breast cancer disease burden than those described above. Many are involved in pathways of DNA repair and maintenance of genome integrity and cell-cycle checkpoints. Mutations in ATM, BRIP1, CHEK2, NBS1, PALB2, and RAD50 are associated with a 2-fold to 4-fold increased risk of breast cancer.[60] Mutation incidence in these genes is low (around 1% or less), with a correspondingly low number of homozygous individuals diagnosed with resulting breast cancer.[52] Studies continue to elucidate the genes responsible for breast cancer tumorigenesis, but it is clear that there is enormous mutation heterogeneity among individual tumors.[66]

## HISTORY OF BENIGN BREAST DISEASE

A personal history of benign breast disease can be associated with an increased risk of subsequent breast cancer depending on the histology. Nonproliferative breast disease, such as simple cyst or fibroadenoma, is associated with slight, if any increased risk of breast cancer (RR 1.3).[67] Interestingly, in a more diverse population, the odds of breast cancer are approximately 35% lower among women with fibroadenoma.[68] Proliferative breast disease without atypia (adenosis, intraductal papilloma, radical scar) carries a relative risk of 1.3 to 1.9.[67,69]

Proliferative breast disease with associated atypia (atypical ductal or lobular hyperplasia) is considered high-risk and is associated with a 4.3-fold increased risk.[67,69] Lobular hyperplasia confers a higher risk than ductal (OR 7.3 vs OR 3.1). With atypical hyperplasia (AH), subsequent breast cancer is more likely in the ipsilateral breast than in the contralateral breast (60% vs 40%), and the ratio of ipsilateral to contralateral disease is highest within the first 5 years after AH diagnosis.[70] Atypical lobular hyperplasia in particular, then, is considered both a cancer precursor and a long-term risk factor.

In addition to histology, factors such as family history and ethnicity also play a role in risk of subsequent cancer. Women with a family history of breast cancer are at a

2.5-fold increased risk than women with no family history and similar histology.[70] African American women with benign breast disease over the age of 50 are 2.28 times more likely to develop breast cancer compared with non-African American women of the same age.[68]

## LIFESTYLE AND DIETARY

### Alcohol and Tobacco

High levels of alcohol intake are associated with an increased risk of breast cancer. Women who drink 3 to 4 servings of alcohol per day have a 32% increased risk compared with nondrinkers.[71] This risk relationship is linear, with each additional serving of alcohol consumed per day increasing risk by 7% to 9%.[71,72] Low levels of alcohol intake are associated with a small increased risk (RR 1.15 for 3–6 servings of alcohol per week), with the most consistent measure being cumulative alcohol intake throughout life. Binge drinking along with alcohol intake both early and late in life are also independent risk factors.[73]

The relationship between tobacco use and breast cancer remains unclear. Some studies suggest that smoking increases breast cancer risk, particularly when women begin early in life, and with high/prolonged use.[74] Unfortunately, it has been difficult to separate the confounding effect of alcohol intake, which often correlates highly with tobacco use. When alcohol intake is controlled for, most studies have been unable to demonstrate a significant association.[71]

### Physical Activity

Numerous studies suggest that physical activity, particularly in adulthood, decreases the risk of developing breast cancer. Among observational and case-control studies, the reported strength of this effect varied considerably, anywhere from 10% to 50% risk reduction with regular moderate to vigorous activity.[75,76] Meta-analysis of prospective studies suggests a more modest effect, with a relative risk around 10% to 12% for subjects engaging in regular physical activity. There seems to be a dose-dependent effect, and the benefit is more substantial for premenopausal women of normal weight and with regard to ER/PR-negative cancer.[77] Ongoing studies are investigating the effects of physical activity on breast cancer recurrence—studies show a benefit in overall mortality (from all causes), and a possible protective effect against recurrence of ER/PR-negative tumors.[78]

Unfortunately, it is difficult to assess the true effect of physical activity on the risk of breast cancer due to confounding bias in study design—physical activity is invariably linked to nutrition, socioeconomic status, and other factors. Nonetheless, it is one of the few modifiable risk factors for breast cancer and worthy of further investigation.

### Dietary

Numerous dietary factors have been studied as potential breast cancer risk factors. Soy has been of particular interest—observational studies demonstrated lower breast cancer rates in regions with high soy intake, and soy contains isoflavones (phytoestrogens) with endogenous ER binding activity.[79] Interestingly, high soy intake seems to be protective in Asian populations, but harmful in Western populations.[80,81] The genetic basis of this dichotomous effect is a topic of interest for future studies.

Many other dietary factors have been studied, including fat, fruit and vegetable intake, antioxidant vitamins (A, C, E and β-carotene), carbohydrate intake, glycemic index, ingestion of dairy products, and others. In observational studies, none of these factors have been definitively linked to a higher or lower risk of breast cancer.[79] A randomized, controlled trial in which the intervention group followed a low-fat, high fruit and vegetable diet also failed to show any statistically significant link with breast cancer risk.[82]

Studies have also failed to show any effect of diet on prognosis or recurrence in women with known breast cancer—a randomized, controlled trial that compared a diet high in fruits, vegetables, and fiber and low in fat failed to show any effect.[83]

### Weight

The effect of obesity on breast cancer risk has been well-studied and depends on menopausal status. Elevated body mass index has significant protective effects before menopause, but has a positive correlation with breast cancer risk after menopause. Obese premenopausal women are half as likely to develop breast cancer compared with women of normal weight, whereas obese postmenopausal women are 25% more likely to develop breast cancer.[84] A meta-analysis of prospective observational studies measured a 12% increased risk of breast cancer in postmenopausal women for each 5 kg/m$^2$ increase.[85] Studies have also demonstrated an 80% higher risk of ER/PR-positive tumors in obese postmenopausal women.[86]

It is hypothesized that the conversion of androgens to estrogen by the aromatase enzyme in adipose tissue increases breast cancer risk in postmenopausal women by increasing circulating estrogen.[87] Premenopausal obese women have decreased serum estradiol, explaining the corresponding protective effect of increased adipose tissue.[88]

## RADIATION EXPOSURE

Significant radiation exposure is a known breast cancer risk factor, including from medical procedures.[89] Age at time of exposure is important, with women exposed at a young age (20 or less) at higher risk compared with women exposed after age 40.[90] In women exposed before age 40, there is a dose-response relationship between amount of exposure and breast cancer risk. Breast cancer in women with significant radiation exposure does not occur until the third decade, but the elevated risk persists for a woman's lifetime.[91] This elevated risk is well-documented among survivors of Hodgkin lymphoma; a 25-year-old woman treated with radiotherapy at a dose of 40 Gy has a 29% chance of developing breast cancer by age 55.[92]

It remains controversial whether low-dose ionizing radiation exposure from chest radiographs or mammography increases breast cancer risk, although evidence does support a link with high cumulative exposure due to repeat imaging taken at a younger age.[93]

## SUMMARY

Breast cancer remains a significant cause of morbidity and mortality, although great strides have been made in improving disease survival. Many of the major risk factors for breast cancer development are not easily modifiable, including reproductive and genetic variables. A thorough understanding of the epidemiology of breast cancer can inform effective screening practices, help clinicians assess risk in individual patients, and assist in management decisions. Although many risk factors have been well-described, ongoing research into the role of ethnicity, genetic predisposition, and tumor histology will further guide screening and treatment moving forward.

**REFERENCES**

1. Howlader N, Noone AM, Krapcho M, et al. SEER cancer statistics review, 1975-2010. Bethesda (MD): National Cancer Institute. Available at: http://seer.cancer.gov/csr/1975_2010/, based on November 2012 SEER data submission. Accessed March 11, 2014.
2. Ferlay J, Shin HR, Bray F, et al. Estimates of worldwide burden of cancer in 2008: GLOBOCAN 2008. Int J Cancer 2010;127:2893–917.
3. Feuer EJ, Wun LM. How much of the recent rise in breast cancer incidence can be explained by increases in mammography utilization? Am J Epidemiol 1992; 136:1423–36.
4. Kumle M. Declining breast cancer incidence and decreased HRT use. Lancet 2008;372:608–10.
5. Lara-Medina F, Perez-Sanchez V, Saavedra-Perez D, et al. Triple-negative breast cancer in Hispanic patients. Cancer 2011;117:3658–69.
6. Cross CK, Harris J, Recht A. Race, socioeconomic status, and breast carcinoma in the U.S. Cancer 2002;95:1988–99.
7. Newman LA, Griffith KA, Jatoi I, et al. Meta-analysis of survival in African American and white American patients with breast cancer: ethnicity compared with socioeconomic status. J Clin Oncol 2006;24:1342–9.
8. Amirikia KC, Mills P, Bush J, et al. Higher population-based incidence rates of triple-negative breast cancer among young African-American women: implications for breast cancer screening recommendations. Cancer 2011;117:2747–53.
9. Yasui Y, Potter JD. The shape of age-incidence curves of female breast cancer by hormone-receptor status. Cancer Causes Control 1999;10:431–7.
10. Hsieh CC, Trichopoulos D, Katsouyanni K, et al. Age at menarche, age at menopause, height and obesity as risk factors for breast cancer: associations and interactions in an international case-control study. Int J Cancer 1990;46(5): 796–800.
11. Kelsey JL, Gammon MD, John EM. Reproductive factors and breast cancer. Epidemiol Rev 1993;15:36–47.
12. MacMahon B, Trichopoulos D, Brown J, et al. Age at menarche, urine estrogens and breast cancer risk. Int J Cancer 1982;30(4):427–31.
13. Apter D, Reinila M, Vihko R. Some endocrine characteristics of early menarche, a risk factor for breast cancer, are preserved into adulthood. Int J Cancer 1989; 44:783–7.
14. Korzeniowski S, Dyba T. Reproductive history and prognosis in patients with operable breast cancer. Cancer 1994;74(5):1591–4.
15. Orgeas CC, Hall P, Rosenberg LU, et al. The influence of menstrual risk factors on tumor characteristics and survival in postmenopausal breast cancer. Breast Cancer Res 2008;10(6):R107.
16. MacMahon B, Cole P, Lin TM, et al. Age at first birth and breast cancer risk. Bull World Health Organ 1970;43(2):209–21.
17. Lee SH, Akuete K, Fulton J, et al. An increased risk of breast cancer after delayed first parity. Am J Surg 2003;186(4):409–12.
18. Nagata C, Hu YH, Shimizu H. Effects of menstrual and reproductive factors on the risk of breast cancer: meta-analysis of the case-control studies in Japan. Jpn J Cancer Res 1995;86(10):910–5.
19. Yang XR, Chang-Claude J, Good EL, et al. Associations of breast cancer risk factors with tumor subtypes: a pooled analysis from the Breast Cancer Association Consortium studies. J Natl Cancer Inst 2011;103(3):250–63.

20. Ma H, Bernstein L, Pike MC, et al. Reproductive factors and breast cancer risk according to joint estrogen and progesterone receptor status: a meta-analysis of epidemiological studies. Breast Cancer Res 2006;8(4):R43.
21. Lambe M, Hsieh C, Trichopoulos D, et al. Transient increase in the risk of breast cancer after giving birth. N Engl J Med 1994;331:5–9.
22. Russo J, Moral R, Balogh GA, et al. The protective role of pregnancy in breast cancer. Breast Cancer Res 2005;7:131–42.
23. Collaborative Group on Hormonal Factors in Breast Cancer. Breast cancer and breastfeeding: collaborative reanalysis of individual data from 47 epidemiological studies in 30 countries, including 50302 women with breast cancer and 96973 women without the disease. Lancet 2002;360:187–95.
24. Lipworth L, Bailey LR, Trichopoulos D. History of breast-feeding in relation to breast cancer risk: a review of the epidemiologic literature. J Natl Cancer Inst 2000;92(4):302–12.
25. Tao SC, Yu MC, Ross RK, et al. Risk factors for breast cancer in Chinese women of Beijing. Int J Cancer 1988;4:495–8.
26. Kotsopoulos J, Lubinski J, Salmena L, et al. Breastfeeding and the risk of breast cancer in BRCA1 and BRCA2 mutation carriers. Breast Cancer Res 2012;14(2): R42.
27. Hildreth NG, Kelsey JL, Eisenfeld AJ, et al. Differences in breast cancer risk factors according to the estrogen receptor level of the tumor. J Natl Cancer Inst 1983;70:1027–31.
28. Byers T, Graham S, Rzepka T, et al. Lactation and breast cancer. Evidence for a negative association in premenopausal women. Am J Epidemiol 1985;12:664–74.
29. Petrakis NL, Wrensch MR, Ernster VL, et al. Influence of pregnancy and lactation on serum and breast fluid estrogen levels: implications for breast cancer risk. Int J Cancer 1987;40:587–91.
30. Russo J, Russo IH. Toward a physiological approach to breast cancer prevention. Cancer Epidemiol Biomarkers Prev 1994;3:353–64.
31. Daling JR, Malone KE, Voigt LF, et al. Risk of breast cancer among young women: relationship to induced abortion. J Natl Cancer Inst 1994;86(21):1584–92.
32. Brind J, Chinchilli VM, Severs WB, et al. Induced abortion as an independent risk factor for breast cancer: a comprehensive review and meta-analysis. J Epidemiol Community Health 1996;50:481–96.
33. Melbye M, Wohlfahrt J, Olsen JH, et al. Induced abortion and the risk of breast cancer. N Engl J Med 1997;336(2):81–5.
34. Collaborative Group on Hormonal Factors in Breast Cancer. Breast cancer and abortion: collaborative reanalysis of data from 53 epidemiological studies, including 83,000 women with breast cancer from 16 countries. Lancet 2004; 363:1007–16.
35. Trichopoulos D, MacMahon B, Cole P. Menopause and breast cancer risk. J Natl Cancer Inst 1972;48:605–13.
36. Collaborative Group on Hormonal Factors in Breast Cancer. Menarche, menopause, and breast cancer risk: individual participant meta-analysis, including 118964 women with breast cancer from 117 epidemiological studies. Lancet Oncol 2012;13(11):1141–51.
37. Rebbeck TR, Lynch HT, Neuhausen SL, et al. Prophylactic oophorectomy in carriers of BRCA1 or BRCA2 mutations. N Engl J Med 2002;346:1616–22.
38. Hunter DJ, Colditz GA, Hankinson SE, et al. Oral contraceptive use and breast cancer: a prospective study of young women. Cancer Epidemiol Biomarkers Prev 2010;19(10):2496–502.

39. Marchbanks PA, McDonald JA, Wilson HG, et al. Oral contraceptives and the risk of breast cancer. N Engl J Med 2002;346:2025–32.

40. Collaborative Group on Hormonal Factors in Breast Cancer. Breast cancer and hormonal contraceptives: collaborative reanalysis of individual data on 53297 women with breast cancer and 100239 women without breast cancer from 54 epidemiological studies. Lancet 1996;347:1713–27.

41. Collaborative Group on Hormonal Factors in Breast Cancer. Breast cancer and hormone replacement therapy: collaborative reanalysis of data from 51 epidemiological studies of 52,705 women with breast cancer and 108,411 women without breast cancer. Lancet 1997;350:1047–59.

42. Chlebowski RT, Kuller LH, Prentice RL, et al. Breast cancer after use of estrogen plus progestin in postmenopausal women. N Engl J Med 2009; 360:573–87.

43. Prentice RL, Chlebowski RT, Stefanick ML, et al. Conjugated equine estrogens and breast cancer risk in the Women's Health Initiative clinical trial and observational study. Am J Epidemiol 2008;167:1407–15.

44. Lee SA, Ross RK, Pike MC. An overview of menopausal oestrogen-progestin hormone therapy and breast cancer risk. Br J Cancer 2005;92:2049–58.

45. Narod SA. Hormone replacement therapy and the risk of breast cancer. Nat Rev Clin Oncol 2011;8:669–76.

46. Saxena T, Lee E, Henderson KD, et al. Menopausal hormone therapy and subsequent risk of specific invasive breast cancer subtypes in the California Teachers Study. Cancer Epidemiol Biomarkers Prev 2010;19:2366–78.

47. Kerlikowske K, Cook AJ, Buist DS, et al. Breast cancer risk by breast density, menopause, and postmenopausal hormone therapy use. J Clin Oncol 2010; 28:3830–7.

48. Eisen A, Lubinski J, Gronwald J, et al. Hormone therapy and the risk of breast cancer in BRCA1 mutation carriers. J Natl Cancer Inst 2008;100:1361–7.

49. Beral V, Reeves G, Bull D, et al. Breast cancer risk in relation to the interval between menopause and starting hormone therapy. J Natl Cancer Inst 2011; 103:296–305.

50. Calle EE, Feigelson HS, Hildenbrand JS, et al. Postmenopausal hormone use and breast cancer associations differ by hormone regimen and histologic subtype. Cancer 2009;115:936–45.

51. Ravdin PM, Cronin KA, Howlader N, et al. The decrease in breast-cancer incidence in 2003 in the United States. N Engl J Med 2007;356:1670–4.

52. Stratton MR, Rahman N. The emerging landscape of breast cancer susceptibility. Nat Genet 2008;40:17–22.

53. Evans JP, Skrzynia C, Susswein L, et al. Genetics and the young woman with breast cancer. Breast Dis 2006;23:17–29.

54. Mavaddat N, Peock S, Frost D, et al. Cancer risks for BRCA1 and BRCA2 mutation carriers: results from the prospective analysis of EMBRACE. J Natl Cancer Inst 2013;11:812–22.

55. Fackenthal JD, Olopade OI. Breast cancer risk associated with BRCA1 and BRCA2 in diverse populations. Nat Rev Cancer 2007;7:937–48.

56. Chen JJ, Silver D, Cantor S, et al. BRCA1, BRCA2, and Rad51 operative in a common DNA damage response pathway. Cancer Res 1999;59:1752–6.

57. Murphy CG, Moynahan ME. BRCA gene structure and function in tumor suppression: a repair-centric perspective. Cancer J 2010;16:39–47.

58. Litton JK, Ready K, Chen H, et al. Earlier age of onset of BRCA mutation-related cancers in subsequent generations. Cancer 2012;118(2):321–5.

59. Palacios J, Robles-Frias MJ, Castilla MA, et al. The molecular pathology of hereditary breast cancer. Pathobiology 2008;75:85–94.
60. Walsh T, King MC. Ten genes for inherited breast cancer. Cancer Cell 2007;11: 103–5.
61. Hwang SJ, Lozano G, Amos CI, et al. Germline p53 mutations in a cohort with childhood sarcoma: sex differences in cancer risk. Am J Hum Genet 2003; 72(4):975–83.
62. Mouchawar J, Korch C, Byers T, et al. Population-based estimate of the contribution of TP53 mutations to subgroups of early-onset breast cancer: Australian Breast Cancer Family Study. Cancer Res 2010;70(12):4795–800.
63. Melhem-Bertrandt A, Bojadzieva J, Ready KJ, et al. Early onset HER2-positive breast cancer is associated with germline TP53 mutations. Cancer 2012; 118(4):908–13.
64. Waite KA, Eng C. Protean PTEN: form and function. Am J Hum Genet 2002; 70(4):829–44.
65. Min-Han T, Mester JL, Ngeow J, et al. Lifetime cancer risks in individuals with germline PTEN mutations. Clin Cancer Res 2012;18(2):400–7.
66. Stephens PJ, Tarpey PS, Davies H, et al. The landscape of cancer genes and mutational processes in breast cancer. Nature 2012;486(7403):400–4.
67. Hartmann LC, Sellers TA, Frost MH, et al. Benign breast disease and the risk of breast cancer. N Engl J Med 2005;353:229–37.
68. Worsham MJ, Raju U, Lu M, et al. Risk factors for breast cancer from benign breast disease in a diverse population. Breast Cancer Res Treat 2009;118: 1–7.
69. Dupont WD, Parl FF, Hartmann WH, et al. Breast cancer risk associated with proliferative breast disease and atypical hyperplasia. Cancer 1993;71:1258–65.
70. Collins LC, Baer HF, Tamimi RM, et al. Magnitude and laterality of breast cancer risk according to histologic type of atypical hyperplasia: results from the Nurses' Health Study. Cancer 2007;109:180–7.
71. Collaborative Group on Hormonal Factors in Breast Cancer. Alcohol, tobacco and breast cancer – collaborative reanalysis of individual data from 53 epidemiological studies, including 58 515 women with breast cancer and 95 067 women without the disease. Br J Cancer 2002;87:1234–45.
72. Smith-Warner SA, Spiegelman D, Yaun SS, et al. Alcohol and breast cancer in women: a pooled analysis of cohort studies. JAMA 1998;279:535–40.
73. Chen WY, Rosner B, Hankinson SE, et al. Moderate alcohol consumption during adult life, drinking patterns, and breast cancer risk. JAMA 2011;306:1884–90.
74. Cui T, Miller AB, Rohan TE. Cigarette smoking and breast cancer risk: update of a prospective cohort study. Breast Cancer Res Treat 2006;100:293–9.
75. Kobayashi LC, Janssen I, Richardson H, et al. Moderate-to-vigorous intensity physical activity across the life course and risk of pre- and post-menopausal breast cancer. Breast Cancer Res Treat 2013;139(3):851–61.
76. Friedenreich CM. Physical activity and cancer prevention: from observational to intervention research. Cancer Epidemiol Biomarkers Prev 2001;10:287–301.
77. Wu Y, Zhang D, Kang S. Physical activity and risk of breast cancer: a meta-analysis of prospective studies. Breast Cancer Res Treat 2013;137(3):869–82.
78. Schmidt ME, Chang-Claude J, Vrieling A, et al. Association of pre-diagnosis physical activity with recurrence and mortality among women with breast cancer. Int J Cancer 2013;133:1431–40.
79. Michels KB, Mohllajee AP, Roset-Bahmanyar E, et al. Diet and breast cancer. Cancer 2007;109:2712–49.

80. Yamamoto S, Sobue T, Kobayashi M, et al. Soy, isoflavones, and breast cancer risk in Japan. J Natl Cancer Inst 2003;95:906–13.
81. Horn-Ross PL, Hoggatt KJ, West DW, et al. Recent diet and breast cancer risk: the California Teachers Study (USA). Cancer Causes Control 2002;13:407–15.
82. Prentice RL, Caan B, Chlebowski RT, et al. Low-fat dietary pattern and risk of invasive breast cancer: the Women's Health Initiative Randomized Controlled Dietary Modification Trial. JAMA 2006;295:629–42.
83. Pierce JP, Natarajan L, Caan BJ, et al. Influence of a diet very high in vegetables, fruit and fiber and low in fat on prognosis following treatment for breast cancer: the Women's Healthy Eating and Living (WHEL) randomized trial. JAMA 2007;298:289–98.
84. Van den Brandt P, Spiegelman D, Yaun S, et al. Pooled analysis of prospective cohort studies on height, weight, and breast cancer risk. Am J Epidemiol 2000; 152:514–27.
85. Renehan AG, Tyson M, Egger M, et al. Body-mass index and incidence of cancer: a systemic review and meta-analysis of prospective observational studies. Lancet 2008;317:569–78.
86. Suzuki R, Orsini N, Saji S, et al. Body weight and incidence of breast cancer defined by estrogen and progesterone receptor status – A meta-analysis. Int J Cancer 2009;124:698–712.
87. Toniolo PG, Levitz M, Zeleniuch-Jacquotte A, et al. A prospective study of endogenous estrogens and breast cancer in postmenopausal women. J Natl Cancer Inst 1995;87:190–7.
88. Thomas HV, Key TJ, Allen DS, et al. Re: reversal of relation between body mass and endogenous estrogen concentrations with menopausal status. J Natl Cancer Inst 1997;89:396–8.
89. John EM, Kelsey JL. Radiation and other environmental exposures and breast cancer. Epidemiol Rev 1993;15:157–62.
90. Land CE, Tokunaga M, Koyama K, et al. Incidence of female breast cancer among atomic bomb survivors, Hiroshima and Nagasaki, 1950-1990. Radiat Res 2003;160:707–17.
91. Preston DL, Mattsson A, Holmberg E, et al. Radiation effects on breast cancer risk: a pooled analysis of eight cohorts. Radiat Res 2002;158:220–35.
92. Travis LB, Hill D, Dores GM, et al. Cumulative absolute breast cancer risk for young women treated for Hodgkin lymphoma. J Natl Cancer Inst 2005;97: 1428–37.
93. Ma H, Hill CK, Bernstein L, et al. Low-dose medical radiation exposure and breast cancer risk in women under age 50 years overall and by estrogen and progesterone receptor status: results from a case-control and case-case comparison. Breast Cancer Res Treat 2008;109:77–90.

# Prophylactic Bilateral Mastectomy and Contralateral Prophylactic Mastectomy

Anees B. Chagpar, MD, MSc, MPH, MA, FRCS(C), FACS

## KEYWORDS

- Prophylactic mastectomy • Risk • Breast cancer • Surgery

## KEY POINTS

- With increasing public awareness of risk of breast cancer and modern techniques of reconstruction, the option of surgical prophylaxis for risk reduction is becoming increasingly popular.
- Bilateral prophylactic mastectomy for women at increased risk of developing breast cancer and contralateral prophylactic mastectomy for those with unilateral breast cancer seeking symmetry, risk reduction and ease of follow-up are acceptable options for many women.
- Prophylactic surgery is not an inconsequential decision, and careful consideration should be given to the risks and benefits of such procedures.

## INTRODUCTION

As women become increasingly aware of their risk of developing breast cancer, many are choosing to undergo prophylactic mastectomy as a means of risk reduction. Although it is clear that this procedure results in a significantly lower incidence rate of breast cancer, the impact on survival has been less well elucidated. For some, the psychological benefit outweighs the potential complications and for others, the desire for symmetry and reduced need for ongoing mammographic surveillance is critical to their decision making. With significant improvements in reconstructive procedures, the cosmetic outcome is acceptable to many women. Nevertheless, careful evaluation of risks and benefits are warranted when considering prophylactic mastectomy.

Financial disclosures pertaining to this work: None.
Department of Surgery, Yale University School of Medicine, 20 York Street, 1st Floor, Suite A, New Haven, CT 06510, USA
*E-mail address:* anees.chagpar@yale.edu

## RISK ASSESSMENT

At the heart of prophylactic surgery is the desire to reduce risk. In this context, the need for accurate risk assessment is of paramount importance. For women with no current history of breast cancer, there are several risk factors that increase the risk of developing breast cancer. Genetic mutations, particularly in BRCA1 and BRCA2, are well known to increase a woman's absolute risk of developing breast cancer to approximately 85%. However, there are several other genetic mutations that also increase risk (**Table 1**). In patients with a significant family history, consultation with a genetic counselor is warranted. Even without a known mutation, patients with a significant family history may opt for prophylactic mastectomy rather than careful surveillance.

It should also be noted that there are several nongenetic risk factors that also increase a patient's risk of developing a future breast cancer. Although most of these benign atypias and classic lobular intraepithelial neoplasias (also known as lobular carcinoma in situ) increase risk, the risk elevation is rarely so significant as to prompt women to opt for prophylactic surgery in the absence of other factors (see **Table 1**).

A variety of risk-assessment tools help to quantitate an individual patient's risk of developing breast cancer, but each has its own limitations. The Gail model is the most often used for patients without a significant genetic risk.[1,2] Though widely accepted, this model has some limitations in terms of not assessing second-degree family history and lack of widespread validation in non-Caucasian populations. Nonetheless, many risk-reducing trials have defined "high risk" as a Gail 5-year risk of 1.67% or greater.[3] Other risk models, such as the Claus model[4] and the Tyrer-Cuzik model,[5] are designed to incorporate family history to a greater degree than Gail. BRACAPRO is often used to estimate the risk of carrying a BRCA gene mutation,[6] and is used to define patients who may benefit from annual magnetic resonance imaging (MRI) screening (>20%–25% lifetime risk).[7]

Quantitative risk estimation is important for patients who are trying to decide between risk-reducing options. For individuals at high risk, several risk-reducing options are available (**Table 2**). Patients who present with an ipsilateral breast cancer also have an increased risk of developing contralateral breast cancer, estimated to be 0.5% to 1.0% per year. For patients who opt for an ipsilateral mastectomy, contralateral prophylactic mastectomy can reduce the contralateral risk of developing breast cancer by 96%[8] while providing symmetry.

## EPIDEMIOLOGY AND DECISION MAKING

Several studies have shown a steady increase in contralateral prophylactic mastectomy rates, but data regarding trends in bilateral prophylactic mastectomy are less

| Table 1 Risk for developing breast cancer | | | |
|---|---|---|---|
| **Genetic Risk Factors** | | **Nongenetic Risk Factors** | |
| Factor | Absolute Lifetime Risk (%) | Factor | Relative Risk |
| BRCA1[39] | 81 | Classic LIN | 7–11× |
| BRCA2[39] | 85 | ADH/ALH | 4–5× |
| p53[40] | 24 | Proliferative change without atypia | 1.9× |
| PTEN[41] | 25 | | |

*Abbreviations:* ADH, atypical ductal hyperplasia; ALH, atypical lobular hyperplasia; LIN, lobular intraepithelial neoplasia.

**Table 2**
**Risk-reducing options**

| Risk-Reducing Measure | Relative Risk (%) |
| --- | --- |
| Tamoxifen | 37[42]–49[3] |
| Raloxifene[a] | 56[43]–59[44] |
| Exemestane[a] | 65[19] |
| Bilateral prophylactic salpingo-oopherectomy | 53[45] |
| Bilateral prophylactic mastectomy | 89.5–100[46–48] |

[a] In postmenopausal women.

common. McLaughlin and colleagues[9] evaluated the 10-year trend for mastectomy procedures in New York and found that whereas contralateral mastectomy rates have been increasing (with a concomitant decline in unilateral mastectomy), the rates of bilateral prophylactic mastectomy remain fairly low (**Fig. 1**). However, in accord with McLaughlin and colleagues, several other investigators have found a significant upward trend in contralateral prophylactic mastectomy rates (**Fig. 2**),[10–14] although interestingly a similar trend has not been seen in Europe.[15]

Several sociodemographic and tumor characteristics have been associated with a higher likelihood of pursuing contralateral prophylactic mastectomy. These factors include younger age,[12,14–17] Caucasian race,[12,14,16] private insurance,[12] a family history of breast cancer,[14–18] and lobular tumor histology.[16,17,19] However, other factors, such as workup with bilateral breast MRI[14,18] and the option of immediate reconstruction,[14,16,18] are independently associated with the decision to pursue contralateral prophylactic mastectomy.

When surveys have asked women about their motivation to pursue contralateral prophylactic mastectomy, women often cite a desire to reduce risk and live longer.[20]

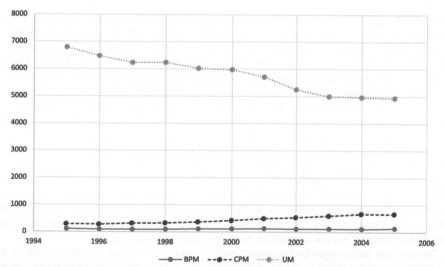

**Fig. 1.** McLaughlin and colleagues' evaluation of the 10-year trend for mastectomy procedures in New York. BPM, bilateral prophylactic mastectomy; CPM, contralateral prophylactic mastectomy; UM, unilateral mastectomy. (*Data from* McLaughlin CC, Lillquist PP, Edge SB. Surveillance of prophylactic mastectomy: trends in use from 1995 through 2005. Cancer 2009;115:5404–12.)

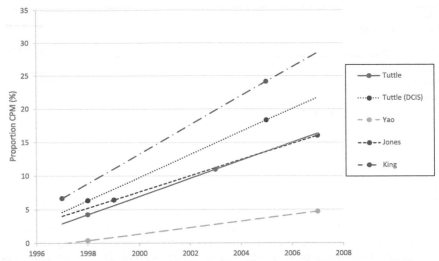

**Fig. 2.** Trends in contralateral prophylactic mastectomy rates. (*Data from* Refs.[10–14])

While it is clear that contralateral prophylactic mastectomy will reduce risk of developing contralateral breast cancer,[21,22] the data regarding survival are more mixed. Whereas some researchers found no impact of contralateral prophylactic mastectomy on disease-specific survival,[22] others, including Bedrosian and colleagues[23] who looked at Surveillance, Epidemiology and End Results data, found that contralateral prophylactic mastectomy was associated with a significantly improved disease-free survival.

## OPERATIVE TECHNIQUE

For patients opting for prophylactic mastectomy, whether bilateral or contralateral, the decisions regarding the operative technique are the same. The first issue is the type of mastectomy: whether conventional (with or without delayed reconstruction), or either skin-sparing or nipple-sparing mastectomy with immediate reconstruction. These techniques are associated with equivalent survival and local recurrence rates.[24] Often the decision is made based on patient preference, taking into consideration the woman's desire for reconstruction. In general, women who opt for bilateral prophylactic mastectomy with immediate reconstruction are ideal candidates for nipple-sparing procedures if they have minimal ptosis, do not smoke, are not obese, and do not have diabetes. Women who are undergoing a conventional or skin-sparing procedure on the ipsilateral breast may opt for the same on the contralateral side for symmetry, although contralateral nipple-sparing mastectomy may be considered if they have the appropriate body habitus and lack comorbidities. Despite the lack of evident disease on the prophylactic side, histopathologic assessment of the subareolar tissue is indicated and, should disease be found, consideration should be given to removing the nipple and converting the procedure to a skin-sparing mastectomy.

The second issue regarding operative technique in this setting is that of whether to perform a concurrent sentinel lymph node biopsy. Some have argued that the risk of this minimally invasive procedure is small, and would preempt the need for axillary evaluation if an occult invasive cancer was found on final pathology.[25] Others, however, argue that the risk of finding metastatic disease warranting axillary staging in patients undergoing prophylactic mastectomy is small and that therefore sentinel node biopsy in these patients can be omitted.[26] For patients undergoing contralateral prophylactic mastectomy, the overall risk of occult invasive disease is approximately 2%.[27] The risk of contralateral positive axillary lymph node metastases is driven primarily by burden of ipsilateral disease, including inflammatory breast cancer and significant ipsilateral lymph node burden.[27]

## SEQUELAE OF PROPHYLACTIC MASTECTOMY

Like all prophylactic surgeries prophylactic mastectomy is elective, and must be considered in the context of balancing the benefits of risk reduction against potential risks. Risks of the surgery include not only common operative risks such as bleeding and infection but also other risks such as reconstructive complications and skin/nipple necrosis. One study found that patients who underwent contralateral prophylactic mastectomy were 1.5 times more likely to have any complication, and 2.7 times more likely to have a major complication, than those who underwent a unilateral mastectomy, after controlling for a variety of potential confounders.[28] Data from the National Surgical Quality Improvement Program database confirmed that overall postoperative complications were 1.9 times more likely in patients who underwent bilateral mastectomy than in those who had unilateral surgery.[29]

For prophylactic mastectomy, one must also consider changes to body image, feelings of femininity and sexuality, self-esteem, and so forth. Several investigators have found that in patients undergoing bilateral prophylactic mastectomy with immediate reconstruction, body image declines after mastectomy, as does sexual satisfaction.[30,31] Negative body image is associated with high preoperative cancer distress.[30]

Similarly, in a study of 269 women undergoing contralateral prophylactic mastectomy who were surveyed at 10.7 years and again at 20.2 years, Frost and colleagues[32] found that 31% reported poorer body image, 24% reported reduced femininity, and 23% reported diminished sexuality. However, the rate of satisfaction and proportion of patients who would choose prophylactic surgery again increased slightly over time.[32] Unukovych and colleagues[33] similarly found no difference in health-related quality of life between women who opted for contralateral prophylactic mastectomy and those in the general population. In addition, no significant differences were identified in health-related quality of life, anxiety, depression, or sexuality before versus after the surgery, although more than half reported at least 1 body-image issue at 2 years postoperatively.[33] It is critical, therefore, to counsel patients about changes in body image and sexuality preoperatively. In a survey of women who had undergone contralateral prophylactic mastectomy, 42% stated that their sense of sexuality was worse than expected, and 31% felt that their self-consciousness about their appearance was also worse than expected.[20] Nevertheless, 80% reported that they were "extremely confident in their decision to have CPM [contralateral prophylactic mastectomy]," and 90% would have made the same decision again.[20] Although one can argue that most patients may be psychologically invested in their previous decisions and would therefore state that they would not do anything differently, one study found that, compared with patients who opted for either bilateral or contralateral prophylactic mastectomy, more patients who opted for unilateral mastectomy would make a different decision ($P = .0007$ and $P = .0005$, respectively).[34]

## COST-EFFECTIVENESS OF PROPHYLACTIC MASTECTOMY

Whereas some have expressed shock regarding the trend of increasing prophylactic mastectomy, others argue that not only is this a manifestation of patient autonomy associated with high patient satisfaction, but it may also be cost-effective from a societal perspective. Several studies have found that bilateral prophylactic mastectomy (when combined with prophylactic oophorectomy) is a cost-effective strategy that dominates other risk-reducing options.[35–37] For patients undergoing contralateral prophylactic mastectomy, Zendejas and colleagues[38] found that in patients with a BRCA mutation, prophylactic surgery is clearly cost-effective. In nonmutation carriers, cost-effectiveness of contralateral prophylactic mastectomy depends on assumptions regarding quality of life for contralateral prophylactic mastectomy versus surveillance.[38] Hence, there is a need to carefully weigh risks and benefits and tailor the risk-reducing strategies for these patients.

## SUMMARY

With growing public awareness of the risk for breast cancer, use of MRI, and newer reconstructive techniques, there has been an increase in prophylactic mastectomies over the past decade. Although it is clear that prophylactic mastectomy can clearly reduce the risk of developing breast cancer, prophylactic mastectomy is also associated with risks that must be carefully considered by the patient and her physician. Nonetheless, most patients who opt for prophylactic mastectomy are pleased with their decision, and, particularly for those with BRCA mutations, this may also be cost-effective.

## REFERENCES

1. Costantino JP, Gail MH, Pee D, et al. Validation studies for models projecting the risk of invasive and total breast cancer incidence. J Natl Cancer Inst 1999;91:1541–8.
2. Gail MH, Brinton LA, Byar DP, et al. Projecting individualized probabilities of developing breast cancer for white females who are being examined annually. J Natl Cancer Inst 1989;81:1879–86.
3. Fisher B, Costantino JP, Wickerham DL, et al. Tamoxifen for prevention of breast cancer: report of the National Surgical Adjuvant Breast and Bowel Project P-1 Study. J Natl Cancer Inst 1998;90:1371–88.
4. Claus EB, Risch N, Thompson WD. Autosomal dominant inheritance of early-onset breast cancer. Implications for risk prediction. Cancer 1994;73:643–51.
5. Tyrer J, Duffy SW, Cuzick J. A breast cancer prediction model incorporating familial and personal risk factors. Stat Med 2004;23:1111–30.
6. Berry DA, Iversen ES Jr, Gudbjartsson DF, et al. BRCAPRO validation, sensitivity of genetic testing of BRCA1/BRCA2, and prevalence of other breast cancer susceptibility genes. J Clin Oncol 2002;20:2701–12.
7. Saslow D, Boetes C, Burke W, et al. American Cancer Society guidelines for breast screening with MRI as an adjunct to mammography. CA Cancer J Clin 2007;57:75–89.
8. McDonnell SK, Schaid DJ, Myers JL, et al. Efficacy of contralateral prophylactic mastectomy in women with a personal and family history of breast cancer. J Clin Oncol 2001;19:3938–43.
9. McLaughlin CC, Lillquist PP, Edge SB. Surveillance of prophylactic mastectomy: trends in use from 1995 through 2005. Cancer 2009;115:5404–12.
10. Tuttle TM, Habermann EB, Grund EH, et al. Increasing use of contralateral prophylactic mastectomy for breast cancer patients: a trend toward more aggressive surgical treatment. J Clin Oncol 2007;25:5203–9.
11. Tuttle TM, Jarosek S, Habermann EB, et al. Increasing rates of contralateral prophylactic mastectomy among patients with ductal carcinoma in situ. J Clin Oncol 2009;27:1362–7.

12. Yao K, Stewart AK, Winchester DJ, et al. Trends in contralateral prophylactic mastectomy for unilateral cancer: a report from the National Cancer Data Base, 1998-2007. Ann Surg Oncol 2010;17:2554–62.
13. Jones NB, Wilson J, Kotur L, et al. Contralateral prophylactic mastectomy for unilateral breast cancer: an increasing trend at a single institution. Ann Surg Oncol 2009;16:2691–6.
14. King TA, Sakr R, Patil S, et al. Clinical management factors contribute to the decision for contralateral prophylactic mastectomy. J Clin Oncol 2011;29:2158–64.
15. Guth U, Myrick ME, Viehl CT, et al. Increasing rates of contralateral prophylactic mastectomy - a trend made in USA? Eur J Surg Oncol 2012;38:296–301.
16. Yi M, Hunt KK, Arun BK, et al. Factors affecting the decision of breast cancer patients to undergo contralateral prophylactic mastectomy. Cancer Prev Res (Phila) 2010;3:1026–34.
17. Arrington AK, Jarosek SL, Virnig BA, et al. Patient and surgeon characteristics associated with increased use of contralateral prophylactic mastectomy in patients with breast cancer. Ann Surg Oncol 2009;16:2697–704.
18. Chung A, Huynh K, Lawrence C, et al. Comparison of patient characteristics and outcomes of contralateral prophylactic mastectomy and unilateral total mastectomy in breast cancer patients. Ann Surg Oncol 2012;19:2600–6.
19. Goss PE, Ingle JN, Ales-Martinez JE, et al. Exemestane for breast-cancer prevention in postmenopausal women. N Engl J Med 2011;364:2381–91.
20. Rosenberg SM, Tracy MS, Meyer ME, et al. Perceptions, knowledge, and satisfaction with contralateral prophylactic mastectomy among young women with breast cancer: a cross-sectional survey. Ann Intern Med 2013;159:373–81.
21. Lostumbo L, Carbine NE, Wallace J. Prophylactic mastectomy for the prevention of breast cancer. Cochrane Database Syst Rev 2010;(11):CD002748.
22. van Sprundel TC, Schmidt MK, Rookus MA, et al. Risk reduction of contralateral breast cancer and survival after contralateral prophylactic mastectomy in BRCA1 or BRCA2 mutation carriers. Br J Cancer 2005;93:287–92.
23. Bedrosian I, Hu CY, Chang GJ. Population-based study of contralateral prophylactic mastectomy and survival outcomes of breast cancer patients. J Natl Cancer Inst 2010;102:401–9.
24. Chagpar AB. Skin-sparing and nipple-sparing mastectomy: preoperative, intraoperative, and postoperative considerations. Am Surg 2004;70:425–32.
25. Burger A, Thurtle D, Owen S, et al. Sentinel lymph node biopsy for risk-reducing mastectomy. Breast J 2013;19:529–32.
26. Murthy V, Chamberlain RS. Prophylactic mastectomy in patients at high risk: is there a role for sentinel lymph node biopsy? Clin Breast Cancer 2013;13:180–7.
27. Nasser SM, Smith SG, Chagpar AB. The role of sentinel node biopsy in women undergoing prophylactic mastectomy. J Surg Res 2010;164:188–92.
28. Miller ME, Czechura T, Martz B, et al. Operative risks associated with contralateral prophylactic mastectomy: a single institution experience. Ann Surg Oncol 2013;20:4113–20.
29. Osman F, Saleh F, Jackson TD, et al. Increased postoperative complications in bilateral mastectomy patients compared to unilateral mastectomy: an analysis of the NSQIP database. Ann Surg Oncol 2013;20:3212–7.
30. Gopie JP, Mureau MA, Seynaeve C, et al. Body image issues after bilateral prophylactic mastectomy with breast reconstruction in healthy women at risk for hereditary breast cancer. Fam Cancer 2013;12:479–87.
31. Brandberg Y, Sandelin K, Erikson S, et al. Psychological reactions, quality of life, and body image after bilateral prophylactic mastectomy in women at high risk for

breast cancer: a prospective 1-year follow-up study. J Clin Oncol 2008;26: 3943–9.

32. Frost MH, Slezak JM, Tran NV, et al. Satisfaction after contralateral prophylactic mastectomy: the significance of mastectomy type, reconstructive complications, and body appearance. J Clin Oncol 2005;23:7849–56.

33. Unukovych D, Sandelin K, Liljegren A, et al. Contralateral prophylactic mastectomy in breast cancer patients with a family history: a prospective 2-years follow-up study of health related quality of life, sexuality and body image. Eur J Cancer 2012;48:3150–6.

34. Han E, Johnson N, Glissmeyer M, et al. Increasing incidence of bilateral mastectomies: the patient perspective. Am J Surg 2011;201:615–8.

35. Anderson K, Jacobson JS, Heitjan DF, et al. Cost-effectiveness of preventive strategies for women with a BRCA1 or a BRCA2 mutation. Ann Intern Med 2006;144: 397–406.

36. Grann VR, Panageas KS, Whang W, et al. Decision analysis of prophylactic mastectomy and oophorectomy in BRCA1-positive or BRCA2-positive patients. J Clin Oncol 1998;16:979–85.

37. Norum J, Hagen AI, Maehle L, et al. Prophylactic bilateral salpingo-oophorectomy (PBSO) with or without prophylactic bilateral mastectomy (PBM) or no intervention in BRCA1 mutation carriers: a cost-effectiveness analysis. Eur J Cancer 2008;44: 963–71.

38. Zendejas B, Moriarty JP, O'Byrne J, et al. Cost-effectiveness of contralateral prophylactic mastectomy versus routine surveillance in patients with unilateral breast cancer. J Clin Oncol 2011;29:2993–3000.

39. King MC, Marks JH, Mandell JB. Breast and ovarian cancer risks due to inherited mutations in BRCA1 and BRCA2. Science 2003;302:643–6.

40. Kleihues P, Schauble B, zur Hausen A, et al. Tumors associated with p53 germline mutations: a synopsis of 91 families. Am J Pathol 1997;150:1–13.

41. Tan MH, Mester JL, Ngeow J, et al. Lifetime cancer risks in individuals with germline PTEN mutations. Clin Cancer Res 2012;18:400–7.

42. Cuzick J, Forbes JF, Sestak I, et al. Long-term results of tamoxifen prophylaxis for breast cancer–96-month follow-up of the randomized IBIS-I trial. J Natl Cancer Inst 2007;99:272–82.

43. Grady D, Cauley JA, Geiger MJ, et al. Reduced incidence of invasive breast cancer with raloxifene among women at increased coronary risk. J Natl Cancer Inst 2008;100:854–61.

44. Martino S, Cauley JA, Barrett-Connor E, et al. Continuing outcomes relevant to Evista: breast cancer incidence in postmenopausal osteoporotic women in a randomized trial of raloxifene. J Natl Cancer Inst 2004;96:1751–61.

45. Rebbeck TR, Lynch HT, Neuhausen SL, et al. Prophylactic oophorectomy in carriers of BRCA1 or BRCA2 mutations. N Engl J Med 2002;346:1616–22.

46. Hartmann LC, Schaid DJ, Woods JE, et al. Efficacy of bilateral prophylactic mastectomy in women with a family history of breast cancer. N Engl J Med 1999;340: 77–84.

47. Hartmann LC, Sellers TA, Schaid DJ, et al. Efficacy of bilateral prophylactic mastectomy in BRCA1 and BRCA2 gene mutation carriers. J Natl Cancer Inst 2001; 93:1633–7.

48. Rebbeck TR, Friebel T, Lynch HT, et al. Bilateral prophylactic mastectomy reduces breast cancer risk in BRCA1 and BRCA2 mutation carriers: the PROSE Study Group. J Clin Oncol 2004;22:1055–62.

# Applications for Breast Magnetic Resonance Imaging

Melissa Pilewskie, MD, Monica Morrow, MD*

## KEYWORDS

- Magnetic resonance imaging • Screening • Breast-conserving therapy
- Local recurrence • Occult cancer

## KEY POINTS

- Magnetic resonance imaging (MRI) screening is supported for specific high-risk populations.
- Data support the use of MRI for imaging women with occult breast cancer.
- MRI has not been shown to improve surgical outcomes in women undergoing breast-conserving surgery.
- Retrospective studies have failed to find significant improvements in breast cancer long-term outcomes with the addition of MRI.

## INTRODUCTION

Mammography is the standard for breast cancer screening, and prospective randomized trials have shown reductions in breast cancer mortality from the implementation of screening mammography.[1] However, screening mammography does have lower sensitivity in women with BRCA gene mutations, high lifetime risk of breast cancer due to family history, and dense breast tissue. Magnetic resonance imaging (MRI) has been evaluated as a screening adjunct given its improved sensitivity in specific subgroups of women and is recommended for screening in high-risk populations.[2–4]

Significant controversy exists regarding the appropriate use of MRI in patients with breast cancer, particularly as part of the preoperative staging work-up. MRI is frequently obtained to exclude the presence of multicentric disease or an occult contralateral breast cancer (CBC) with the presumed benefit of improving patient selection for breast conservation as well as decreasing ipsilateral breast tumor

The authors have nothing to disclose.
Breast Service, Department of Surgery, Memorial Sloan Kettering Cancer Center, 300 East 66th Street, New York, NY 10065, USA
* Corresponding author.
E-mail address: morrowm@mskcc.org

recurrence (IBTR) and CBC rates. A survey sent to the American Society of Breast Surgeons in 2010 reported that 41% of responders routinely order breast MRI for newly diagnosed patients with breast cancer.[5]

This article reviews the relevant data on MRI use in screening, the short-term and long-term outcomes associated with the use of MRI for cancer staging, the use of MRI in occult primary breast cancer, and MRI imaging to assess eligibility for accelerated partial breast irradiation (APBI) and to evaluate tumor response after neoadjuvant chemotherapy (NAC).

## MRI FOR SCREENING
### MRI Screening in BRCA Mutation Carriers and Other High-Risk Women

Mammography remains the gold standard for breast cancer screening and is the only imaging modality to have shown a breast cancer mortality benefit.[6–8] However, mammography has lower sensitivity in women with BRCA mutations, those with elevated lifetime risk based on family history, and those with dense breast tissue,[3,9–13] whereas MRI has improved sensitivity for the detection of breast cancer regardless of breast density.[14] Studies examining the use of MRI for screening have been done in high-risk women with a known or suspected BRCA mutation or those with a family history of breast cancer and an elevated lifetime risk of developing breast cancer. In 2008, in a systematic review, Warner and colleagues[10] reported on 4983 women from 11 prospective MRI screening studies. There was substantial heterogeneity in the study inclusion criteria, including study design, number of screens, use of ultrasound or clinical breast examination, exclusion of patients with prior breast cancer, patient age, and method of risk assessment. The proportion of women in each study with a known BRCA mutation ranged from 8% to 100%, but all studies included women considered high risk because of an elevated annual or lifetime breast cancer risk. All studies reported improved sensitivity (with a positive test defined as Breast Imaging-Reporting and Data System [BIRADS] 4 or 5) with MRI (range 51%–100%) compared with mammography (range 14%–59%). A meta-analysis performed on 10 studies found an overall sensitivity of mammography of 32% (95% confidence interval [CI] 23–41) compared with 75% (95% CI 62–88) for MRI. Combining the 2 screening tests had the highest sensitivity for BIRADS 4 or 5 lesions at 84% (95% CI 70–97). Specificity of mammography (98.5%, 95% CI 97.8–99.2) was slightly higher than that of MRI (96.1%, 95% CI 93.7–96.6). Subsequently, similar results were reported from the multicenter high breast cancer–risk Italian 1 study, which prospectively enrolled 501 women with either a BRCA mutation, or a strong family history of breast or ovarian cancer, to undergo annual evaluation with clinical breast examination, mammography, ultrasound, and MRI. The median age of screened women was 45 years (range 22–79). A total of 52 cancers were identified: 94% screen detected, 6% interval cancers, and 28% node positive. The overall sensitivity of screening modalities was as follows: clinical breast examination 18% (95% CI 8.4–30.9), mammography 50% (95% CI 35.5–64.5), ultrasound 52% (95% CI 37.4–66.3), and MRI 91% (95% CI 79.2–97.6). The addition of mammography or ultrasound to MRI increased the sensitivity only slightly, to 93%. The specificity was again lower for MRI (96.7%, 95% CI 95.4–97.7) compared with mammography (99.0%, 95% CI 98.2–99.5).[11]

### Outcomes in BRCA carriers and high-risk women screened with MRI
Although the sensitivity of MRI exceeds that of mammography for cancer detection in these high-risk women, the ultimate goal of screening is to improve patient outcomes. Warner and colleagues[15] examined the stage of breast cancer identified in 2 groups of BRCA-positive women: those screened with MRI (n = 445) and those who had

conventional screening alone (n = 830). The cumulative incidence of invasive cancer at 6 years was not different between the MRI and no-MRI groups (10.6% and 12.2%, respectively; $P$ = .7). However, the cumulative incidence of ductal carcinoma in situ (DCIS) or stage I breast cancer was significantly higher in the MRI-screened group (13.8%) compared with 7.2% in the conventional imaging group ($P$ = .01). Conversely, the incidence of stages II to IV breast cancer at 6 years was lower in the MRI-screened cohort (1.9%) compared with 6.6% in the conventional imaging group ($P$ = .02). Similarly, the average size of MRI detected invasive tumors was smaller (0.9 cm) than the conventional imaging group (1.8 cm) ($P<.001$). On multivariate analysis, after controlling for age, oophorectomy, parity, prior history of breast cancer, tamoxifen use, oral contraceptive use, and hormone replacement therapy, the adjusted hazard ratio (HR) for the development of stage II to IV breast cancer in the MRI cohort was 0.30 (95% CI 0.12–0.72).

Whether MRI screening is associated with improved survival in BRCA mutation carriers remains unclear. The Dutch MRI screening study prospectively followed 2157 high-risk women, defined as BRCA mutation carriers or those with an estimated cumulative lifetime risk of breast cancer of 15% or more, in a screening program with clinical breast examination, annual mammography, and MRI. At a median follow-up of 4.9 years, significant differences in outcomes and tumor characteristics among the BRCA1, BRCA2, and non-mutation high-risk groups were noted. The BRCA1 group had the highest rate of interval cancer development (32.3%) compared with 6.3% for the BRCA2 group (high-risk group 3.7%, moderate-risk group 6.3%; $P$ = .01). Patients with BRCA1-associated cancer were also diagnosed at younger ages, had fewer DCIS lesions, had larger tumor size at diagnosis, and had more grade 3 tumors and more hormone receptor-negative tumors. The cumulative distant metastasis–free survival at 6 years for the patients with BRCA cancer was 83.9% compared with 100% for the non-mutation high-risk patients.[13] A Norwegian surveillance program for women with BRCA1 mutations followed 802 women screened with MRI and mammogram for a mean of 4.2 years. During the follow-up period, 68 women developed breast cancer and 10 patients died of their disease. The 5-year and 10-year breast cancer–specific survivals in this MRI-screened BRCA1 population were 75% and 69%, respectively. The 5-year survival for stage I breast cancer in this group was 82%, which is significantly lower than the 98% survival reported by the Norwegian Cancer Registry ($P<.05$).[16] These findings raise important questions regarding improvements in outcomes of BRCA1-associated cancers even when detected at smaller sizes with MRI screening. In contrast, Passaperuma and colleagues[12] reported long-term outcomes in 496 BRCA mutation carriers followed in a prospective single-institution screening program of annual MRI, mammography, ultrasound, and clinical breast examination. Fifty-seven cancers were diagnosed, 65% invasive and 35% DCIS, with no statistically significant difference noted in tumor size (mean invasive cancer size, 1.02 cm), tumor grade, or nodal status between BRCA1 and BRCA2 cancers. Of those women with no prior history of breast or ovarian cancer, at a median follow-up of 8.4 years, there was 1 breast cancer-related death, for an annual breast cancer–specific mortality rate of 0.5%. With mixed data on survival benefit seen in women with BRCA mutations or familial risk screened with MRI, additional long-term follow-up is needed to determine the true added benefit of MRI screening in this population.

## MRI Screening in Women with a History of Chest Irradiation

The current guidelines from the American Cancer Society[4] and the American College of Radiology[2] support the use of MRI screening in addition to mammography for

BRCA mutation carriers and untested first-degree relatives of BRCA mutation carriers, those with a lifetime breast cancer risk estimated at 20% to 25% or more, as well as carriers of other genetic mutations associated with increased breast cancer risk or a history of chest wall irradiation between 10 and 30 years of age (**Box 1**). The last group listed is based on expert opinion as women with a history of chest wall irradiation have a significantly elevated breast cancer risk, but there are limited data on the utility of MRI screening in this group.[17]

One prospective and 2 retrospective studies have assessed the utility of MRI screening in women with a history of chest wall irradiation (**Table 1**). Retrospective reviews by Sung and colleagues[18] and Freitas and colleagues[19] reported on 91 and 98 women with a history of chest irradiation, respectively. Both studies reported an additional cancer detection rate of 4% with the addition of MRI and non-significant differences in the sensitivity of MRI and mammography. Ng and colleagues[20] reported a prospective screening study of annual mammography and MRI in 148 women previously treated with mantle radiation for Hodgkin lymphoma. In contrast to the screening studies in high-risk women based on BRCA mutations and family history, this study did not find MRI to be more sensitive than mammography (year 1: MRI 57%, mammography 71%), whereas the combination of the 2 studies had a sensitivity of 100%. There were no interval cancers in this cohort. Eighteen malignancies were detected and included 7 node-negative invasive cancers, 1 node-positive invasive cancer, 9 DCIS lesions, and 1 phyllodes tumor. The carcinomas had an overall low-risk profile, with 88% estrogen receptor (ER) positive, 75% low to intermediate grade, and all 12 mm or less. The 5 cancers detected by MRI alone consisted of 4 DCIS lesions and one 7-mm invasive cancer. A similar lack of benefit for MRI screening has been reported for women at an increased risk from lobular carcinoma in situ.[21] These studies make the important point that most women at increased risk of breast cancer development do not share the unique phenotype of BRCA1 mutation carriers, whereby cancers are likely to be ER negative and lack DCIS, so the results of MRI screening studies in known or suspected BRCA mutation carriers should not be extrapolated to all other high-risk groups.

## Future MRI Screening Studies

To date, there have been no completed randomized MRI screening trials in high-risk women. The ongoing familial MRI screening study (FaMRIsc) trial is a multicenter

---

**Box 1**
**Recommended groups for MRI screening in addition to annual mammography[a]**

- BRCA mutation carriers
- Untested first-degree relatives of BRCA mutation carriers
- Lifetime risk of breast cancer estimated at 20% to 25% or more
- Chest wall irradiation between 10 and 30 years of age
- Women with other genetic syndromes resulting in elevated breast cancer risk[b]

[a] Recommended by the American Cancer Society and the American College of Radiology.
[b] Including Li-Fraumeni, Cowden, and Bannayan-Riley-Ruvalcaba syndromes.
*Data from* Saslow D, Boetes C, Burke W, et al. American Cancer Society guidelines for breast screening with MRI as an adjunct to mammography. CA Cancer J Clin 2007;57(2):75–89; and Mainiero MB, Lourenco A, Mahoney MC, et al. ACR appropriateness criteria: breast cancer screening. J Am Coll Radiol 2013;10(1):11–4.

**Table 1**
MRI screening in women with a history of chest wall irradiation

| Author, Year | No. of Women Screened | Malignancies Detected by MRI Alone | Detected by Mammography Alone | Detected by MRI and Mammography | Incremental Cancer Detection Rate with Addition of MRI (%) | Mammography Sensitivity, Specificity (%) | MRI Sensitivity, Specificity (%) |
|---|---|---|---|---|---|---|---|
| Sung et al,[18] 2011 | 91 | 40% (4/10) | 30% (3/10) | 30% (3/10) | 4.4 | 67, 93 | 67, 82 |
| Freitas et al,[19] 2013 | 98 | 31% (4/13) | 8% (1/13) | 62% (8/13) | 4.1 | 69, 98 | 92, 94 |
| Ng et al,[20] 2013 | 148 | 28% (5/18) | 33% (6/18) | 39% (7/18) | 3.4 | 68, 93[a] | 67, 94[a] |

[a] Sensitivity and specificity after excluding first screen.

randomized controlled trial enrolling women 30 to 55 years of age with a cumulative life-time breast cancer risk of more than 20% according to the modified Claus model or as assessed by a clinical genetics center. Women with BRCA1 or BRCA2 mutations are excluded. Women will be randomized to annual mammography and clinical breast examination, or annual MRI and clinical breast examination with mammography in years 1 and 3. The primary outcome is breast cancer detection, with secondary end points of false-positive rates, sensitivity, positive predictive value, cost-effectiveness, and breast cancer mortality. Breast density will be measured in both groups with the aim to discriminate optimal screening in these high-risk women based on risk factors and mammographic density.[22]

## MRI FOR TREATMENT SELECTION

Breast cancer assessed clinically and by mammography is found to be unicentric in more than 90% of cases.[23] However, pathology studies examining serial sectioning of mastectomy specimens have documented that there are often foci of tumor in either the same quadrant (multifocal) or other quadrants of the breast (multicentric) that were clinically and mammographically occult. Holland and colleagues[24] found additional tumor foci in 63% of mastectomy specimens in patients with unicentric tumors of 5 cm or less; 20% were found within 2 cm of the index lesion and the remaining 43% at a distance greater than 2 cm away, although often within 4 cm of the primary cancer. The likelihood of identifying additional cancer was not related to the size of the primary tumor. Additional studies have identified multifocal or multicentric disease in 21% to 63% of cases, including 44% of mammographically detected tumors.[24–30] Although it is known that these tumor foci often remain in the breast following breast-conserving surgery, multiple prospective randomized trials have proven survival equivalence between lumpectomy with whole-breast radiation therapy (RT) and mastectomy.[31,32] Furthermore, in the current era, IBTR rates following breast-conserving therapy (BCT) at 10 years are less than 10% and as low as 3% to 7% in women treated with adjuvant systemic therapy.[33,34] This finding is far lower than the rates of multifocal and multicentric disease noted in the previously mentioned pathology studies, suggesting that these tumor foci are effectively treated with radiotherapy and systemic therapy, and that they do not require surgical removal.

The utility of MRI for extent-of-disease work-up in women with a known breast cancer hinges on a clinical benefit of finding additional foci of cancer in the unilateral or contralateral breast, not simply the identification of additional cancer. Perioperative breast MRI does identify additional cancer that is not apparent on clinical examination, mammogram, or ultrasound. A meta-analysis reporting on 2610 patients with breast cancer undergoing MRI found that additional disease was identified in 16% of patients, with a range of 6% to 34% in individual studies. The impact of these MRI findings was a reported increase from wide-local excision to mastectomy in 8.1% of women (95% CI 5.9–11.3) and a larger local excision in 11.3% of women (95% CI 6.8–18.3).[35] This finding raises the question of whether the identification of occult tumor foci by MRI improves surgical outcomes by identifying patients requiring mastectomy because of excessive disease burden, or reduces re-excision rates following breast-conserving surgery by more accurately identifying the disease extent. Improved patient selection might also improve long-term outcomes by decreasing the rate of IBTR.

### Surgical Outcomes

Re-excision caused by positive margins is a common occurrence, and recent data show that approximately 25% of all women successfully treated with BCT undergo a re-excision.[36,37] Re-excision is traumatic to patients, impacts cosmesis, is costly to the health care system, and may delay the initiation of adjuvant therapy. Strategies to reduce the need for re-excision would address a substantial problem in breast cancer surgery.

Two prospective randomized trials assessed the effect of MRI on surgical outcomes in patients with breast cancer, with a primary end point of re-operation rates (both re-excision and conversion to mastectomy).[38,39] The comparative effectiveness of MRI in breast cancer (COMICE) trial randomized 1625 patients with breast cancer deemed eligible for breast conservation by clinical examination and standard imaging (mammography and ultrasound) to MRI or no additional evaluation. There was no difference in re-operation rates in the MRI (19%) or no-MRI group (19%) (odds ratio [OR] 0.96, 95% CI 0.75–1.24, $P = .77$). Before the breast-conservation attempt, 1% (n = 10) of women in the no-MRI group were converted to mastectomy compared with 7% (n = 58) in the MRI group. Twenty-eight percent (16 of 58) of mastectomies in the MRI group were deemed pathologically avoidable.[39] Although this trial has been criticized for inclusion of low-volume MRI centers and lack of a requirement for biopsy of all MRI-detected abnormalities, the lack of benefit of MRI on short-term surgical outcomes is supported by the results of the MR mammography of non-palpable breast tumors (MONET) trial and the retrospective studies discussed later. The MONET trial randomized 418 women with a BIRADS 3 to BIRADS 5 lesion to routine imaging with mammography and ultrasound followed by biopsy or the addition of MRI before biopsy. One hundred sixty-three women were diagnosed with a malignant lesion. There was a paradoxic increase in the re-excision rate in the MRI group (34%) compared with the no-MRI group (12%, $P = .008$) and no difference in conversion to mastectomy (11% in the MRI group compared with 14% in the no-MRI group, $P = .49$).[38] A meta-analysis by Houssami and colleagues[40] included 3112 patients with breast cancer from 7 comparative cohort studies evaluating surgical outcomes with the addition of breast MRI as well as the aforementioned prospective randomized studies. A significant increase in both the initial and overall mastectomy rates was seen in the MRI group (16.4% and 25.5%, respectively) compared with the no-MRI group (8.1% and 18.2%, respectively), with a consistent increase in mastectomy rates after adjusting for age (initial mastectomy adjusted OR 3.06, 95% CI 2.03–4.62, $P<.001$; overall mastectomy adjusted OR 1.51, 95% CI 1.21–1.89, $P<.001$). Furthermore, there was no difference in the rate of re-excision following an initial breast-conservation attempt, with a rate of 11.6% in the MRI group compared with 11.4% in the no-MRI group ($P = .87$).

In addition, studies examining factors associated with contralateral prophylactic mastectomy have found increased utilization when patients have undergone MRI evaluation. Studies by King and colleagues[41] and Sorbero and colleagues[42] found MRI imaging to be a significant predictor of undergoing a contralateral prophylactic mastectomy on multivariate analysis. Together, these studies provide a large body of evidence indicating no significant improvement in the rates of re-excision for women undergoing breast conservation but a concerning increase in the use of mastectomy for both cancer treatment as well as contralateral risk reduction in those imaged with MRI.

## Long-Term Outcomes

### IBTR
Although improvements in surgical outcomes are not evident with the addition of MRI, the benefit of detecting and managing additional foci of disease may be in improved long-term outcomes, such as decreased rates of IBTR or CBC development. As

mentioned, rates of IBTR following BCT are low and have declined substantially over time, with reports showing a decrease in IBTR from 8% to 20% in the 1980s to 1% to 5% in the 1990s.[43,44] In the National Surgical Adjuvant Breast and Bowel Project (NSABP) trials conducted since the 1990s, rates of IBTR at 10 years were less than 8% in both node-positive and node-negative women receiving systemic therapy.[33,34] The explanation for the decrease in rates of IBTR is likely multifactorial, including improved surgical and pathologic techniques as well as the increased use of systemic therapy for small node-negative breast cancers. In contrast, rates of local recurrence after mastectomy did not decrease during this same period.[44] These observations suggest 2 mechanisms for local recurrence: an excessive tumor burden unable to be controlled with RT or biologically aggressive disease. MRI is another technique available to identify patients with excessive tumor burden who are not appropriate candidates for breast conservation. However, 3 retrospective studies[45–47] have demonstrated that rates of local recurrence do not differ in patients with ER-negative, progesterone receptor–negative, and HER2-negative breast cancer (triple-negative breast cancer) treated by BCT or mastectomy, suggesting that most of the recurrences seen today (as opposed to 30 years ago during the initial experience with breast conservation) are secondary to aggressive biology and not a large residual disease burden.

There are no prospective randomized trials assessing the effect of MRI on rates of IBTR, but 5 retrospective studies have addressed this question. The study by Fischer and colleagues[48] is the only one to show reduced IBTR with the addition of MRI. This study retrospectively compared 121 patients with preoperative MRI to 225 without. At a mean follow-up of 40 months, IBTR occurred in 1.2% of the MRI group and 6.8% of the no-MRI group (P<.001). The 6.8% incidence of IBTR at less than 5 years of follow-up is unusually high by current standards, making the outcome of this study difficult to interpret. In addition, no statistical adjustments for differences between the MRI and no-MRI groups were made. The MRI group had a higher percentage of DCIS patients (12% vs 3%); more T1 tumors (64% vs 48%); more node-negative tumors (61% vs 54%); fewer high-grade lesions (13% vs 28%); and, paradoxically, a higher percentage of patients treated with chemotherapy (95% vs 82%).[48] Four additional retrospective studies have all reported no difference in rates of IBTR with the addition of perioperative MRI. Studies by Solin and colleagues,[49] Hwang and colleagues,[50] Shin and colleagues,[51] and Ko and colleagues[52] all reported low IBTR rates (<4%) at 5 to 8 years in both women with and without MRI treated with breast conservation (**Table 2**). There is no reason to think that the use of MRI will have an impact on breast cancer–specific survival, as the Early Breast Cancer Trialists' overview[53] demonstrated a need to reduce local failure rates by 10% or more at 5 years in order to observe a statistically significant survival difference at 15 years, and it is not possible to identify a subgroup of patients with breast cancer excised to negative margins with 5-year IBTR rates in excess of 10%. Not surprisingly, the aforementioned retrospective studies by Solin and colleagues,[49] Shin and colleagues,[51] and Ko and colleagues[52] found no improvement in survival for those women imaged with MRI.

## CBC

Detection of a contralateral cancer is the second long-term outcome with the potential to be impacted by the use of MRI. Although women with unilateral breast carcinoma do have an increased risk for the development of second cancers, the absolute risk is relatively low in the absence of a BRCA mutation. In 134,501 women with unilateral DCIS, stage 1 breast carcinoma, or stage 2 breast carcinoma reported to the Surveillance, Epidemiology, and End Results Program database between 1973 and 1996, the

**Table 2**
Studies evaluating association of MRI and IBTR

| Author, Year | Total No. of Patients | Patients with MRI | Variables Controlled for on MV Analysis | Reported Time Interval for IBTR (y) | IBTR Rates (%) | | |
|---|---|---|---|---|---|---|---|
| | | | | | MRI | No MRI | P Value |
| Fischer et al,[48] 2004 | 346 | 121 (35%) | Not done | 3.4 | 1.2 | 6.5 | <.001 |
| Solin et al,[49] 2008 | 756 | 215 (28%) | Age, treatment year | 8.0 | 3.0 | 4.0 | .51 |
| Hwang et al,[50] 2009 | 463 | 127 (27%) | Age, year, chemotherapy, endocrine therapy, tumor grade, LVI, HR status, HER2 status | 8.0 | 1.8 | 2.5 | .67 |
| Shin et al,[51] 2012 | 794 | 572 (72%) | Not done | 5.0 | 1.2 | 2.3 | .33 |
| Ko et al,[52] 2013 | 615 | 229 (37%) | Nuclear grade, HR status, tumor size[a] | 5.7 | 0.4 | 3.6 | .013 |

*Abbreviations:* HR, hormone receptor; LVI, lymphovascular invasion; MV, multivariate.
[a] Adjusted OR for IBTR 6.37, $P = .076$.

actuarial 10-year risk of CBC development was 6.1%.[54] Additionally, the incidence of CBC has been decreasing by 3% per year since 1985 primarily because of the use of endocrine therapy following a diagnosis of ER-positive breast cancer.[55] Based on these low incidence rates, it is difficult to argue that more intensive surveillance of the contralateral breast added to annual mammogram is a cost-effective strategy for the general population of women with breast cancer. A meta-analysis addressing the rate of contralateral cancer detection by MRI in women with unilateral breast cancer reported on 22 studies including 3253 patients. MRI found a synchronous contralateral cancer in 4.1% of patients: 35% were DCIS and 65% were invasive cancers (mean size 9.3 mm).[56] If MRIs were detecting clinically relevant synchronous contralateral malignancies, then that should translate into reduced rates of metachronous CBC. To date, 4 retrospective studies have reported rates of metachronous CBC development in women imaged with MRI versus those without.[48,49,52,57] These results are summarized in **Table 3**. Criticisms of the Fischer study were discussed previously.

**Table 3**
Studies evaluating association of MRI and CBC

| Author, Year | Total No. of Patients | Patients with MRI | Reported Time Interval for CBC (y) | CBC Rates (%) | | |
|---|---|---|---|---|---|---|
| | | | | MRI | No MRI | P Value |
| Fischer et al,[48] 2004 | 346 | 121 (35%) | 3.4 | 1.7 | 4.0 | <.001 |
| Solin et al,[49] 2008 | 756 | 215 (28%) | 8.0 | 6.0 | 6.0 | .39 |
| Kim et al,[57] 2013 | 3094 | 1771 (57%)[a] | 3.8 | 0.5 | 1.4 | .02 |
| Ko et al,[52] 2013 | 615 | 229 (37%) | 5.7 | 2.2 | 1.3 | .51 |

[a] A total of 1771 women had bilateral MRI; the remaining 1323 women underwent unilateral MRI at time of the index cancer diagnosis.

In all studies, rates of CBC were low (0.5%–6.0%) in both groups. The 2 studies reporting a significant decrease in CBC rates with the addition of MRI found an absolute difference in CBC between the MRI and no-MRI groups of 1% to 2%.[48,57] The similarly low rates of CBC development in patients with or without MRI raise the possibility that MRI is detecting lesions that would never become clinically relevant either because of tumor biology or because of the appropriate use of systemic therapy, which has shown to decrease rates of clinically apparent CBC.[53] Similar to the situation with the use of MRI for determining the extent of cancer in the index breast, this raises the possibility of overtreatment.

## Special Populations

### Lobular carcinoma

Attempts to identify subgroups of patients who may benefit from MRI imaging have focused on lobular carcinoma and DCIS. A review of MRI in lobular carcinoma, which included 18 studies and 450 cancers, reported additional disease detected by MRI in 32% of cases (95% CI 22%–44%) and a subsequent change in surgical management in 28.3% of women. The mean sensitivity for MRI in infiltrating lobular carcinoma was 93.3% (95% CI 88%–96%).[58] Two retrospective studies have focused on the effects of MRI on surgical management in women with infiltrating lobular carcinoma and report conflicting results. McGhan and colleagues[59] compared women with infiltrating lobular carcinoma who did (n = 72) and did not (n = 109) undergo MRI. They reported a sensitivity of MRI for cancer detection of 99% and no significant difference in rates of re-excision or conversion to mastectomy.[59] In comparison, Mann and colleagues[60] performed a retrospective review of 99 patients with infiltrating lobular carcinoma who underwent MRI compared with 168 women with no MRI and found a significant decrease in the rate of re-excision in women undergoing breast conservation with the addition of MRI (9% MRI, 27% no MRI, P = .01). In the meta-analysis of Houssami and colleagues[40] examining the effect of MRI on rates of re-excision, there was a non-significant trend toward a decreased rate of re-excision in patients with invasive lobular cancer undergoing MRI (adjusted OR 0.56, 95% CI 0.29–1.09, P = .09); but this was achieved at the expense of an increased age-adjusted mastectomy rate (OR 1.64, 95% CI 1.04–2.59, P = .034).

### DCIS

Literature on the performance of MRI for the detection of DCIS is conflicting. Sardanelli and colleagues[14] reported a sensitivity of only 40% for the detection of DCIS by MRI when the results of pathologic serial sectioning were used as the standard, which was similar to the 37% sensitivity seen with mammography. In contrast, studies by Kuhl and colleagues[61] and Menell and colleagues[62] observed significantly improved sensitivity for DCIS with MRI (92% and 88%, respectively) compared with mammography (56% and 27%, respectively; P<.0001) when conventional pathologic evaluation was used.

Four retrospective single-institution studies have all failed to report improved rates of positive margins or re-excision in women with DCIS imaged with MRI (**Table 4**).[63–66] These studies report conflicting rates of conversion to mastectomy for women with DCIS, with Itakura and colleagues[64] and Kropcho and colleagues[65] showing a significant increase in the mastectomy rate for women undergoing MRI. A large single-institution study reported outcomes for 2321 women undergoing BCT for DCIS with and without perioperative MRI at a median follow-up of 4.9 years. Rates of locoregional recurrence (LRR) did not differ between the groups, with 5- and 8-year rates of 8.5% and 14.6%, respectively, in the MRI group, and 7.2% and 10.2%, respectively, in the no-MRI

**Table 4**
**Studies evaluating the effect of MRI on surgical outcomes in DCIS**

| Author, Year | Total No. of Patients | Patients with MRI | Mastectomy Rate (%) | | | Positive Margin/ Re-excision Rate (%) | | |
|---|---|---|---|---|---|---|---|---|
| | | | MRI | No MRI | P Value | MRI | No MRI | P Value |
| Allen et al,[63] 2010 | 98 | 63 (64%) | 20.3[a] | 25.7[a] | .62 | 21.2 | 30.8 | .41 |
| Itakura et al,[64] 2011 | 149 | 38 (26%) | 45.0[b] | 14.0[b] | <.001 | 16.0 | 11.0 | .42 |
| Kropcho et al,[65] 2012 | 158 | 60 (38%) | 17.7[c] | 4.1[c] | .0004 | 30.7 | 24.7 | .40 |
| Pilewskie et al,[66] 2013 | 352 | 217 (62%) | 34.6[b] | 27.4[b] | .20 | 14.3 | 20.0 | .19 |

[a] Overall mastectomy rate.
[b] Initial mastectomy rate.
[c] Mastectomy rate following attempted breast conservation.

group ($P = .52$). On multivariate analysis, there was no association of MRI and improved LRR rates (HR 1.18, 95% CI 0.79–1.78, $P = .42$). This finding persisted in the 904 women who did not receive adjuvant RT (HR 1.36, 95% CI 0.78–2.39, $P = .28$). There were also no differences in CBC rates with or without MRI at 5 years (no MRI 3.5% vs MRI 3.5%) or 8 years (no MRI 5.1% vs MRI 3.5%, log rank $P$ value .86).[67]

## MRI FOR OCCULT BREAST CANCER

Less than 1% of breast cancers present as axillary nodal metastases with an occult primary tumor, which cannot be detected by physical examination, mammography, or ultrasound. Traditionally, these cases have been treated with mastectomy to ensure removal of the primary tumor, but in approximately one-third of the breast specimens, cancer is not identified by pathologic evaluation.[68] Although breast conservation has been successfully carried out in patients with occult tumors using whole-breast irradiation without surgical excision,[69] this deprives patients of the benefit of a boost dose of radiation to the primary tumor site. The use of MRI to identify the primary tumor, allowing both surgical excision and the use of a radiation boost, is a clinically valuable tool in this uncommon circumstance.

Studies evaluating the use of MRI in cases of occult breast cancer have been small and retrospective, but typically demonstrate the detection of tumor in more than two-thirds of these cases with low false-negative rates.[70–77] A meta-analysis by de Bresser and colleagues[78] summarized the results of 220 patients in 8 studies. MRI identified a suspicious lesion in 72% of cases, with a sensitivity of 90% and a specificity of 31% (range 22%–50%). The mean size of tumors identified on pathologic examination ranged from 5 to 16 mm, and more than 90% (pooled mean 96%) were invasive carcinomas.

Based on these data, MRI is a standard part of the evaluation of patients with occult breast cancer and identifies the primary tumor in approximately 60% of cases. Patients with small unifocal tumors are candidates for conventional BCT, whereas a negative MRI provides reassurance that a large tumor burden is unlikely and that patients may be adequately treated with axillary dissection and whole-breast irradiation.

## MRI TO SELECT PATIENTS FOR APBI

The use of a short course of RT limited to the region of the tumor bed, known as APBI, is currently a subject of great interest. APBI is not thought to be a more effective method of radiotherapy than conventional whole-breast RT, but is intended to increase the convenience of RT by reducing the 6.0- to 6.5-week treatment time of standard RT to 5 days or less. In addition to convenience, APBI offers the theoretical advantage of decreasing the radiation dose delivered to areas of the breast not involved with carcinoma and decreasing the radiation dose to adjacent organs.[79]

Significant heterogeneity exists between methods of APBI delivery and study inclusion criteria. The current American Society for Therapeutic Radiology and Oncology (ASTRO) guidelines for patients deemed suitable for APBI include 60 years of age or older, and unicentric invasive ER-positive lymph node-negative tumors 2 cm or less in size, with margins greater than 2 mm, and no extensive intraductal component.[79] The potential of MRI to improve on these selection criteria is uncertain. Two prospective studies reported the impact of MRI in women deemed eligible for APBI based on physical examination, mammography, and ultrasound. Both studies reported loss of eligibility for APBI in 12% of patients based on the identification of additional disease on MRI.[80,81] However, there are no data as to whether the identification of additional disease translates into lower rates of IBTR in women treated with APBI. This situation may be clarified as further follow-up becomes available, but at present, the ASTRO consensus panel concluded that "there are insufficient data to justify the routine use of MRI."[82] It is also worth noting that APBI is not the standard approach to irradiation in BCT, but one that is reserved for women with favorable tumors at relatively low risk for local recurrence, so the possibility of APBI does not provide a rationale for the use of MRI in all women with newly diagnosed breast cancer.

## MRI-NAC

A meta-analysis of 14 prospective randomized trials assessing the effectiveness of NAC found that the use of breast-conserving surgery increased by 16.6% (95% CI 15.1–18.1) in patients receiving chemotherapy first, which is likely an underestimate of the benefit of NAC because many of the patients included in these trials were candidates for breast conservation from the onset. Approximately 80% of patients will respond with a 50% or greater reduction in tumor diameter after neoadjuvant therapy, with 6% to 19% demonstrating a pathologic complete response (pCR) in initial studies.[83] With newer combinations of anthracyclines and taxanes, pCR is seen in approximately 25% of patients[84,85]; the combination of chemotherapy and trastuzumab is associated with pCR in 55% to 65% of cases.[85]

The assessment of residual tumor burden following NAC is important both for surgical planning and for future research aims to address the proper management of the breast following a pCR. Physical examination, mammography, and ultrasound are not particularly accurate in evaluating the response of the tumor to chemotherapy. In one study of 189 patients treated with NAC, the correlation coefficients for residual tumor size as estimated by physical examination, ultrasound, and mammography were 0.42, 0.42, and 0.41, respectively. More importantly, from the perspective of clinical decision making, tumor size as estimated by each of these modalities was within 1 cm of the actual pathologic size in only 66% to 75% of cases.[86] Similar results were reported by Peintinger and colleagues[87] who observed that the accuracy of mammography and sonography in predicting pCR was 89% and that pathologic tumor size was within 0.5 cm of the predicted size in 69% of patients. In light of this, it is not particularly surprising that in the NSABP B27 study, although the addition of a taxane to doxorubicin-cyclophosphamide NAC increased the rate of pCR from 13% to 26%, the rate of BCT did not change.[84] Improved methods of evaluating the extent of viable tumor after neoadjuvant therapy would address a significant clinical need. Multiple studies have addressed whether MRI improves the evaluation of the extent of residual disease following NAC. A meta-analysis of 44 studies including 2050 patients reported on the ability of MRI to identify residual disease following NAC for women with predominately stage II and III invasive ductal carcinoma treated between 1990 and 2008. Most NAC regimens consisted of anthracycline and taxane regimens, and 11 studies included the use of trastuzumab. Surgical pathology was the reference standard for all but 2 studies. The median sensitivity of MRI (correctly identifying residual disease) was 0.92, and the specificity (correct identification of pCR) was 0.60. The overall area under the curve (AUC) of MRI predicting pCR was 0.88. The accuracy of MRI in detecting a pCR varied based on the definition of a pCR, with lower accuracy seen when the definition of pCR allowed residual DCIS. Corresponding AUC for pCR definitions were as follows: 0.83 when defined as the absence of invasive disease (DCIS permitted), 0.86 when defined as the absence of invasive disease and DCIS, 0.90 for non-specific pCR definitions, and 0.91 for near pCR (allowing small clusters of microscopic invasive cells). In comparing MRI with other tests, on univariate analysis, MRI had improved accuracy over mammography (relative diagnosis OR [RDOR] 0.27, $P = .02$) and was not significantly better than clinical examination (RDOR 0.53, $P = .10$) or ultrasound (RDOR 0.54, $P = .15$).[88]

The Translational Breast Cancer Research Consortium Trial 017 was a multicenter retrospective study with the aim of estimating the accuracy of MRI in predicting a pCR following NAC.[89] A total of 770 women from 8 National Cancer Institute–designated comprehensive cancer institutes were included, and a pCR was defined as no residual invasive or in situ disease. The overall accuracy of MRI for predicting a pCR was 74%, although MRI accuracy differed significantly by tumor subtype. Triple-negative and HER2-positive tumors had the highest negative predictive values at 60% and 62%, respectively. With negative predictive values of MRI for detecting a pCR between 33% and 62% between subtypes, MRI alone does not seem to be sufficient to alter therapy following NAC at this time. None of these studies address the accuracy of MRI in determining when a woman is a candidate for BCT after NAC, an end point of greater clinical interest than the predication of pCR because women who do not achieve pCR may still be able to undergo breast conservation if the residual disease is confined to a limited area of the breast.

## SUMMARY

The current evidence supports the selective use of breast MRI for screening-specific high-risk populations, namely, women with known or suspected BRCA1 and BRCA2 mutations, a family history consistent with genetic breast cancer, or a history of chest wall irradiation during childhood or adolescence. There is also evidence that MRI is beneficial for imaging women with occult breast cancer to identify an index tumor and dictate proper surgical therapy. MRI is superior to mammography in assessing the response to NAC, but does not always exclude the presence of significant amounts of microscopic residual disease.

The evidence to support the routine use of MRI in the preoperative work-up of invasive or in situ breast cancer is lacking. Most of the data demonstrate no improvement in short-term surgical outcomes, such as margin status, or in long-term outcomes, such as IBTR or CBC development. There is mixed evidence regarding the use of MRI in the work-up of infiltrating lobular carcinoma in regard to surgical outcomes; but outcomes in this group of luminal A–type cancers are favorable and equivalent to those seen with ductal cancer, so it is not clear that further study of this question is a priority for limited research resources. Future research in this field would be most beneficial in areas addressing clinical problems, such as the need for excision following NAC in the setting of a radiologic and pCR, or the ability to identify populations of patients either appropriate for partial breast irradiation or the elimination of RT following BCT.

## REFERENCES

1. Gotzsche PC, Nielsen M. Screening for breast cancer with mammography. Cochrane Database Syst Rev 2011;(1):CD001877.
2. Mainiero MB, Lourenco A, Mahoney MC, et al. ACR appropriateness criteria breast cancer screening. J Am Coll Radiol 2013;10(1):11–4.
3. Kuhl CK, Schrading S, Leutner CC, et al. Mammography, breast ultrasound, and magnetic resonance imaging for surveillance of women at high familial risk for breast cancer. J Clin Oncol 2005;23(33):8469–76.
4. Saslow D, Boetes C, Burke W, et al. American Cancer Society guidelines for breast screening with MRI as an adjunct to mammography. CA Cancer J Clin 2007;57(2):75–89.
5. Parker A, Schroen AT, Brenin DR. MRI utilization in newly diagnosed breast cancer: a survey of practicing surgeons. Ann Surg Oncol 2013;20(8):2600–6.
6. Swedish Organised Service Screening Evaluation Group. Reduction in breast cancer mortality from organized service screening with mammography: 1. further confirmation with extended data. Cancer Epidemiol Biomarkers Prev 2006;15(1):45–51.
7. Hendrick RE, Smith RA, Rutledge JH 3rd, et al. Benefit of screening mammography in women aged 40-49: a new meta-analysis of randomized controlled trials. J Natl Cancer Inst Monogr 1997;(22):87–92.
8. Tabar L, Vitak B, Chen HH, et al. Beyond randomized controlled trials: organized mammographic screening substantially reduces breast carcinoma mortality. Cancer 2001;91(9):1724–31.
9. Boyd NF, Guo H, Martin LJ, et al. Mammographic density and the risk and detection of breast cancer. N Engl J Med 2007;356(3):227–36.
10. Warner E, Messersmith H, Causer P, et al. Systematic review: using magnetic resonance imaging to screen women at high risk for breast cancer. Ann Intern Med 2008;148(9):671–9.
11. Sardanelli F, Podo F, Santoro F, et al. Multicenter surveillance of women at high genetic breast cancer risk using mammography, ultrasonography, and contrast-enhanced magnetic resonance imaging (the high breast cancer risk Italian 1 study): final results. Invest Radiol 2011;46(2):94–105.
12. Passaperuma K, Warner E, Causer PA, et al. Long-term results of screening with magnetic resonance imaging in women with BRCA mutations. Br J Cancer 2012; 107(1):24–30.
13. Rijnsburger AJ, Obdeijn IM, Kaas R, et al. BRCA1-associated breast cancers present differently from BRCA2-associated and familial cases: long-term follow-up of the Dutch MRISC Screening Study. J Clin Oncol 2010;28(36):5265–73.
14. Sardanelli F, Giuseppetti GM, Panizza P, et al. Sensitivity of MRI versus mammography for detecting foci of multifocal, multicentric breast cancer in Fatty and dense breasts using the whole-breast pathologic examination as a gold standard. AJR Am J Roentgenol 2004;183(4):1149–57.
15. Warner E, Hill K, Causer P, et al. Prospective study of breast cancer incidence in women with a BRCA1 or BRCA2 mutation under surveillance with and without magnetic resonance imaging. J Clin Oncol 2011;29(13):1664–9.

16. Moller P, Stormorken A, Jonsrud C, et al. Survival of patients with BRCA1-associated breast cancer diagnosed in an MRI-based surveillance program. Breast Cancer Res Treat 2013;139(1):155–61.
17. Henderson TO, Amsterdam A, Bhatia S, et al. Systematic review: surveillance for breast cancer in women treated with chest radiation for childhood, adolescent, or young adult cancer. Ann Intern Med 2010;152(7):444–55 W144–54.
18. Sung JS, Lee CH, Morris EA, et al. Screening breast MR imaging in women with a history of chest irradiation. Radiology 2011;259(1):65–71.
19. Freitas V, Scaranelo A, Menezes R, et al. Added cancer yield of breast magnetic resonance imaging screening in women with a prior history of chest radiation therapy. Cancer 2013;119(3):495–503.
20. Ng AK, Garber JE, Diller LR, et al. Prospective study of the efficacy of breast magnetic resonance imaging and mammographic screening in survivors of Hodgkin lymphoma. J Clin Oncol 2013;31(18):2282–8.
21. Oppong BA, King TA. Recommendations for women with lobular carcinoma in situ (LCIS). Oncology (Williston Park) 2011;25(11):1051–6, 1058.
22. Saadatmand S, Rutgers EJ, Tollenaar RA, et al. Breast density as indicator for the use of mammography or MRI to screen women with familial risk for breast cancer (FaMRIsc): a multicentre randomized controlled trial. BMC Cancer 2012;12:440.
23. Morrow M, Bucci C, Rademaker A. Medical contraindications are not a major factor in the underutilization of breast conserving therapy. J Am Coll Surg 1998;186(3):269–74.
24. Holland R, Veling SH, Mravunac M, et al. Histologic multifocality of Tis, T1-2 breast carcinomas. Implications for clinical trials of breast-conserving surgery. Cancer 1985;56(5):979–90.
25. Anastassiades O, Iakovou E, Stavridou N, et al. Multicentricity in breast cancer. A study of 366 cases. Am J Clin Pathol 1993;99(3):238–43.
26. Egan RL. Multicentric breast carcinomas: clinical-radiographic-pathologic whole organ studies and 10-year survival. Cancer 1982;49(6):1123–30.
27. Lagios MD. Multicentricity of breast carcinoma demonstrated by routine correlated serial subgross and radiographic examination. Cancer 1977;40(4):1726–34.
28. Qualheim RE, Gall EA. Breast carcinoma with multiple sites of origin. Cancer 1957;10(3):460–8.
29. Rosen PP, Fracchia AA, Urban JA, et al. "Residual" mammary carcinoma following simulated partial mastectomy. Cancer 1975;35(3):739–47.
30. Schwartz GF, Patchesfsky AS, Feig SA, et al. Multicentricity of non-palpable breast cancer. Cancer 1980;45(12):2913–6.
31. Fisher B, Anderson S, Bryant J, et al. Twenty-year follow-up of a randomized trial comparing total mastectomy, lumpectomy, and lumpectomy plus irradiation for the treatment of invasive breast cancer. N Engl J Med 2002;347(16):1233–41.
32. Veronesi U, Cascinelli N, Mariani L, et al. Twenty-year follow-up of a randomized study comparing breast-conserving surgery with radical mastectomy for early breast cancer. N Engl J Med 2002;347(16):1227–32.
33. Anderson SJ, Wapnir I, Dignam JJ, et al. Prognosis after ipsilateral breast tumor recurrence and locoregional recurrences in patients treated by breast-conserving therapy in five National Surgical Adjuvant Breast and Bowel Project protocols of node-negative breast cancer. J Clin Oncol 2009;27(15):2466–73.
34. Wapnir IL, Anderson SJ, Mamounas EP, et al. Prognosis after ipsilateral breast tumor recurrence and locoregional recurrences in five National Surgical

Adjuvant Breast and Bowel Project node-positive adjuvant breast cancer trials. J Clin Oncol 2006;24(13):2028–37.

35. Houssami N, Ciatto S, Macaskill P, et al. Accuracy and surgical impact of magnetic resonance imaging in breast cancer staging: systematic review and meta-analysis in detection of multifocal and multicentric cancer. J Clin Oncol 2008; 26(19):3248–58.

36. Morrow M, Jagsi R, Alderman AK, et al. Surgeon recommendations and receipt of mastectomy for treatment of breast cancer. JAMA 2009;302(14):1551–6.

37. McCahill LE, Single RM, Aiello Bowles EJ, et al. Variability in reexcision following breast conservation surgery. JAMA 2012;307(5):467–75.

38. Peters NH, van Esser S, van den Bosch MA, et al. Preoperative MRI and surgical management in patients with nonpalpable breast cancer: the MONET - randomised controlled trial. Eur J Cancer 2011;47(6):879–86.

39. Turnbull L, Brown S, Harvey I, et al. Comparative effectiveness of MRI in breast cancer (COMICE) trial: a randomised controlled trial. Lancet 2010;375(9714): 563–71.

40. Houssami N, Turner R, Morrow M. Preoperative magnetic resonance imaging in breast cancer: meta-analysis of surgical outcomes. Ann Surg 2013;257(2): 249–55.

41. King TA, Sakr R, Patil S, et al. Clinical management factors contribute to the decision for contralateral prophylactic mastectomy. J Clin Oncol 2011;29(16): 2158–64.

42. Sorbero ME, Dick AW, Beckjord EB, et al. Diagnostic breast magnetic resonance imaging and contralateral prophylactic mastectomy. Ann Surg Oncol 2009;16(6):1597–605.

43. Pass H, Vicini FA, Kestin LL, et al. Changes in management techniques and patterns of disease recurrence over time in patients with breast carcinoma treated with breast-conserving therapy at a single institution. Cancer 2004;101(4):713–20.

44. Ernst MF, Voogd AC, Coebergh JW, et al. Using loco-regional recurrence as an indicator of the quality of breast cancer treatment. Eur J Cancer 2004;40(4): 487–93.

45. Adkins FC, Gonzalez-Angulo AM, Lei X, et al. Triple-negative breast cancer is not a contraindication for breast conservation. Ann Surg Oncol 2011;18(11): 3164–73.

46. Parker CC, Ampil F, Burton G, et al. Is breast conservation therapy a viable option for patients with triple-receptor negative breast cancer? Surgery 2010; 148(2):386–91.

47. Zumsteg ZS, Morrow M, Arnold B, et al. Breast-conserving therapy achieves locoregional outcomes comparable to mastectomy in women with T1-2N0 triple-negative breast cancer. Ann Surg Oncol 2013;20(11):3469–76.

48. Fischer U, Zachariae O, Baum F, et al. The influence of preoperative MRI of the breasts on recurrence rate in patients with breast cancer. Eur Radiol 2004; 14(10):1725–31.

49. Solin LJ, Orel SG, Hwang WT, et al. Relationship of breast magnetic resonance imaging to outcome after breast-conservation treatment with radiation for women with early-stage invasive breast carcinoma or ductal carcinoma in situ. J Clin Oncol 2008;26(3):386–91.

50. Hwang N, Schiller DE, Crystal P, et al. Magnetic resonance imaging in the planning of initial lumpectomy for invasive breast carcinoma: its effect on ipsilateral breast tumor recurrence after breast-conservation therapy. Ann Surg Oncol 2009;16(11):3000–9.

51. Shin HC, Han W, Moon HG, et al. Limited value and utility of breast MRI in patients undergoing breast-conserving cancer surgery. Ann Surg Oncol 2012; 19(8):2572–9.

52. Ko ES, Han BK, Kim RB, et al. Analysis of the effect of breast magnetic resonance imaging on the outcome in women undergoing breast conservation surgery with radiation therapy. J Surg Oncol 2013;107(8):815–21.

53. Clarke M, Collins R, Darby S, et al. Effects of radiotherapy and of differences in the extent of surgery for early breast cancer on local recurrence and 15-year survival: an overview of the randomised trials. Lancet 2005;366(9503): 2087–106.

54. Gao X, Fisher SG, Emami B. Risk of second primary cancer in the contralateral breast in women treated for early-stage breast cancer: a population-based study. Int J Radiat Oncol Biol Phys 2003;56(4):1038–45.

55. Nichols HB, Berrington de Gonzalez A, Lacey JV Jr, et al. Declining incidence of contralateral breast cancer in the United States from 1975 to 2006. J Clin Oncol 2011;29(12):1564–9.

56. Brennan ME, Houssami N, Lord S, et al. Magnetic resonance imaging screening of the contralateral breast in women with newly diagnosed breast cancer: systematic review and meta-analysis of incremental cancer detection and impact on surgical management. J Clin Oncol 2009;27(33):5640–9.

57. Kim JY, Cho N, Koo HR, et al. Unilateral breast cancer: screening of contralateral breast by using preoperative MR imaging reduces incidence of metachronous cancer. Radiology 2013;267(1):57–66.

58. Mann RM, Hoogeveen YL, Blickman JG, et al. MRI compared to conventional diagnostic work-up in the detection and evaluation of invasive lobular carcinoma of the breast: a review of existing literature. Breast Cancer Res Treat 2008; 107(1):1–14.

59. McGhan LJ, Wasif N, Gray RJ, et al. Use of preoperative magnetic resonance imaging for invasive lobular cancer: good, better, but maybe not the best? Ann Surg Oncol 2010;17(Suppl 3):255–62.

60. Mann RM, Loo CE, Wobbes T, et al. The impact of preoperative breast MRI on the re-excision rate in invasive lobular carcinoma of the breast. Breast Cancer Res Treat 2010;119(2):415–22.

61. Kuhl CK, Schrading S, Bieling HB, et al. MRI for diagnosis of pure ductal carcinoma in situ: a prospective observational study. Lancet 2007;370(9586):485–92.

62. Menell JH, Morris EA, Dershaw DD, et al. Determination of the presence and extent of pure ductal carcinoma in situ by mammography and magnetic resonance imaging. Breast J 2005;11(6):382–90.

63. Allen LR, Lago-Toro CE, Hughes JH, et al. Is there a role for MRI in the preoperative assessment of patients with DCIS? Ann Surg Oncol 2010;17(9): 2395–400.

64. Itakura K, Lessing J, Sakata T, et al. The impact of preoperative magnetic resonance imaging on surgical treatment and outcomes for ductal carcinoma in situ. Clin Breast Cancer 2011;11(1):33–8.

65. Kropcho LC, Steen ST, Chung AP, et al. Preoperative breast MRI in the surgical treatment of ductal carcinoma in situ. Breast J 2012;18(2):151–6.

66. Pilewskie M, Kennedy C, Shappell C, et al. Effect of MRI on the management of ductal carcinoma in situ of the breast. Ann Surg Oncol 2013;20(5):1522–9.

67. Pilewskie M, Olcese C, Eaton A, et al. Perioperative breast MRI is not associated with lower locoregional recurrence rates in DCIS patients treated with or without radiation. Ann Surg Oncol 2014. [Epub ahead of print].

68. Fourquet A, Kirova YM, Campana F. Occult primary cancer with axillary metastases. In: Harris JR, Lippman ME, Morrow M, et al, editors. Diseases of the breast. 4th edition. Philadelphia: Lippincott Williams & Wilkins; 2010. p. 817–21.

69. Varadarajan R, Edge SB, Yu J, et al. Prognosis of occult breast carcinoma presenting as isolated axillary nodal metastasis. Oncology 2006;71(5–6):456–9.

70. Buchanan CL, Morris EA, Dorn PL, et al. Utility of breast magnetic resonance imaging in patients with occult primary breast cancer. Ann Surg Oncol 2005; 12(12):1045–53.

71. Henry-Tillman RS, Harms SE, Westbrook KC, et al. Role of breast magnetic resonance imaging in determining breast as a source of unknown metastatic lymphadenopathy. Am J Surg 1999;178(6):496–500.

72. Ko EY, Han BK, Shin JH, et al. Breast MRI for evaluating patients with metastatic axillary lymph node and initially negative mammography and sonography. Korean J Radiol 2007;8(5):382–9.

73. McMahon K, Medoro L, Kennedy D. Breast magnetic resonance imaging: an essential role in malignant axillary lymphadenopathy of unknown origin. Australas Radiol 2005;49(5):382–9.

74. Morris EA, Schwartz LH, Dershaw DD, et al. MR imaging of the breast in patients with occult primary breast carcinoma. Radiology 1997;205(2):437–40.

75. Olson JA Jr, Morris EA, Van Zee KJ, et al. Magnetic resonance imaging facilitates breast conservation for occult breast cancer. Ann Surg Oncol 2000;7(6): 411–5.

76. Orel SG, Weinstein SP, Schnall MD, et al. Breast MR imaging in patients with axillary node metastases and unknown primary malignancy. Radiology 1999; 212(2):543–9.

77. Lu H, Xu YL, Zhang SP, et al. Breast magnetic resonance imaging in patients with occult breast carcinoma: evaluation on feasibility and correlation with histopathological findings. Chin Med J (Engl) 2011;124(12):1790–5.

78. de Bresser J, de Vos B, van der Ent F, et al. Breast MRI in clinically and mammographically occult breast cancer presenting with an axillary metastasis: a systematic review. Eur J Surg Oncol 2010;36(2):114–9.

79. Smith BD, Smith GL, Roberts KB, et al. Baseline utilization of breast radiotherapy before institution of the Medicare practice quality reporting initiative. Int J Radiat Oncol Biol Phys 2009;74(5):1506–12.

80. Dorn PL, Al-Hallaq HA, Haq F, et al. A prospective study of the utility of magnetic resonance imaging in determining candidacy for partial breast irradiation. Int J Radiat Oncol Biol Phys 2013;85(3):615–22.

81. Horst KC, Fero KE, Ikeda DM, et al. Defining an optimal role for breast magnetic resonance imaging when evaluating patients otherwise eligible for accelerated partial breast irradiation. Radiother Oncol 2013;108(2):220–5.

82. Smith BD, Arthur DW, Buchholz TA, et al. Accelerated partial breast irradiation consensus statement from the American Society for Radiation Oncology (ASTRO). Int J Radiat Oncol Biol Phys 2009;74(4):987–1001.

83. Kaufmann M, von Minckwitz G, Smith R, et al. International expert panel on the use of primary (preoperative) systemic treatment of operable breast cancer: review and recommendations. J Clin Oncol 2003;21(13):2600–8.

84. Bear HD, Anderson S, Brown A, et al. The effect on tumor response of adding sequential preoperative docetaxel to preoperative doxorubicin and cyclophosphamide: preliminary results from National Surgical Adjuvant Breast and Bowel Project Protocol B-27. J Clin Oncol 2003;21(22):4165–74.

85. Buzdar AU, Valero V, Ibrahim NK, et al. Neoadjuvant therapy with paclitaxel followed by 5-fluorouracil, epirubicin, and cyclophosphamide chemotherapy and concurrent trastuzumab in human epidermal growth factor receptor 2-positive operable breast cancer: an update of the initial randomized study population and data of additional patients treated with the same regimen. Clin Cancer Res 2007;13(1):228–33.
86. Chagpar AB, Middleton LP, Sahin AA, et al. Accuracy of physical examination, ultrasonography, and mammography in predicting residual pathologic tumor size in patients treated with neoadjuvant chemotherapy. Ann Surg 2006; 243(2):257–64.
87. Peintinger F, Kuerer HM, Anderson K, et al. Accuracy of the combination of mammography and sonography in predicting tumor response in breast cancer patients after neoadjuvant chemotherapy. Ann Surg Oncol 2006;13(11):1443–9.
88. Marinovich ML, Houssami N, Macaskill P, et al. Meta-analysis of magnetic resonance imaging in detecting residual breast cancer after neoadjuvant therapy. J Natl Cancer Inst 2013;105(5):321–33.
89. De Los Santos JF, Cantor A, Amos KD, et al. Magnetic resonance imaging as a predictor of pathologic response in patients treated with neoadjuvant systemic treatment for operable breast cancer. Translational Breast Cancer Research Consortium trial 017. Cancer 2013;119(10):1776–83.

# Molecular Profiling of Breast Cancer

Amy E. Cyr, MD, Julie A. Margenthaler, MD*

## KEYWORDS

- Breast cancer • Molecular profiling • Molecular diagnostics • Prognostication
- Genome

## KEY POINTS

- Molecular profiling has identified at least 4 distinct subtypes of breast cancer: luminal, HER2-enriched, basal-like, and normal breast–like.
- Patients with ductal carcinoma in situ who have undergone surgical excision to margins of 3 mm or more and who have a low-risk 12-gene recurrence score may safely omit adjuvant radiation therapy.
- The 21-gene recurrence score, 70-gene signature, and PAM50 risk of recurrence score are all useful tools for determining prognosis beyond standard clinicopathologic features and in predicting response to chemotherapy for patients with ER-positive, node-negative, and node-positive invasive breast cancer.
- Molecular diagnostic tools should not replace standard clinicopathologic features but rather provide complementary information to aid in the complex decision-making process of adjuvant treatment recommendations in patients with breast cancer.
- Prospective clinical trials are needed to determine the impact of gene assays on outcomes for patients with breast cancer.

## MOLECULAR PROFILING OF INTRINSIC SUBTYPES OF BREAST CANCER
### Cluster Analysis and Subtypes

Molecular studies have demonstrated the great heterogeneity of breast cancer.[1–4] One of the first applications of microarray-based gene-expression profiling analysis in breast cancer was the landmark work by Perou and colleagues[5] and Sorlie and colleagues.[6] These studies were the first to demonstrate that estrogen receptor (ER)-positive and ER-negative breast cancers are biologically distinct diseases with respect to their molecular analysis.[6] In addition, cluster analysis of genes revealed that there are at least 4 molecular subtypes of breast cancer, including luminal, human

Disclosures: None.
Department of Surgery, Washington University School of Medicine, 660 South Euclid Avenue, Campus Box 8109, St Louis, MO 63110, USA
* Corresponding author.
E-mail address: margenthalerj@wudosis.wustl.edu

Surg Oncol Clin N Am 23 (2014) 451–462
http://dx.doi.org/10.1016/j.soc.2014.03.004
1055-3207/14/$ – see front matter © 2014 Elsevier Inc. All rights reserved.

epidermal growth factor receptor 2 (HER2)-enriched, basal-like, and normal breast–like.[5] Luminal A (~40% of all breast cancers) and luminal B (~20% of all breast cancers) are the most common subtypes, and are characterized by the expression of ER, progesterone receptor (PR), and other genes associated with ER activation. Although luminal A and luminal B constitute most ER-positive breast cancers, there are important molecular distinctions between the two. Luminal A tumors typically have high expression of ER-related genes, low expression of HER2 genes, and low expression of proliferation-related genes.[7,8] In comparison with luminal A tumors, luminal B tumors have lower expression of ER-related genes, variable expression of HER2 genes, and higher expression of the proliferation-related genes.[9] The HER2-enriched subtype (~10%–15% of all breast cancers) is characterized by high expression of the HER2 and proliferation-related genes, and low expression of the luminal and basal-like genes.[10] Importantly not all HER2-enriched subtypes translate to clinically HER2-positive breast cancer, and vice versa. Thus, not all HER2 mutations result in HER2 amplification and protein overexpression. Furthermore, approximately 50% of clinically HER2-positive breast cancers are not HER-enriched at a molecular level, but are characterized as HER2-positive luminal subtypes.[11] The basal-like subtype (~15%–20% of all breast cancers) is characterized by low expression of the luminal and HER2 genes and high expression of the proliferation cluster of genes.[12] Although most basal-like breast cancers are triple-negative (ER-negative, PR-negative, HER2-negative), not all triple-negative breast cancers are basal-like. Finally, the normal-like subtype is characterized by gene expression similar to that of normal breast tissue. It remains unclear whether this represents a separate subtype with clinical significance or a technical artifact of the molecular analysis.[11]

### Subtype Prognostication and Treatment Recommendations

It must be borne in mind that the molecular analysis of intrinsic subtypes of breast cancer identifies relevant biology. These studies were not designed for prognostication. However, subtype analysis does correlate with prognosis in multiple large data sets.[10,11,13–15] Overall, patients with luminal A breast cancer have the best prognosis, followed by patients with luminal B breast cancer. Patients with either HER2-enriched or basal-like subtypes have the worst overall survival. However, more recent advances in targeted therapies (eg, trastuzumab) hold significant promise in the ability to alter that natural history.[16] A consensus conference was held to discuss the role of molecular subtype analysis in clinical decision making.[13] The panel concluded that ER/PR/HER2 measurements should not be used as surrogates for assigning patients into molecular groups, and that molecular subtype analysis was insufficient at present to incorporate into the decision-making algorithm for treatment recommendations.[13]

## MOLECULAR PREDICTION AND PROGNOSTICATION FOR TREATMENT DECISION MAKING
### Overview

Concurrent with the evolution of molecular subtype classification of breast cancers, several researchers and industry sponsors have developed multiple gene prognostic signatures, several of which have been validated and are in clinical use. The 3 most commonly used molecular prognostic profiles are the Recurrence Score (RS), derived from Oncotype Dx, the Amsterdam 70-gene signature (Mammaprint), and the Risk of Recurrence Score (ROR), derived from PAM50. The RS was validated in an independent data set from samples collected from node-negative, ER-positive patients treated with tamoxifen in the large multicenter National Surgical Adjuvant Breast and Bowel Project (NSABP) B-14 trial.[17] A recurrence score from zero to 100 is reported, with 3 categories of risk: low (scored 0–18), medium (scored 19–30), and high (scored 31–100). The test also reports ER, PR, and HER2 status. The 70-gene signature was developed using a supervised DNA microarray analysis of gene-expression arrays on frozen tissue from 98 primary breast tumors, followed by validation in multiple studies.[18–21] It is approved for use in both ER-positive and ER-negative tumors, and reports either a low-risk or high-risk result. The PAM50 ROR is a 50-gene test that characterizes an individual tumor by intrinsic subtype and generates a ROR; it has also been validated in several studies.[22–24] Although several other genomic signatures are available, the remainder of this review refers only to published data related to these 3 validated signatures. Furthermore, because ER/PR-negative tumors of all sizes are candidates for adjuvant chemotherapy, with or without the addition of trastuzumab depending on HER2 expression, this article focuses on the evidence surrounding the use of molecular prognostic tools for patients with ductal carcinoma in situ (DCIS) and ER-positive invasive breast cancer.

## Ductal Carcinoma in Situ

Breast-conserving therapy, which includes wide local excision of the tumor followed by irradiation, has become a standard treatment option for women with DCIS.[25] Local recurrence has been shown to be affected by several patient and tumor characteristics, including patient's age, extent of disease, nuclear grade, margin status, presence of comedonecrosis, and utilization of adjuvant radiation.[26] The National Comprehensive Cancer Network (NCCN) included excision alone as an acceptable treatment option for patients with DCIS in the 2008 practice guidelines, but they did not define which subgroup of patients for which excision alone is appropriate.[27] In 2003, Silverstein[28] updated his Van Nuys Prognostic Index, which describes the use of nuclear grade, necrosis, size, margin width, and patient's age to predict recurrence following excision of DCIS. Excision alone is recommended for those with scores of 4 to 6; excision plus adjuvant radiation therapy is recommended for those with scores of 7 to 9; and mastectomy is recommended for those with scores of 10 to 12.[28] This scoring translated to a less than 20% local recurrence rate at 12 years when these criteria were followed.[28] However, the primary limitation for the Van Nuys Prognostic Index is the lack of an ability to account for the wide heterogeneity of DCIS.

Molecular and biological markers that provide prognostic and predictive information hold the most promise for tailoring therapy on an individual level. Expression of p16, cyclooxygenase-2, and Ki-67, which indicate an abrogated response to cellular stress, have been shown to delineate which DCIS lesions are more likely to confer a high risk for recurrence.[29] The 21-gene RS for ER-positive invasive breast cancer was used as a benchmark for the development of a 12-gene subset that has been used to develop and validate a DCIS score that divides patients into low risk, intermediate risk, and high risk for 10-year local in-breast recurrence.[30] The DCIS score was prospectively evaluated using archived tumor samples from the Eastern Cooperative Oncology Group E5194 study.[31] This prospective, nonrandomized study investigated the risk of local recurrence in 670 patients with DCIS following wide local excision alone. Patients were required to have negative margin widths of 3 mm or more and were divided into 2 treatment arms consisting of grade 1 or 2, size 2.5 cm or smaller, or grade 3, size 1.0 cm or smaller. Radiation was not allowed, but approximately 30% of patients did receive optional adjuvant tamoxifen.

The relationship between the DCIS score risk group and 10-year risk of an ipsilateral breast event (IBE), whether in situ or invasive, was highly statistically significant ($P = .006$ for any IBE and $P = .003$ for an invasive IBE).[30] Multivariable modeling of risk for IBE, both excluding and including the DCIS score, were also performed. When the DCIS score was excluded, tumor size and postmenopausal status were the only factors significantly associated with risk for IBE (hazard ratio [HR] 1.54, $P = .006$ and HR 0.49, $P = .02$, respectively). However, when the DCIS score was included in the model, the 12-gene score was statistically significant (HR 2.37, $P = .02$), in addition to tumor size and menopausal status. Thus, patients who have undergone wide local excision for DCIS who have a low-risk score could reasonably elect to omit radiation therapy, whereas patients in the intermediate or high-risk groups should consider adjuvant radiation therapy and tamoxifen following wide local excision.

One significant limitation in the application of the DCIS score to clinical practice is that the patients have to fit the specific profile of the patients in the E5194 study; this is challenging with regard to margin status, whereby many clinicians commonly consider margins of less than 3 mm sufficient. Patients with close or positive margins following wide local excision of DCIS are not appropriate candidates for molecular profiling at present. One must also consider a patient's age, comorbidities, tumor size, tamoxifen therapy eligibility, and other clinical factors when making adjuvant radiation decisions.

### ER-Positive, Node-Negative Invasive Breast Cancer

Adjuvant chemotherapy has been in widespread use for ER-positive, lymph node–negative breast cancers, even for small Stage I tumors, since the 1988 National Institutes of Health guidelines were published.[32] Patients have been assigned to high-risk and low-risk groups based on clinical and pathologic characteristics in an attempt to personalize the treatment approach.[33,34] The emergence of genomic techniques and the ability to measure the expression of many disparate genes have extended our ability to tailor therapy to the individual patient beyond that offered by standard clinical and pathologic parameters. Furthermore, molecular assays can provide both prognostic information (projected clinical outcome at the time of diagnosis independent of therapy) and predictive information (likelihood of response to a given therapeutic modality).

In a landmark study, Paik and colleagues[35] validated the 21-gene RS as a predictor of the prospectively defined primary end point of distant recurrence-free survival in a large cohort of ER-positive, node-negative, tamoxifen-treated patients with breast cancer enrolled in the NSABP B-14 trial. The RS was calculated for each patient; 51% of the patient population fell into the low-risk group (n = 338), 22% fell into the intermediate-risk group (n = 149), and 27% fell into the high-risk group (n = 181). The rates of distant recurrence at 10 years were 6.8% for the low-risk group, 14.3% for the intermediate-risk group, and 30.5% for the high-risk group ($P<.001$ low-risk vs high-risk).

In a subsequent validation study, the 21-gene RS was strongly associated with the risk of death from breast cancer in a similar cohort and also in patients who did not receive adjuvant systemic therapy.[36] The objective of this additional study of the NSABP B-20 patients was to determine the magnitude of the chemotherapy benefit with methotrexate and fluorouracil (MF) or cyclophosphamide, methotrexate, and fluorouracil (CMF) as a function of the RS. The primary analysis was predetermined to compare the tamoxifen-treated patients with both chemotherapy arms combined. Patients with a low RS showed no evidence of benefit from CMF-like chemotherapy, and patients with an intermediate RS also did not show clear benefit from adjuvant CMF-like chemotherapy. By contrast, those patients with a high recurrence score treated with adjuvant CMF-like chemotherapy, in addition to endocrine therapy, experienced a significant improvement in distant relapse-free survival, with a 28% absolute benefit for adjuvant chemotherapy and tamoxifen (P<.001).[36] Furthermore, this association with RS and survival were independent from standard clinical and pathologic variables, supporting the utility of this molecular analysis beyond ER and HER2 status, tumor grade, and stage. One interesting subanalysis from the NSABP B-20 validation study is that 44% of the patients younger than 40 years had low-risk RS results.[37] Although younger patients do worse overall and are probably more likely to benefit from chemotherapy, there is a large fraction of younger patients for whom the RS is low and benefits of chemotherapy may be minimal.

The 21-gene RS has been endorsed by American Society of Clinical Oncology and 2 expert panels (NCCN Breast Cancer Clinical Practice Guidelines and the 2011 St Gallen International Expert Consensus).[38–40] These panels consider RS to be useful for patients with ER-positive, node-negative breast cancer as an aid to decision-making for administering adjuvant chemotherapy. The management of patients with intermediate-risk RS is being studied in the TAILORx (Trial Assigning IndividuaLized Options for Treatment) trial, where patients with ER-positive, node-negative breast cancer and intermediate-risk RS were randomized to either endocrine therapy alone or endocrine therapy with adjuvant chemotherapy.[41] The study has completed accrual, but the survival data will not be available for several years.

The RS assay has also been shown to predict the likelihood of locoregional recurrence.[42] In an analysis of patients from the NSABP B-14 and B-20 trials, there was a statistically significant association between the RS and locoregional recurrence regardless of the treatment group. In patients treated with tamoxifen alone, the rate of locoregional recurrence at 10 years was only 4.3% for those with a low-risk RS compared with 7.2% for those with an intermediate-risk RS and 15.8% for those with a high-risk RS (P<.001).[42] There were also significant associations between the RS and locoregional recurrence in placebo-treated patients from NSABP B-14 (P = .022) and in chemotherapy plus tamoxifen-treated patients from NSABP B-20 (P = .028). The RS was an independent predictor of locoregional recurrence in multivariate analysis, in addition to patient's age and type of initial treatment. What remains unanswered is whether the recommendations for adjuvant radiation therapy should be altered based on these molecular data. The omission of adjuvant radiation for patients with a low-risk RS is a potential future area of research interest.

The 70-gene signature has been approved by the Food and Drug Administration for the prognostication of patients with Stage I or II, node-negative, invasive breast cancer of tumor size less than 5 cm. This profile was based on an empirical microarray analysis of 78 breast cancers from patients who were younger than 55 years, who had tumors that were 5 cm or less and node-negative, and who had not received any adjuvant systemic therapy.[43] The patients were stratified into poor-prognosis disease if distant metastasis occurred within 5 years and good prognosis if no metastasis occurred within 5 years. The optimum threshold between these disparate outcomes was identified and applied to a cohort of 295 retrospectively accrued invasive breast cancers, of which 61 were node-negative in the initial study.[18] This analysis revealed that the 70-gene signature was an independent prognostic marker of outcome. Subsequent studies have shown that the 70-gene signature also correlates with chemotherapy sensitivity, whereby patients with poor prognosis signatures derive the greatest benefit from adjuvant chemotherapy.[44] There is also Level II evidence that the 70-gene signature more accurately predicts outcome in cases where there is disagreement between the 70-gene signature and standard clinical and pathologic features.[18] The MINDACT (Microarray In Node-Negative and 1 to 3 positive lymph node Disease may Avoid Chemo Therapy) is a prospective, randomized phase 3 trial that was designed to answer this question, comparing the 70-gene signature with the common clinicopathologic characteristics in selecting patients with breast cancer with 0 to 3 positive nodes for adjuvant chemotherapy.[45]

The PAM50 assay provides a ROR prognostic for relapse-free survival in patients with node-negative tumors who did not receive adjuvant systemic therapy.[46] The ability of the ROR to predict prognosis was confirmed in a subsequent study of 786 patients with ER-positive disease treated only with adjuvant tamoxifen.[22] When combined with tumor size, the ROR was more predictive of outcome when compared with standard clinicopathologic variables, including tumor grade, PR status, and Ki-67 proliferation marker. Dowsett and colleagues[24] showed that the ROR outperformed the RS in its ability to stratify patients with ER-positive, node-negative breast cancer. More patients were scored as high risk and fewer as intermediate risk by ROR in comparison with RS, suggesting that the ROR may be a better prognostic indicator than the RS among this population.

### ER-Positive, Node-Positive Invasive Breast Cancer

Node positivity continues to be an indication for cytotoxic therapy in patients with ER-positive, node-positive breast cancer, and this recommendation is included in the current NCCN guidelines.[39] It is well known that an increasing amount of lymph node disease is associated with poorer outcomes.[47–49] However, there is a recognized subset of node-positive women who never develop metastatic disease despite not being treated with cytotoxic therapy. Therefore, within this population of node-positive patients, multigene assays are being used to further stratify patients in terms of prognosis; similarly to patients with node-negative disease, those with higher risk of distant recurrence could be treated more aggressively.

Multiple studies have evaluated the prognostic capability of gene-expression signatures in the setting of node-positive breast cancer, although many of these studies are small and have limited follow-up. A subset analysis of the Southwestern Oncology Group (SWOG) 8814 trial[50] was performed to determine whether the RS could provide prognostic information for patients with node-positive disease as it does for node-negative disease. In the original SWOG trial, postmenopausal women with hormone receptor–positive, node-positive breast cancer were randomized to tamoxifen alone, cyclophosphamide, doxorubicin, fluorouracil (CAF) chemotherapy with sequential tamoxifen, or CAF with concurrent tamoxifen. The addition of CAF to tamoxifen improved disease-free and overall survival for patients with 1 to 3 positive nodes and for patients with 4 or more positive nodes. Oncotype DX was performed on banked tissue samples from the trial (148 in the tamoxifen-alone arm and 219 in the sequential CAF-tamoxifen arm). The RS significantly predicted 10-year disease-free and overall survival for patients in the tamoxifen-alone arm after adjusting for the amount of nodal disease: 10-year disease-free survival was 60%, 49%, and 43%, respectively, for patients with low-, intermediate-, and high-risk RS ($P = .017$). Overall survival was 77%, 68%, and 51% ($P = .003$) for the same groups.[50]

Dowsett and colleagues[51] analyzed tissue samples from the ATAC (Arimidex, Tamoxifen, Alone or in Combination) trial to determine whether the RS could predict distant recurrence in both node-negative and node-positive patients. For 872 node-negative patients, 9-year distant recurrence rates were 4%, 12%, and 25% for the low-, intermediate-, and high-risk RS groups, respectively. A similar trend was seen for the 306 node-positive patients, for whom distant recurrence rates were 17%, 28%, and 49% ($P = .002$). These rates reflect adjustment for tumor size, grade, patient's age, and treatment (tamoxifen vs anastrozole). Tumor size and amount of lymph node disease remained significant predictors of time to distant recurrence on multivariate analysis. The HR between low and high RS was more pronounced in the node-negative group (5.2) when compared with the node-positive group (2.7). Overall survival for node-negative patients with low-, intermediate-, and high-risk RS were 88%, 84%, and 73%, respectively. For node-positive patients, overall survival was 74%, 69%, and 54%. It is worth noting that this is one of the only studies evaluating a gene assay on patients treated with aromatase inhibitors (rather than tamoxifen, as was used in most trials).[51]

Distant disease and overall survival are also predicted by the Mammaprint 70-gene signature. Van de Vijver and colleagues[18] reported a consecutive series of 295 patients with Stage I and II breast cancer, all younger than 53 years, and half node-positive. One hundred twenty of the 144 node-positive patients included received systemic therapy: chemotherapy, endocrine therapy, or both. Distant metastatic events and overall survival were significantly predicted by the 70-gene signature among all patients and among the node-positive subgroup (all $P<.001$). On multivariate analysis, poor prognosis signature, tumor size, and nonuse of chemotherapy remained the most significant predictors of distant metastasis (all $P<.001$).[18] Similarly, Mook and colleagues[52] applied the 70-gene signature to 241 patients with 1 to 3 positive nodes. Ten-year distant metastasis–free survival and breast cancer–specific survival were 91% and 96%, respectively, for women with good prognosis signatures, and 76% and 76% for women with poor prognosis signatures. On multivariate analysis, the gene signature predicted disease-specific survival better than traditional prognostic factors ($P = .005$).[52]

Genetic signatures can also provide prognostic information regarding local-regional disease. Mamounas and colleagues[53] reported that RS predicts local-regional recurrence in node-positive patients. Node-positive, ER-positive patients included in the NSABP B-28 trial were treated with both chemotherapy and tamoxifen. RS significantly predicted local-regional recurrence for patients undergoing mastectomy ($P = .004$) or lumpectomy with radiation ($P = .022$), and for patients with 4 or more positive nodes ($P = .001$); there was a nonsignificant trend for patients with 1 to 3 positive nodes ($P = .12$).[53]

Several molecular diagnostic tests, including Oncotype DX, the Mammaprint 70-gene signature, and PAM50, were compared by Prat and colleagues.[54] A data set was created of ER-positive patients, both node-negative and node-positive, treated with tamoxifen. The investigators concluded that multiple gene-expression signatures were prognostic for node-negative, ER-positive cancers, but that this prognostic capability was significantly worse for node-positive cancers. In addition, a paucity of node-positive tumors, specifically those with low-risk and intermediate-risk RS, had at least 90% distant recurrence-free survival at 8.5 years' follow-up, and therefore only a small minority of these patients would receive little benefit from chemotherapy.[54]

In addition to providing this prognostic information in the setting of node-positive disease, molecular diagnostics can also provide predictive information. In the SWOG subanalysis performed by Albain and colleagues,[50] RS was seen to predict survival benefit with chemotherapy over tamoxifen alone; no significant disease-free or overall survival improvement was seen with CAF for patients with low-risk and intermediate-risk RS, but CAF did improve these survival rates for patients with high-risk RS.[50]

To provide more robust data on the predictive power of these molecular assays in the setting of node-positive, ER-positive disease, several large prospective trials are under way. MINDACT includes multiple treatment arms; clinical and pathologic factors and the 70-gene signature are used to stratify patients. Poor-prognosis patients are given chemotherapy and, if they are ER-positive, endocrine therapy.

Good-prognosis patients are treated with endocrine therapy if they are ER-positive. Patients whose clinicopathologic features and gene signature are discordant are randomized; either the clinicopathologic feature or the gene signature is used to determine treatment recommendations.[45,55] SWOG S1007 (the RxPonder [Rx for POsitive NoDe Endocrine Responsive] Trial) includes women with hormone receptor–positive, HER2-negative breast cancer and 1 to 3 positive nodes. Patients with an RS less than or equal to 25 are randomized to chemotherapy plus endocrine therapy or to endocrine therapy alone. Patients with an RS greater than 25 are not randomized, but treatment is determined by the treating physician.[55]

## IMPACT OF MOLECULAR PROFILING ON PRACTICE PATTERNS

Given that there are multiple such tests recently available, and given their cost, many investigators have evaluated the impact of these molecular diagnostics on clinical practice and on health care economics. Several retrospective studies have demonstrated that use of the RS is associated with less chemotherapy than clinicians would have recommended before knowing the RS results.[56–58] Chen and colleagues[59] reported that chemotherapy was used for 6% of low-risk patients, 42% of intermediate-risk patients, and 84% of high-risk patients. Oncotype DX testing was associated with younger patient age, better performance status, and higher tumor grade.[59] Most of these studies are limited by their retrospective nature. Lo and colleagues[60] created a prospective multicenter trial examining the impact of the RS on systemic therapy recommendations, and found that medical oncologists changed their recommendations for 31% of a cohort of 89 patients after obtaining the RS.[60]

The RASTER (MicroarRAay PrognoSTics in Breast CancER) trial was a prospective trial designed to assess the feasibility of implementing use of the 70-gene assay in community-based practice, and to assess its effect on adjuvant therapy recommendations. Eight hundred twelve node-negative women in the Netherlands were enrolled in this study over a 3-year period, and concordance between the gene assay results and traditionally used clinicopathologic guidelines was assessed. Genetic signatures were available for 427 patients. The genetic signature was discordant with national treatment guidelines, with Adjuvant! Online, and with St Gallen criteria for 30%, 37%, and 39% of patients, respectively. This feasibility study concluded that additional studies were warranted to determine the impact of these molecular diagnostics on patient outcomes.[61]

The use of chemotherapy is costly for the health care system. Several investigators have quantified the economic impact of the use of these diagnostic tests. These studies quantify dollars saved with the use of gene assays, specifically resulting from fewer recommendations for chemotherapy, therefore saving costs for the drugs themselves, supportive care, and management of complications.[62] Other studies have concluded that the tests are cost-effective as defined by cost per quality-adjusted life-year (QALY) gained. For instance, Lamond and colleagues[63] found the RS to be cost-effective in both node-negative and node-positive patients in a Canadian model, although the cost per QALY was higher for node-positive patients ($14,844 per QALY for node-positive women vs $9591 for node-negative patients).[63]

## SUMMARY

Greater understanding of tumor biology allows targeted, personalized therapies for breast cancer. In addition to recognizing different histologies, it has become standard practice to classify breast cancers by grade and by their intrinsic subtypes. The molecular diagnostic tests discussed in this article represent the evolution in our ability to tailor therapeutic recommendations to individual patients. Although these tests were developed and validated on tissue samples from prospective clinical trials, the current data regarding application of these tests to clinical practice are still retrospective in nature. Results from the ongoing TAILORx, MINDACT, and RxPonder trials are not yet available, and other clinical trials incorporating these genetic signatures are under way or in development. Currently recruiting trials include the MINT (Multi Institutional Neoadjuvant Therapy) Mammaprint Project, which will assess the ability of the 70-gene signature, along with other genomic assays and traditional clinicopathologic features, to predict response to neoadjuvant chemotherapy for locally advanced breast cancers as measured by pathologic complete response. Investigators are also comparing these gene assays with each other: in RxPonder, the RS will be compared with the PAM-50 ROR,[55] and the PROMIS (Prospective Registry of Mammaprint in breast cancer patients with an Intermediate recurrence Score) observational study will use the 70-gene signature in patients with intermediate-risk RS.[64] These diagnostic tests hold great promise and are anticipated to improve patient outcomes and health care costs, but until such prospective data are available, their impact remains speculative.

# REFERENCES

1. Reis-Filho JS, Weigelt B, Fumagalli D, et al. Molecular profiling: moving away from tumor philately. Sci Transl Med 2010;2:47ps43.
2. Sotiriou C, Pusztai L. Gene-expression signatures in breast cancer. N Engl J Med 2009;360:790–800.
3. Weigelt B, Baehner FL, Reis-Filho JS. The contribution of gene expression profiling to breast cancer classification, prognostication, and prediction: a retrospective of the last decade. J Pathol 2010;220:263–80.
4. Iwamoto T, Pusztai L. Predicting prognosis of breast cancer with gene signatures: are we lost in a sea of data? Genome Med 2010;2:81.
5. Perou CM, Sorlie T, Eisen MB, et al. Molecular portraits of human breast tumours. Nature 2000;406:747–52.
6. Sorlie T, Perou CM, Tibshirani R, et al. Gene expression patterns of breast carcinomas distinguish tumor subclasses with clinical implications. Proc Natl Acad Sci U S A 2001;98:10869–74.
7. Fan C, Oh DS, Wessels L, et al. Concordance among gene-expression-based predictors for breast cancer. N Engl J Med 2006;355:560–9.
8. Hu Z, Fan C, Oh DS, et al. The molecular portraits of breast tumors are conserved across microarray platforms. BMC Genomics 2006;7:96.
9. Voduc KD, Cheang MC, Tyldesley S, et al. Breast cancer subtypes and the risk of local and regional relapse. J Clin Oncol 2010;28:1684–91.
10. Reis-Filho JS, Pusztai L. Gene expression profiling in breast cancer: classification, prognostication, and prediction. Lancet 2011;378:1812–23.
11. Prat A, Ellis MJ, Perou CM. Practical implications of gene-expression-based assays for breast oncologists. Nature 2012;9:48–57.
12. Reis-Filho JS, Tutt AN. Triple negative tumours: a critical review. Histopathology 2008;52:108–18.
13. Schwartz GF, Bartelink H, Burstein HJ, et al. Adjuvant therapy in Stage I carcinoma of the breast: the influence of multigene analyses and molecular phenotyping. Breast J 2012;118:2031–8.
14. Carey LA, Perou CM, Livasy CA, et al. Race, breast cancer subtypes, and survival in the Carolina Breast Cancer Study. JAMA 2006;295:2492–502.

15. Prat A, Adamo B, Cheang MC, et al. Molecular characterization of basal-like and non-basal-like triple-negative breast cancer. Oncologist 2013;18:123–33.
16. Slamon DJ, Leyland-Jones B, Shak S, et al. Use of chemotherapy plus a monoclonal antibody against HER2 for metastatic breast cancer that overexpresses HER2. N Engl J Med 2001;344:783–92.
17. Paik S. Development and clinical utility of a 21-gene recurrence score prognostic assay in patients with early breast cancer treated with tamoxifen. Oncologist 2007;12:631–5.
18. Van de Vijver MJ, He YD, Van't Veer LJ, et al. A gene-expression signature as a predictor of survival in breast cancer. N Engl J Med 2002;347:1999–2009.
19. Buyse M, Loi S, Van't Veer L, et al. Validation and clinical utility of a 70-gene prognostic signature for women with node-negative breast cancer. J Natl cancer Inst 2006;98:1183–92.
20. Mook S, Schmidt MK, Weigelt B, et al. The 70-gene prognosis signature predicts early metastasis in breast cancer patients between 55 and 70 years of age. Ann Oncol 2010;21:717–22.
21. Mook S, Knauer M, Bueno-de-Mesquita JM, et al. Metastatic potential of T1 breast cancer can be predicted by the 70-gene MammaPrint signature. Ann Surg Oncol 2010;17:1406–13.
22. Nielsen TO, Parker JS, Leung S, et al. A comparison of PAM50 intrinsic subtyping with immunohistochemistry and clinical prognostic factors in tamoxifen-treated estrogen receptor-positive breast cancer. Clin Cancer Res 2010;16:5222–32.
23. Chia SK, Bramwell VH, Tu D, et al. A 50-gene intrinsic subtype classifier for prognosis and prediction of benefit from adjuvant tamoxifen. Clin Cancer Res 2012;18:4465–72.
24. Dowsett M, Lopez-Knowles E, Sidhu K. Comparison of PAM50 risk of recurrence score with oncotypeDx and IHC4 for predicting risk of distant recurrence after endocrine therapy. J Clin Oncol 2013;31:2783–90.
25. Fisher B, Anderson S, Bryant J, et al. Twenty-year follow-up of a randomized trial comparing total mastectomy, lumpectomy, and lumpectomy plus irradiation for the treatment of invasive breast cancer. N Engl J Med 2002;347:1233–41.
26. Benson JR, Wishart GC. Predictors of recurrence for ductal carcinoma in situ after breast-conserving surgery. Lancet Oncol 2013;14:e348–57.
27. Carlson RW, Allred DC, Anderson BO, et al. NCCN clinical practice guidelines in oncology: breast cancer. Fort Washington (PA): National Comprehensive Cancer Network; 2008. Available at: www.nccnorg. Accessed August 23, 2013.
28. Silverstein MJ. The University of Southern California/Van Nuys prognostic index for ductal carcinoma in situ of the breast. Am J Surg 2003;186:337–43.
29. Gauthier ML, Berman HK, Miller C, et al. Abrogated response to cellular stress identifies DCIS associated with subsequent tumor events and defines basal-like breast tumours. Cancer Cell 2007;12:479–91.
30. Solin L, Gray R, Baehner F, et al. A quantitative multigene RT-PCR assay for predicting recurrence risk after surgical excision alone without irradiation for ductal carcinoma in situ (DCIS): a prospective validation study of the DCIS Score from the ECOG E5194. J Natl Cancer Inst 2013;105:701–10.
31. Hughes LL, Wang M, Page DL, et al. Local excision alone without irradiation for ductal carcinoma in situ of the breast: a trial of the Eastern Cooperative Oncology Group. J Clin Oncol 2009;27:5319–24.
32. National Cancer Institute. Clinical alert. Bethesda (MD): National Cancer Institute; 1988.

33. Dignam JJ, Dukic V, Anderson SJ, et al. Hazard of recurrence and adjuvant treatment effects over time in lymph node-negative breast cancer. Breast Cancer Res Treat 2009;116:595–602.
34. Boyages J, Taylor R, Chua B, et al. A risk index for early node-negative breast cancer. Br J Surg 2006;93:564–71.
35. Paik S, Shak S, Tang G, et al. A multigene assay to predict recurrence of tamoxifen-treated, node-negative breast cancer. N Engl J Med 2004;351:2817–26.
36. Habel LA, Shak S, Jacobs MK, et al. A population-based study of tumor gene expression and risk of breast cancer death among lymph node-negative patients. Breast Cancer Res 2006;8:R25.
37. Paik S, Tang G, Shak S, et al. Gene expression and benefit of chemotherapy in women with node-negative, estrogen receptor-positive breast cancer. J Clin Oncol 2006;24:3726–34.
38. Harris L, Fritsche H, Mennel R, et al. American Society of Clinical Oncology 2007 update of recommendations for the use of tumor markers in breast cancer. J Clin Oncol 2007;25:5287–312.
39. NCCN clinical practice guidelines in oncology: breast cancer. Available at: http://www.nccn.org/professionals/physician_gls/pdf/breast.pdf. Accessed August 24–25, 2013.
40. Goldhirsch A, Wood WC, Coates AS. Strategies for subtypes—dealing with the diversity of breast cancer: highlights of the St. Gallen International Expert Consensus on the primary therapy of early breast cancer 2011. Ann Oncol 2011;22:1736–47.
41. Zujewski JA, Kamin L. Trial assessing individualized options for treatment for breast cancer: the TAILORx trial. Future Oncol 2008;4:603–10.
42. Mamounas EP, Tang G, Fisher B, et al. Association between the 21-gene recurrence score assay and risk of locoregional recurrence in node-negative, estrogen receptor-positive breast cancer: results from NSABP B-14 and NSABP B-20. J Clin Oncol 2010;28:1677–83.
43. Van't Veer LJ, Dai H, Van de Vijver MJ, et al. Gene expression profiling predicts clinical outcome of breast cancer. Nature 2002;415:530–6.
44. Knauer M, Mook S, Rutgers EJ, et al. The predictive value of the 70-gene signature for adjuvant chemotherapy in early breast cancer. Breast Cancer Res Treat 2010;120:655–61.
45. Rutgers E, Piccart-Gebhart MJ, Bogaerts J, et al. The EORTC 10041/BIG 03-04 MINDACT trial is feasible: results of the pilot phase. Eur J Cancer 2011;47:2742–9.
46. Parker JS, Mullins M, Cheang MC, et al. Supervised risk predictor of breast cancer based on intrinsic subtypes. J Clin Oncol 2009;27:1160–7.
47. Dent DM. Axillary lymphadenectomy for breast cancer. Arch Surg 1996;131:1125–7.
48. Fisher B, Jeong JH, Anderson S, et al. Twenty-five-year follow-up of a randomized trial comparing radical mastectomy, total mastectomy, and total mastectomy followed by radiation. N Engl J Med 2002;347:567–75.
49. Tan LK, Giri D, Hummer AJ, et al. Occult axillary node metastases in breast cancer are prognostically significant: results in 368 node-negative patients with 20-year follow-up. J Clin Oncol 2008;26:1803–9.
50. Albain KS, Barlow WE, Shak S, et al. Prognostic and predictive value of the 21-gene recurrence score assay in a randomized trial of chemotherapy for postmenopausal, node-positive, estrogen receptor-positive breast cancer. Lancet Oncol 2010;11:55–65.

51. Dowsett M, Cuzick J, Wale C, et al. Prediction of risk of distant recurrence using the 21-gene recurrence score in node-negative and node-positive postmenopausal patients with breast cancer treated with anastrozole or tamoxifen: a TransATAC study. J Clin Oncol 2010;28:1829–34.

52. Mook S, Schmidt MK, Viale G, et al. The 70-gene prognosis-signature predicts disease outcome in breast cancer patients with 1-3 positive lymph nodes in an independent validation study. Breast Cancer Res Treat 2009;116:295–302.

53. Mamounas EP, Tang G, Paik S, et al. The 21-gene recurrence score predicts risk of loco-regional recurrence in node (+), ER (+) breast cancer after adjuvant chemotherapy and tamoxifen: results from the NSABP B-28. Abstract #2, Social of Surgical Oncology Annual Cancer Symposium. 2013.

54. Prat A, Parker JS, Fan C, et al. Concordance among gene-expression based predictors for ER-positive breast cancer treated with adjuvant tamoxifen. Ann Oncol 2012;23:2866–73.

55. Goncalves R, Bose R. Using multigene tests to select treatment for early-stage breast cancer. J Natl Compr Canc Netw 2013;11:174–82.

56. Ademuyiwa FO, Miller A, O'Connor T, et al. The effects of Oncotype DX recurrence scores on chemotherapy utilization on a multi-institutional breast cancer cohort. Breast Cancer Res Treat 2011;126:797–802.

57. Asad J, Jacobson AF, Estabrook A, et al. Does Oncotype DX recurrence score affect the management of patients with early-stage breast cancer? Am J Surg 2008;196:527–9.

58. Klang SH, Hammerman A, Liebermann N, et al. Economic implications of 21-gene breast cancer risk assay from the perspective of an Israeli-managed health care organization. Value Health 2010;13:381–7.

59. Chen C, Dhanda R, Tseng WY, et al. Evaluating use characteristics for the Oncotype dx 21-gene recurrence score and concordance with chemotherapy use in early-stage breast cancer. J Oncol Pract 2013;9:182–7.

60. Lo SS, Mumby PB, Norton J, et al. Prospective multicenter study of the impact of the 21-gene recurrence score assay on medical oncologist and patient adjuvant breast cancer treatment selection. J Clin Oncol 2010;28:1671–7.

61. Bueno-de-Mesquita JM, van Harten WH, Retel VP, et al. Use of 70-gene signature to predict prognosis of patients with node-negative breast cancer: a prospective community-based feasibility study (RASTER). Lancet Oncol 2007;8:1079–87.

62. Hornberger J, Chien R, Krebs K, et al. US insurance program's experience with a multigene assay for early-stage breast cancer. J Oncol Pract 2011;7:e38s–45s.

63. Lamond NW, Skedgel C, Rayson D, et al. Cost-utility of the 21-gene recurrence score assay in node-negative and node-positive breast cancer. Breast Cancer Res Treat 2012;133:1115–23.

64. Available at: www.Clinicaltrials.gov. Accessed August 27, 2013.

# Management of the Clinically Node-Negative Axilla in Primary and Locally Recurrent Breast Cancer

 CrossMark

Ashley C. McGinity, MD, Meeghan A. Lautner, MD, Ismail Jatoi, MD, PhD*

## KEYWORDS

- Sentinel lymph node • Recurrence • Breast cancer • Axilla

## KEY POINTS

- Axillary lymph node dissection should be performed in clinically node-negative axilla only when sentinel lymph node biopsy (SLNB) shows metastatic disease.
- Performing immunohistochemistry on routine SLNBs is not recommended.
- Sentinel lymph node biopsy on ipsilateral breast tumor recurrences is feasible and seems reliable.
- Lymphoscintigraphy provides useful information for accurately identifying the sentinel lymph node.

## INTRODUCTION

For patients with primary breast cancer, nodal status remains a key determinant of overall prognosis. Thus, patients who present with metastasis to the axillary lymph nodes have a worse prognosis than those who do not. To reduce the morbidity of axillary surgery, the sentinel lymph node biopsy (SLNB) technology was introduced in the 1990s. Since then, SLNB has become the standard of care for staging patients with clinically node-negative disease. However, with the widespread implementation of SLNB technology during the past 15 years, a new dilemma has arisen: how to manage the clinically node-negative axilla in patients with ipsilateral breast tumor recurrences (IBTRs). No clear answer exists because no randomized trials have addressed the effect of SLNB remapping on locoregional recurrences and mortality. Yet, some investigators advocate for repeat SLNB in patients with an IBTR with clinically node-negative axilla.

---

The authors have nothing to disclose.
Department of Surgery, University of Texas Health Science Center San Antonio, 7703 Floyd Curl Drive, MC 7738, San Antonio, TX 78229-3900, USA
* Corresponding author.
E-mail address: jatoi@uthscsa.edu

This article therefore discusses 2 separate issues: (1) management of the axilla in patients with clinically node-negative primary breast cancer, and (2) management of the clinically node-negative axilla in patients with IBTRs.

## SENTINEL LYMPH NODE BIOPSY IN CLINICALLY NODE-NEGATIVE PRIMARY BREAST CANCER

Patients with clinically node-positive primary breast cancer should undergo axillary clearance. Sentinel lymph node biopsy is an option only for those with clinically node-negative breast cancer.

For patients with primary breast cancer, the management of the axilla has been a topic of considerable interest and controversy for many years. In the late 19th century, William Halsted[1] argued that the axillary lymph nodes were the gateway for the distant spread of breast cancer. Thus, he maintained that extirpation of the breast, underlying pectoralis muscle, and the adjacent axillary lymphatics en bloc (radical mastectomy) was the optimal treatment of primary breast cancer.

The results of large randomized trials conducted under the auspices of the National Surgical Adjuvant Breast and Bowel Project (NSABP) and the Cancer Research Campaign Working Party (King's/Cambridge) have challenged this hypothesis. The NSABP B-04 trial randomized patients with clinically node-negative breast cancer to radical mastectomy versus total mastectomy with postoperative axillary radiation versus total mastectomy followed by axillary dissection only in patients who subsequently developed clinically positive nodes.[2] In the King's/Cambridge trial, women with clinically node-negative early breast cancer were randomized to total mastectomy with immediate axillary radiation versus total mastectomy and observation of the axilla (with delayed treatment of the axilla in patients who subsequently developed axillary recurrences).[3]

Both of these trials demonstrated that the delayed treatment of the axilla did not adversely affect survival, and therefore called into question the notion that the axillary nodes served as the nidus for the distant spread of breast cancer.[2,3] However, the NSABP B-04 and King's/Cambridge trials do indicate that treatment of the axilla (with either surgery or radiotherapy) in patients with clinically node-negative breast cancer substantially reduces the risk of axillary recurrences. Moreover, surgery is the preferred method of treating the axilla because it also enables staging of the patient (as either node-positive or node-negative). However, patients without metastasis to the axilla needlessly undergo axillary surgery, and incur the potential morbidity associated with axillary surgery. Thus, SLNB technology was developed to reduce the risk of morbidity associated with unnecessary axillary surgery.

In 1970, Kett and colleagues[4] published results of lymphatic mapping of the breast after periareolar injection of blue dye. This procedure identified an isolated blue node that was commonly adjacent to the axillary vein. In 1993, Krag and colleagues[5] reported the identification of an isolated node using technetium sulfur and a gamma probe. Giuliano and colleagues[6] described the technique of blue dye mapping of sentinel lymph nodes (SNLs) of the breast, and reported that SLNB was 95.6% accurate in predicting the status of the axilla. Albertini and colleagues[7] combined the 2 methods (blue dye and radiocolloid), and reported a similar sentinel node identification rate of 92.0%. A randomized prospective trial by Morrow and colleagues[8] in 1999 compared the combination of blue dye and radioactive colloid versus the use of blue dye alone and showed equivalent sentinel node identification rates.

Considerable evidence now shows that SLNB is a much less morbid procedure than the standard ALND, and that the 2 procedures are associated with similar survival rates and risk of local recurrences. The NSABP B-32 trial randomized 5611 women with clinically node-negative breast cancer to ALND versus SLNB plus ALND (with ALND performed only if evidence showed metastasis to the SLN). The study used both blue dye and radiotracer to identify the SLN. Patients in the SLNB arm of the trial had equivalent survival and regional control to those in the standard ALND arm.[9] In addition, patients in the SLNB arm had a lower risk of morbidity compared with those in the standard ALND arm.[10] Significantly fewer shoulder abduction deficits (75% vs 41%; P<.001), lymphedema (7%–9% vs 13%–14%), arm numbness (31.0% vs 8.1%; P<.001), and tingling (13.5% vs 7.5%; P<.001) were associated with SLNB versus ALND.

Several other randomized control trials have demonstrated the reduced morbidity of SLNB compared with ALND. In the Axillary Lymphatic Mapping Against Nodal Axillary Clearance (ALMANAC) trial, Mansel and colleagues[11] showed that the SLNB group had a lower incidence of lymphedema, shorter time of drain usage, shorter hospital stay, and faster resumption of everyday activities compared with the ALND group. The absolute risk of developing lymphedema 12 months after SLNB was 5% versus 13% (relative risk [RR], 0.37; 95% CI, 0.23–0.60) in those who underwent an ALND. Similarly, the absolute risk of experiencing sensory loss at 12 months after SLNB was 11% compared with 31% of patients who had ALND (RR, 0.37; 95% CI, 0.27–0.50).

Veronesi and colleagues[12] reported the results of their trial undertaken in Milan, which randomized 512 patients to ALND versus SLNB (with ALND only in patients with positive SLNs) and followed them for 24 months after surgery. The patients randomized to the SLNB arm of the trial had significantly less axillary pain (8% vs 39%), less numbness (1% vs 68%), and better overall arm mobility (0% vs 21%) than those randomized to the ALND arm of the trial.

Purushotham and colleagues[13] randomized 298 patients with tumors smaller than 3 cm to similar groups (ALND vs SLNB followed by ALND if sentinel node–positive). They reported decreased sensory deficits, decreased seroma occurrence, and reduction in lymphedema in the SLNB arm. Similarly, the GIVOM (Gruppo Interdisciplinare Veneto di Oncologia Mammaria) trial in Italy randomized 697 patients to ALND versus SLNB (with ALND in node-positive cases). In addition to the decrease in lymphedema and numbness and better range of motion, they noted improved quality of life for patients randomized to SLNB.[14]

The Sentinel Node versus Axillary Clearance (SNAC) trial randomized 1083 patients either to SLNB followed by axillary clearance if the SLN was positive or not detected, or to routine axillary clearance. A significant decrease in wound infection, seroma formation, impairment of range of motion, and numbness was seen in the group randomized to SLNB.[15]

Kell and colleagues[16] published a meta-analysis of 7 randomized controlled trials with a total of 9608 patients comparing standard ALND versus SLNB. The goal of this overview was to determine morbidity reduction with SLNB versus standard ALND. This meta-analysis showed a reduction in risk of infection (odds ratio [OR], 0.58; 95% CI, 0.42–0.80; $P = .0011$), seroma (OR, 0.40; 95% CI, 0.31–0.51; $P = .0071$), arm swelling (OR, 0.30; 95% CI, 0.14–0.66; $P = .0028$), and numbness (OR, 0.25; 95% CI, 0.1–0.59; $P = .0018$) in patients in the SLNB arm compared with those in the standard ALND arm.

These results indicate that standard ALND can no longer be justified as the standard means of staging patients with clinically node-negative primary breast cancer (**Table 1**). Rather, SLNB is the standard method of staging these patients.

However, the results of the American College of Surgeons Oncology Group (ACSOG) Z0011 trial suggests that not all patients with positive SLNs need to proceed with

**Table 1**
**Outcomes of randomized controlled trials comparing rate of complications with SLNB versus ALND**

| | Number of Patients | Limb Swelling (%) | Numbness (%) | Abduction Deficits (%) | Seroma (%) |
|---|---|---|---|---|---|
| NSABP-B32 | N = 5611 | | | | |
| SLNB | 2697 | 8.0 | 8.1 | 13.0 | N/A |
| ALND | 2619 | 14.0 | 31.1 | 19.0 | |
| ALMANAC | N = 954 | | | | |
| SLNB | 478 | 5.0 | 11.0 | N/A | N/A |
| ALND | 476 | 13.0 | 31.0 | | |
| Milan | N = 516 | | | | |
| SLNB | 259 | 7.0 | 1.0 | 0 | N/A |
| ALND | 257 | 75.0 | 68.0 | 21.0 | |
| Purushotham et al | N = 298 | | | | |
| SLNB | 143 | N/A | 66.0 | N/A | 14.0 |
| ALND | 155 | | 84.0 | | 21.0 |
| SNAC | N = 1083 | | | | |
| SLNB | 544 | 2.8 | N/A | 2.5 | 17.0 |
| ALND | 539 | 4.2 | | 4.4 | 36.0 |
| GIVOM | N = 697 | | | | |
| SLNB | 345 | 10.0 | 8.0 | N/A | N/A |
| ALND | 352 | 5.0 | 15.0 | | |
| Z0011 | N = 744 | | | | |
| SLNB | 371 | 6.0 | 9.0 | N/A | 6.0 |
| ALND | 373 | 11.0 | 39.0 | | 14.0 |

*Abbreviation:* N/A, not available.

axillary lymph node dissection.[17] Specifically, this trial suggests that selected patients with SLN-positive disease who undergo lumpectomy and radiotherapy may not require a formal axillary clearance. Although this study has limitations (the study did not meet its targeted accrual goal; follow-up was only 6 years; and a disproportionately large number of patients in this study had estrogen receptor–positive tumors), it does suggest that selected patients with sentinel node–positive tumors can avoid ALND.

Another conundrum is the presence of micrometastases in the SLN. The American Joint Committee on Cancer (AJCC) defines macrometastases as foci of tumor cells greater than 2.0 mm, micrometastases are those foci measuring between 0.2 and 2.0 mm (pN1mi), and isolated tumor cells (pN0(i+)) foci measuring 0.2 mm or less. Micrometastases are found using deeper cross-sections and immunohistochemistry (IHC), and their significance has been investigated in patients from the NSABP B-32 trial.[18] The occult metastases or micrometastases were found using deeper cuts and IHC, whereas the standard metastases were found using standard 2-mm intervals and hematoxylin-eosin (H&E) staining. The 5-year overall survival rate among patients with occult metastases detected was 94.6% using the Kaplan-Meier method, compared with 95.8% in patients without detectable metastases. Although this difference attains statistical significance, it has little clinical relevance.

The relevance of micrometastases in the SLN detected with IHC was further investigated in the ACOSOG Z0010 study.[19] The study enrolled 5210 patients with early-stage breast cancer who were treated with breast-conservation therapy and SLNB. In 10.5% of patients (349 of 3326 patients) whose SLNs were negative on H&E

staining, micrometastases were detected by IHC. However, the presence of these micrometastases did not alter the 5-year survival rates (95.7%; 95% CI, 95.0%–96.5% for IHC-negative, and 95.1%; 95% CI, 92.7%–97.5% for IHC-positive disease).

The International Breast Cancer Study Group (IBCSG) recently reported the results of a large trial randomizing 934 patients with sentinel node micrometastasis to undergo either axillary dissection or not. The 5-year disease-free survival rate was 87.8% in the group who did not undergo axillary dissection (95% CI, 84.4–91.2), and 84.4% (95% CI, 80.7–88.1) in the group who did. More long-term surgical complications were seen in the axillary dissection group (lymphedema, neuropathy).[20] These results suggest that ALND can be avoided in patients with micrometastasis to the sentinel node. Moreover, one might argue that standard H&E staining of the sentinel nodes is sufficient, and that IHC staining should be avoided because it leads to potential overstaging.

## MANAGEMENT OF THE CLINICALLY NODE-NEGATIVE AXILLA IN LOCALLY RECURRENT BREAST CANCER

As women with breast cancer continue to live longer, new challenges are arising regarding the management of the axilla in patients with an IBTR after breast-conservation therapy. With the more widespread use of SLNB, management of the axilla in patients with IBTR after breast-conservation therapy has generated controversy. Approximately 10% to 15% of all patients treated with breast-conservation therapy will experience an IBTR within a 10-year period, although these rates are decreasing with improvements in adjuvant systemic therapy.[21] The standard management of IBTR after breast-conservation therapy has been a salvage mastectomy.[22] However, the question has arisen whether sentinel node remapping should be undertaken in patients with clinically node-negative breast cancer who present with IBTR. To date, no randomized controlled trials have addressed this issue. Thus, whether sentinel node remapping ultimately results in improved outcomes (reduction in risk of mortality or recurrences) for these patients is currently unknown. However, several observational studies suggest that a repeat SLNB is feasible in patients who subsequently experience an IBTR after surgery for primary breast cancer.

Cox and colleagues[23] at the H. Lee Moffitt Cancer Center and Research Institute performed a retrospective review of their dataset for patients from 1994 to 2006 who underwent SLNB and then underwent reoperative SLNB. This study identified 56 patients with IBTR who had a previous lumpectomy and a negative SLNB, and 52 of these underwent a repeat SLNB. In this study, the SLN was successfully identified in 80.4% of cases using both blue dye and radiocolloid. Of the patients with clinically node-negative breast cancer who underwent successful remapping, 9 of 45 (20%) had positive SLNs and underwent formal ALND, whereas the remaining 80% were spared ALND. At 26 months of mean follow-up, no axillary recurrences were seen, suggesting that ALND could be avoided in patients who are SLNB-negative after IBTR.

Port and colleagues[24] undertook a retrospective study at Memorial Sloan-Kettering Cancer Center of 117 patients who experienced IBTR after breast-conservation therapy (previously treated with either SLNB or ALND). All of these patients underwent SLNB, irrespective of whether they had previously undergone SLNB or ALND. Their SLN remapping success rate was 55% (64 of 117). Because of the larger sample size, the investigators were able to detect a significant difference in the success rate of the remapping between patients who underwent previous SLNB alone versus ALND. The success rate of identifying an SLN after a previous SLNB was significantly higher than if the patient had undergone an ALND at the time of primary diagnosis

(74% vs 38%; $P = .0002$). No axillary recurrences were seen in any of these patients at a mean follow-up of 2.2 years, suggesting that ALND can be avoided in patients who undergo remapping with SLNB. These investigators performed lymphoscintigraphy preoperatively on most patients undergoing remapping, and found that the success of the reoperative SLNB correlated with a positive lymphoscintigraphy (79% vs 24%; $P<.0001$). In the earlier study, lymphoscintigraphy showed that 30% of the patients with IBTR had drainage to other nodal basins, such as the internal mammary or supraclavicular basins.

Axelsson and Jonsson[25] undertook a nonrandomized prospective trial in Denmark of 50 patients with IBTR after either lumpectomy or mastectomy who were all mapped preoperatively with lymphoscintigraphy. In this study, 45% of patients had SLNs detected at surgery (and 83% of these had a positive preoperative lymphoscintigraphy). Sentinel lymph nodes contained metastases in 16%, and these patients went on to completion ALND.

The use of preoperative lymphoscintigraphy was further supported by Taback and colleagues,[26] who reviewed 15 patients who developed an IBTR after undergoing breast-conservation surgery, SLNB and/or ALND, and adjuvant breast radiation therapy. All patients underwent preoperative lymphoscintigraphy, and 7 cases of aberrant nodal drainage were reported. These basins include the internal mammary, supraclavicular, interpectoral, and contralateral axilla. The authors postulated that this is likely because of the combination of prior axillary surgery and breast irradiation, which can alter the drainage pathways. Not surprisingly, 2 of the 3 patients who had the SLN identified in the contralateral axilla had undergone ipsilateral ALND as part of their initial treatment. Thus, preoperative lymphoscintigraphy may provide useful information regarding ipsilateral axillary SLN identification.

The sentinel node and recurrent breast cancer (SNARB) study undertaken in the Netherlands reviewed 150 patients who had locally recurrent breast cancer after undergoing either lumpectomy or mastectomy.[27] The SLN was successfully identified in most patients, and preoperative lymphoscintigraphy was also performed. Aberrant drainage pathways were visualized in 58.9% patients, and were significantly more frequent in patients who had undergone previous ALND versus SLNB (79.3% vs 25.0%; $P<.0001$). The lymphoscintigraphy-directed repeat SLNB altered treatment plans in 16.5% of patients, and 50.0% of patients with previous negative SLNB results were spared ALND.

Maaskant-Braat and colleagues[28] undertook a meta-analysis of SLNBs in patients with IBTR, involving a total of 692 patients from 25 studies. In this study, 301 patients had previous SLNB, 361 with previous ALND, and 30 had no previous axillary surgery. Sentinel node was identified in 65.3%. Higher identification rates were reported in patients with previous SLNB compared with previous ALND (81.0% vs 52.2%; $P<.0001$). Aberrant drainage pathways were identified on lymphoscintigraphy in 43.2%.

These studies raise an important issue: what impact does SLN identification have on the ultimate outcome in patients with IBTR? In these studies, patients with clinically node-negative IBTR who were SLN-positive underwent ALND (whereas those who were SLN-negative did not), but whether this strategy has any overall benefit on local recurrence or mortality is unknown. Ultimately, this question can only be resolved through a large randomized prospective trial with long-term follow-up.

## SUMMARY

In patients with primary breast cancer, axillary surgery is an important staging tool, and substantially reduces the risk of axillary recurrences. The SLNB is the preferred

**Table 2**
Outcomes of observational studies in patients with IBTR undergoing repeat SLNB

| | Number of Patients | Success Rate of Mapping (%) | Repeat SLN Positive for Disease (%) | Axillary Recurrence at Follow-up (n) |
|---|---|---|---|---|
| Cox et al,[23] 2008 | 56 | 80.4 | 20.0 | 0 at 2.2 y |
| Port et al,[24] 2007 | 117 | 54.7 | 16.0 | 0 at 2.2 y |
| Axelsson & Jonsson,[25] 2008 | 50 | 45.0 | 16.0 | N/A |
| Taback et al,[26] 2006 | 15 | 79.0 | 27.0 | 0 at 3.1 y |
| Maaskant-Braat et al,[27] 2013 | 150 | 52.6 | 11.4 | N/A |
| Total | 388 | 62.3 | 18.1 | |

*Abbreviation:* N/A, not available.

method of staging the axilla compared with standard ALND, because it results in significantly less morbidity. In the years ahead, the number of breast cancer survivors will continue to increase as treatment modalities improve. Moreover, larger numbers of patients who experience IBTR after surgery for primary breast cancer will likely be seen, and the role of SLN remapping in this setting remains controversial. No randomized controlled trial exists to define the exact algorithm that should be followed, but observational studies have indicated that SLNB is feasible in the setting of IBTR (**Table 2**). Most studies would also suggest the use of lymphoscintigraphy to help guide the remapping of the lymphatic drainage, particularly in those who have undergone prior ALND. This information may allow more patients to continue to avoid the morbidity associated with ALND, even in the setting of IBTR. However, the overall impact of SLNB (on mortality and local recurrence) in the setting of IBTR is not known, as no randomized trials have addressed this issue.

## REFERENCES

1. Halstead W. The results of radical operations for the cure of carcinoma of the breast. Ann Surg 1907;46(1):1–19.
2. Fisher B, Montague E, Redmond C, et al. Comparison of radical mastectomy with alternative treatments for primary breast cancer. A first report of results from a prospective randomized clinical trial. Cancer 1977;39(6):2827–39.
3. Cancer Research Campaign Working Party. Cancer research campaign (King's/Cambridge) trial for early breast cancer. A detailed update at the tenth year. Lancet 1980;2(8185):55–60.
4. Kett K, Varga G, Lukacs L. Direct lymphography of the breast. Lymphology 1970; 3(1):2–12.
5. Krag D, Weaver D, Alex J, et al. Surgical resection and radiolocalization of the sentinel lymph node in breast cancer using a gamma probe. Surg Oncol 1993; 2:335–40.
6. Giuliano A, Kirgan D, Guenther J, et al. Lymphatic mapping and sentinel lymphadenectomy for breast cancer. Ann Surg 1994;220(3):391–401.
7. Albertini J, Lyman G, Cox C, et al. Lymphatic mapping and sentinel node biopsy in the patient with breast cancer. JAMA 1996;276(22):1818–22.
8. Morrow M, Rademaker AW, Bethke K, et al. Learning sentinel node biopsy: results of prospective randomized trial of two techniques. Surgery 1999;126(4):714–20.

9. Krag D, Anderson S, Julian T, et al. Sentinel-lymph-node resection compared with conventional axillary-lymph-node dissection in clinically node-negative patients with breast cancer: overall survival findings from the NSABP B-32 randomised phase 3 trial. Lancet 2010;11:927–33.

10. Ahikaga T, Krag D, Land S, et al. Morbidity results from the NSABP B-32 trial comparing sentinel lymph node dissection versus axillary dissection. J Surg Oncol 2010;102:111–8.

11. Mansel RE, Fallowfield L, Kissin M, et al. Randomized multicenter trial of sentinel lymph node biopsy versus standard axillary treatment in operable breast cancer: the ALMANAC trial. J Natl Cancer Inst 2006;98(9):599–609.

12. Veronesi U, Paganelli G, Viale G, et al. A randomized comparison of sentinel-node biopsy with routine axillary dissection in breast cancer. N Engl J Med 2003;349(6):546–53.

13. Purushotham A, Upponi S, Klevesath MB, et al. Morbidity after sentinel lymph node biopsy in primary breast cancer: results from a randomized controlled trial. J Clin Oncol 2005;23(19):4312–21.

14. Del Bianco P, Zavagno G, Burelli P, et al. Morbidity comparison of sentinel lymph node biopsy versus axillary lymph node dissection in breast cancer patients: results of the sentinella-GIVOM Italian randomised clinical trial. Eur J Surg Oncol 2008;34(5):508–13.

15. Gill G. Sentinel-lymph-node-based management or routine axillary clearance? One year outcomes of sentinel node biopsy versus axillary clearance (SNAC): a randomized controlled surgical trial. Ann Surg Oncol 2008;16(2):266–75.

16. Kell M, Burke JM, Barry M, et al. Outcome of axillary staging in early breast cancer: a meta-analysis. Breast Cancer Res Treat 2010;120(2):441–7.

17. Giuliano A, Hunt K, Ballman K, et al. Axillary dissection vs no axillary dissection in women with invasive breast cancer and sentinel node metastasis. JAMA 2011;305(6):569–75.

18. Weaver D, Ashikaga T, Krag D, et al. Effect of occult metastases on survival in node-negative breast cancer. N Engl J Med 2011;364(4):412–21.

19. Giuliano A, Hawes D, Ballman K, et al. Association of occult metastases in sentinel lymph nodes and bone marrow with survival among women with early-stage invasive breast cancer. JAMA 2011;306(4):385–93.

20. Galimberti V, Cole B, Zurrida S, et al. Axillary dissection versus no axillary dissection in patients with sentinel node micrometastases (IBCSG 23-01): a phase 3 randomised controlled trial. Lancet Oncol 2013;14(4):297–305.

21. Fisher B, Redmond C, Poisson R, et al. Eight-year results of a randomized clinical trial comparing total mastectomy and lumpectomy with or without irradiation in the treatment of breast cancer. N Engl J Med 1989;320:822–8.

22. Burger A, Pain S, Peley G. Treatment of recurrent breast cancer following breast conserving surgery. Breast J 2013;19(3):310–8.

23. Cox CE, Furman BT, Kiluk JV, et al. Use of reoperative sentinel lymph node biopsy in breast cancer patients. J Am Coll Surg 2008;207(1):57–61.

24. Port ER, Garcia-Etienne CA, Park J, et al. Reoperative sentinel lymph node biopsy: a new frontier in the management of ipsilateral breast tumor recurrence. Ann Surg Oncol 2007;14(8):2209–14.

25. Axelsson C, Jonsson P. Sentinel lymph node biopsy in operations for recurrent breast cancer. Eur J Surg Oncol 2008;34:626–30.

26. Taback B, Nguyen P, Hansen N, et al. Sentinel lymph node biopsy for local recurrence of breast cancer after breast-conserving therapy. Ann Surg Oncol 2006;13(8):1099–104.

27. Maaskant-Braat A, Roumen R, Voogd A, et al. Sentinel node and recurrent breast cancer (SNARB): results of a nationwide registration study. Ann Surg Oncol 2013; 20:620–6.
28. Maaskant-Braat A, Voogd A, Rudi M, et al. Repeat sentinel node biopsy in patients with locally recurrent breast cancer: a systemic review and meta-analysis of the literature. Breast Cancer Res Treat 2013;138:13–20.

# Management of Axillary Disease

Abigail S. Caudle, MD, MS, Julie A. Cupp, MD, Henry M. Kuerer, MD, PhD*

## KEYWORDS

- Breast cancer • Nodal metastasis • Sentinel lymph node
- Axillary lymphadenectomy • Neoadjuvant chemotherapy

## KEY POINTS

- Accurate staging of the axillary lymph nodes is critical to defining prognosis and for planning therapy.
- In patients with clinically negative axillary lymph nodes, sentinel lymph node dissection (SLND) is the standard approach to surgically staging the axillary nodes and has been shown to be technically feasible and accurate in multi-institutional randomized studies.
- The ACOSOG Z0011 trial demonstrated that carefully selected clinically node-negative women undergoing breast conservation therapy who have 1 or 2 positive sentinel lymph nodes may safely omit axillary lymph node dissection (ALND) without impact on oncologic outcomes.
- SLND can be performed successfully after neoadjuvant chemotherapy in clinically node-negative patients and allows for a single surgical procedure for patients as well as a lower proportion of patients requiring ALND.
- ALND remains the standard approach for clinically node-positive patients who undergo neoadjuvant chemotherapy. Emerging data from trials such as the ACOSOG Z1071 study may soon change this practice.

## INTRODUCTION

The presence of axillary lymph node metastases is the most significant predictor of cancer outcomes in breast cancer, and remains an important aspect of diagnosis and management of these patients.[1–3] Nodal status is often the key determinant of extent of surgery as well as systemic therapy and radiation. In the past, women diagnosed with breast cancer underwent axillary lymph node dissection (ALND) in order to stage the axilla. The introduction of sentinel lymph node dissection (SLND) as a validated staging procedure allowed clinicians to gain the same information while minimizing morbidity with no difference in oncologic outcomes.[4] Although all patients

There are no conflicts of interest to report.
Department of Surgical Oncology, The University of Texas MD Anderson Cancer Center, 1515 Holcombe Boulevard, Unit 1484, Houston, TX 77230-1402, USA
* Corresponding author.
E-mail address: hkuerer@mdanderson.org

Surg Oncol Clin N Am 23 (2014) 473–486
http://dx.doi.org/10.1016/j.soc.2014.03.007
1055-3207/14/$ – see front matter © 2014 Elsevier Inc. All rights reserved.

surgonc.theclinics.com

with positive lymph nodes underwent ALND in the past, recent data have changed this approach, and have allowed for highly selected women to omit ALND. Emerging data will potentially broaden this approach in growing populations of patients. Therefore, surgeons must be able to accurately assess the axillary nodes for the presence of metastases, delineate the extent of nodal disease, and understand the impact on oncologic outcomes in order to design operations that are effective but also minimize morbidity.

## STAGING OF AXILLARY NODAL REGION

Physical examination of breast cancer patients should always include specific attention to the regional nodal basins such as the axillary, infraclavicular, and supraclavicular regions. When axillary adenopathy is noted, clinicians should record the size of the palpable lymph node as well as whether the nodes feel matted together. Unfortunately, physical examination is not sensitive or specific, as involved nodes may not be palpable, and palpable nodes may actually be reactive, especially after breast biopsies. The false-negative rate for physical examination is as high as 45% in some series.[5] For this reason, clinical examination is complemented by nodal ultrasonography. Axillary lymph nodes can be assessed for features associated with malignancy such as enlarged size, thickened or eccentric cortex, or compression of the fatty hilum.[6] Suspicious nodes routinely undergo fine needle aspiration (FNA) or core biopsy to provide pathologic confirmation of involvement with a subsequent sensitivity of 86% to 89% and specificity as high as 100%.[7,8] This information can then be used in designing a treatment plan.

The American Join Committee on Cancer (AJCC) staging classification has different parameters for nodal staging based on clinical versus pathologic evaluation.[3] Clinically identified axillary lymph nodes (either by examination or imaging studies) are designated as N1 if they are in the ipsilateral nodal basin and are mobile, or N2 if they are fixed or matted to each other or other structures. Contralateral axillary metastases are classified as distant metastases. The pathologic staging system has more variation. Metastases that are less than or equal to 0.2 mm are classified as isolated tumor cells and are designated at pN0(i+). Metastases in 1 to 3 axillary lymph nodes are categorized as N1, with a designation of "mi" if the metastases are micrometastases (>0.2 mm but ≤2 mm). Involvement of 4 to 9 axillary lymph nodes is staged as pN2, and at least 10 involved nodes are defined as pN3.

## CLINICALLY NODE-NEGATIVE PATIENT
### SLND Technique

SLND is based on the concept that the breast has an orderly pattern of lymphatic drainage, with specific lymph nodes, or sentinel nodes, that drain the breast first, followed by drainage to the remaining nodal basin. This idea was first reported by Braithwaite over 100 years ago after observing the lymphatic drainage pattern of a gangrenous appendix. The first clinical applications were presented in the 1970s for penile cancer, although the technique did not become widely used because of its difficulty.[9] In the early 1990s, a more feasible technique was created for melanoma that allowed for widespread implementation into practice.[10] Before this point, women standardly underwent ALND for staging of axillary nodes, with the associated morbidities of the procedure including functional deficits, chronic pain, and development of lymphedema. Unfortunately, many of these patients had no nodal metastases and thus suffered the morbidities without an oncologic benefit. Thus there was tremendous interest in applying the technique to breast cancer patients. SLND was quickly validated as an accurate technique for staging nodal basins in breast cancer patients with increased sensitivity and decreased risks.[11–14]

In clinically node-negative patients who undergo surgery as the first component of their breast cancer treatment, SLND is the standard surgical approach to axillary staging. Multiple studies have demonstrated that an SLN can be identified in 93% to 99% of patients, with a false-negative rate (ie, number of patients with axillary metastases in which no cancer is seen in the SLN) of 5% to 11%.[11,15] If the SLN is negative for metastases, then no further axillary surgery is required, and the remaining lymph nodes can be left in place.

## Sentinel Node-Positive Patients

With the development of SLND, pathologists began to perform more detailed evaluation, because fewer lymph nodes were removed, leading to increased sensitivity and a growing population of women identified with micrometastatic (<0.2 mm) or low-volume nodal metastases. Although the American Society of Clinical Oncology[16] and the National Comprehensive Cancer Network[15] guidelines recommended completion of ALND for any patient with a positive SLN, regardless of size, many clinicians questioned this paradigm, pointing to data that only 20% of patients with micrometastases and 12% of those with isolated tumor cells (ITCs) had additional positive non-SLNs.[17,18] An analysis of the Surveillance, Epidemiology, and End Results (SEER) data from 1998 to 2004 showed that 16% of SLN-positive patients did not undergo completion ALND. This proportion rose to 38% in those with micrometastases.[19] A similar study of national patterns using the National Cancer Data Base (NCDB) showed that 20.8% of patients with a positive SLN between 1998 and 2005 did not undergo ALND.[20] There were no differences in the incidence of axillary recurrence or in overall survival (OS) between patients who underwent ALND compared with those who did not, although selection bias must be considered in these retrospective accounts. However, these studies showed that clinicians believed that ALND could be omitted in select SLN-positive patients, although there were no prospective data to support this.

Several phase 3, multicenter trials have been reported in the last 5 years designed to answer this question; all have slight variations in trial design and eligibility criteria. The American College of Surgeons Oncology Group (ACOSOG) Z0011 trial was a multi-institutional, prospective trial with a noninferiority design.[21,22] It enrolled clinically node-negative patients with T1 or T2 tumors who were treated with breast conservation therapy (BCT) and adjuvant radiotherapy who were found to have 1 or 2 positive SLN on standard pathologic examination with hematoxylin and eosin (H&E) staining. Patients were randomized to completion ALND versus SLN alone and followed for evidence of disease recurrence and for overall survival. After opening in 1999 with a planned accrual of 1900 patients, the trial closed early in 2004 with 891 enrolled patients secondary to slow accrual and a low event rate. In an intent-to-treat analysis, there were 420 patients in the ALND arm and 436 in the SLND alone arm, with similar clinicopathologic features between the 2 groups. At median follow-up of 6.3 years, local recurrence was seen in 3.6% of the ALND group versus 1.8% of the SLND alone group ($P = .11$). Axillary recurrences were also similar between the 2 groups (0.5% in ALND cohort vs 0.9% in ALND alone, $P = .45$). There were no differences in 5-year overall survival (91.9% in ALND vs 92.5% in SLND alone, $P = .24$) or disease-free survival (82.2% vs 83.8%, $P = .13$). The investigators concluded that ALND could be safely omitted in clinically node-negative patients with T1 or T2 tumors undergoing BCT with 1 or 2 positive lymph nodes. Twenty-seven percent of the ALND group was found to have metastases in non-SLN. Of the patients with micrometastases in the SLN, only 10% had additional positive non-SLN. The study design in depicted in **Fig. 1**.

A similar European trial, the EORTC 10981-22023 AMAROS (After Mapping of the Axilla, Radiotherapy or Surgery?) trial was also a multi-institutional trial enrolling clinically node-negative patients with T1 or T2 tumors with a positive SLN. In contrast to the ACOSOG Z0011 trial, patients were randomized to ALND or axillary radiotherapy (the Z0011 trial did not allow third field nodal irradiation). The results were reported at the 2013 American Society of Clinical Oncology (ASCO) Annual meeting describing 744 subjects in the ALND arm and 681 in the axillary radiation arm.[15] At median 6.1 years follow-up, the axillary recurrence rates were 0.54% (4 cases of 744) in the ALND group and 1.03% (7 of 681) in the axillary radiation group. In comparison, they also followed 3131 patients with a negative SLN and found an axillary recurrence rate of 0.8%. There were no statistical differences in 5-year overall survival (93.3% ALND vs 92.5% axillary radiation, $P = .3386$) or disease-free survival (86.9% ALND vs 82.7% axillary radiation, $P = .1788$).

Finally, the IBCSG 23-01 trial corroborates the findings that patients with small-volume nodal disease do not need completion ALND.[23] This phase 3 noninferiority trial randomized clinically node-negative patients with T1 or T2 tumors who had only

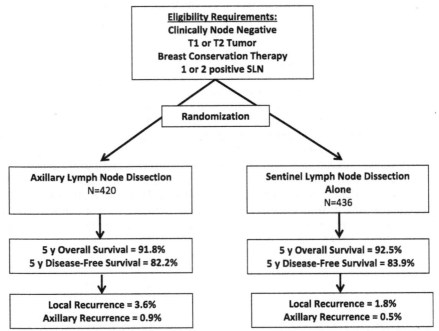

**Fig. 1.** Schema for the ACOSOG Z0011 Trial. The ACOSOG Z0011 trial was designed to determine whether there was a difference in overall survival or locoregional recurrence in patients with early breast cancer and 1 or 2 positive SLN who underwent axillary lymph node dissection versus those that had no further axillary therapy. (*Data from* Giuliano A, Hunt K, Ballman K, et al. Axillary dissection vs no axillary dissection in women with invasive breast cancer and sentinel node metastasis: a randomized clinical trial. JAMA 2011;305(6):569–75; and Giuliano A, McCall L, Beitsch P, et al. Locoregional recurrence after sentinel lymph node dissection with or without axillary dissection in patients with sentinel lymph node metastases: the American College of Surgeons Oncology Group Z0011 randomized trial. Ann Surg 2010;252(3):426–32.)

micrometastases identified in SLNs. Unlike the Z0011 trial, subjects could undergo mastectomy or BCT and could have any number of positive SLNs as long as all metastases were no more than 2 mm (micrometastases were seen in 37.5% of the ALND cohort and 44.8% of the SLND cohort in the Z0011 trial).[22] Radiation fields were not defined in the trial design so patients had heterogeneous radiation administration. Only 9% of patients in each group underwent mastectomy; none received adjuvant radiation. In the remaining 91% of patients who underwent BCT, 19% of both groups received intraoperative radiotherapy alone, and 70% received standard adjuvant whole breast radiation therapy (WBRT). Nine percent of the ALND group and 8% of the no ALND group received a combination of intraoperative and WBRT, while 2% to 3% of the groups did not receive adjuvant WBRT. Locoregional recurrences were seen in 2.4% (11 of 464) of the ALND group versus 2.8% (13 of 467) of patients without ALND. Five-year disease-free survival was 84.4% in the ALND cohort compared with 87.8% in the group without ALND ($P = .16$). Once again, the authors concluded that patients with nodal disease limited to micrometastases might safely omit ALND without compromising oncologic outcomes.

These trials have been widely discussed in the breast cancer community and have led to a change in practice patterns in the United States.[24] Investigators from MD Anderson Cancer Center reviewed the practice patterns in patients meeting the Z0011 inclusion criteria treated in the year before the release of the Z0011 results compared with those treated the year after an institutional multidisciplinary meeting discussing the results. Before Z011, 85% (53 of 62) of SLN-positive patients underwent ALND compared with 24% (10 of 42) treated after Z0011. In addition, surgeons were less likely to perform intraoperative nodal assessment after Z0011 (26% vs 69%, $P<.001$) and had a decrease in mean operative time to 79 minutes compared with 92 minutes before Z0011 ($P<.001$), representing possible cost-saving results.[25] The potential for cost savings was estimated by 1 group to be a 64% reduction in inpatient hospital stays and an 18% reduction in perioperative costs when Z0011 criteria were applied to SLN-positive patients undergoing BCT.[26] On the national scale, a survey of 849 American Society of Breast Surgeons members reported that 57% would not routinely perform ALND in sentinel node-positive patients meeting the Z0011 criteria.[27]

### Management of Isolated Tumor Cells

As pathologic analysis of SLNs has evolved, the addition of immunohistochemical (IHC) staining has allowed for characterization of isolated tumor cells (ITCs), defined as clusters of cells no more than 0.2 mm, single tumor cells, or clusters of less than 200 cells in a single cross-section.[3] The discovery of these occult metastases that were previously unrecognized when only standard H&E evaluation was performed left clinicians wondering what, if any, effect this extremely small amount of metastasis has on clinical outcomes. The ACOSOG Z0010 trial was a prospective observation trial enrolling women who underwent BCT who had a negative SLND by routine H&E staining. IHC staining was then performed on the SLN blocks at a central laboratory with the treating clinicians blinded to the results (thus they treated all patients based on the negative H&E result). Of 3326 specimens reported to be negative by H&E staining, 10.5% (349) had metastases identified by IHC. Five-year OS was similar between IHC-negative (95.7%) and IHC-positive (95.1%) patients ($P = .64$), validating the practice of treating these patients as node negative.[28] Additionally, in a subgroup analysis of the NSABP B-32 trial, occult metastases were identified by IHC in 15.9% of patients with negative H&E results. Similar to the Z0010 trial, treating clinicians were blinded to the IHC results and thus considered the patients node negative when making therapeutic decisions. In contrast to the ACOSOG Z0010 trial, they did show a small, but statistically significant difference in 5-year OS (94.6% in the IHC-positive patients compared with 95.8% in IHC-negative patients, $P = .03$). However, the authors concluded that an absolute survival difference of 1.2% did not warrant a change in adjuvant therapy based on the IHC results alone.[29]

The exception to this may be patients with tumors with lobular histology. Lobular cancer cells grow in noncohesive patterns, and are more likely to be seen as widely dispersed isolated tumor cells in lymph nodes.[30,31] Not only are patients with lobular tumors more likely to have ITCs, they are also more likely to have additional positive lymph nodes when ITCs are identified.[31,32] In a study from MD Anderson Cancer Center, 17% of patients with lobular tumors had additional positive lymph nodes when ITCs were seen in the SLN.[30] Based on these data, many surgeons still recommend ALND when ITCs are seen in patients with lobular tumors.[25,30]

### Timing of SLND in Patients Undergoing Neoadjuvant Chemotherapy

Neoadjuvant chemotherapy (NCT) is increasingly used in breast cancer patients with the benefits of allowing for in situ assessment of tumor response, as well as downsizing the tumor, which may facilitate breast conservation therapy. Another benefit of NCT is that 40% to 75% of patients presenting with clinically involved lymph nodes will convert to pathologic lymph node negative.[33–35] Thus, SLND can lead to different results (and resulting adjuvant therapies) depending on whether it is performed before or after NCT. Some clinicians have advocated for upfront SLND before initiating chemotherapy, arguing that SLN identification is more successful before chemotherapy and the knowledge of nodal status is important to treatment planning.[36] However, this approach commits all women, even if the SLN is negative, to 2 surgical procedures. It also commits women with small-volume nodal disease that would have been easily eradicated with chemotherapy to ALND. Data from MD Anderson Cancer institution have demonstrated that the SLN identification rate is not altered by NCT (98.7% if surgery first vs 97.4% if SLN was performed after NCT) with similar false-negative rates (4.1% in surgery first cohort vs 5.8% in NCT). After stratification for tumor size, the number of positive SLNs was lower if performed after NCT as opposed to before chemotherapy, which resulted in fewer ALNDs.[37] In addition to sparing patients, performing SLND after NCT prioritizes the nodal status after NCT, which is a better prognostic indicator than the identification of occult nodal metastases before NCT.[38]

## CLINICALLY NODE-POSITIVE PATIENTS
### Axillary Lymph Node Dissection

ALND is now only performed if there is confirmation of axillary metastases, either by ultrasound and needle biopsy or by SLND. It is also indicated in cases in which an SLN cannot be identified or there is a contraindication to SLND such as in inflammatory breast cancer. ALND allows for a more thorough staging of the axillary nodes since all nodes are removed, and the total number of involved nodes can be counted, and therefore remains the gold standard for comparing less invasive surgical approaches. Standard ALND involves the removal of the level 1 and 2 axillary lymph nodes. Level 3 nodes are not routinely removed unless there is evidence of their involvement.

Unfortunately, ALND is associated with significant short- and long-term morbidities. Short-term effects include the need for uncomfortable postoperative drains and potential for seromas. Ligation of intercostobrachial nerves, which often occurs during the resection, can lead to pain and neuropathies that can be permanent. Functional limitations of arm abduction are common in the immediate postoperative period and can be persistent even with aggressive physical therapy. Perhaps the most significant impact is the possibility of lymphedema, which requires aggressive and time-consuming therapy with physical therapy, diet modifications, compression garments, and carries an increased risk of cellulitis. In 1 study of patients who underwent ALND, 70% of patients had at least 1 complaint, including 21% with decreased strength, 20% with intercostobrachial neuralgias, 9% requiring compression garments, and 6% who had to change their vocational status because of surgical morbidity.[39]

The recent prospective trials randomizing patients to SLND alone versus ALND has allowed for more precise data collection to evaluate the differences in morbidity between the procedures. The ACOSOG Z0011 trial reported adverse surgical effects in 70% of patients after ALND versus 22% after SLND alone with more wound infections (7% vs 3%, $P = .0016$), seromas (14% vs 6%, $P = .001$), and parasthesia at 1 year (39% vs 9%, $P<.0001$) in the ALND group. At 1 year, patients undergoing ALND subjectively reported more lymphedema than those who underwent SLND alone (19% vs 6%, $P<.001$); however the proportion with lymphedema by actual arm measurements was similar (11% vs 6%, $P = .08$).[14] The AMOROS trial also reported significant differences in between patients who underwent ALND versus axillary radiation, with increased lymphedema rates at 1 year in the ALND group (40% vs 22%, $P<.0001$).[15]

### Neoadjuvant Chemotherapy

The role of SLND in patients who present with clinically involved lymph nodes and have a clinical response to NCT is currently under review. Because 40% to 75% of patients have eradication of their nodal disease, there is considerable interest in finding reliable methods to restage the axilla in hope of sparing these patients the morbidity of ALND. There are concerns, however, that SLND may not be accurate in this setting; single institution reports have shown unacceptable false-negative rates of 15% to 30%.[40–42] The ACOSOG Z1071 trial enrolled women with clinically positive lymph nodes confirmed by FNA who then underwent NCT.[43] At the completion of chemotherapy, participants had an SLND followed by completion ALND, and the results of the SLND were then compared with the pathologic assessment of all lymph nodes (shown in **Fig. 2**). The primary endpoint of the study was to determine the false-negative rate of SLND in this setting. Eradication of all nodal disease was seen in 40% of the patients, and an SLN could be identified in 92.5% of subjects. In N1 patients with at least 2 SLNs examined, researchers found a false-negative rate of 12.8%, slightly higher than the prespecified study endpoint of 10%. In subgroup analysis, use of dual-agent mapping and retrieval of an increased number of SLN were associated with lower false-negative rates.[44]

The SENTINA (SENTinel NeoAdjuvant) study was designed to evaluate the optimal timing of SLND in patients receiving NCT.[45] There were 4 arms in the trial: (A) clinically node-negative patients who underwent SLND before NCT, a portion of whom were then moved to arm (B) if they had a positive SLN then had a second SLND after NCT. The third arm (C) consisted of clinically node-positive patients who converted to clinically negative after NCT and then underwent SLND to restage the axilla followed by ALND. The remaining arm (D) consisted of clinically node-positive patients who remained clinically positive after NCT and underwent ALND. The authors showed that SLNs could be detected in 99.1% of patients before NCT; however, a second SLND procedure was only successful in 60.8% of patients, demonstrating that

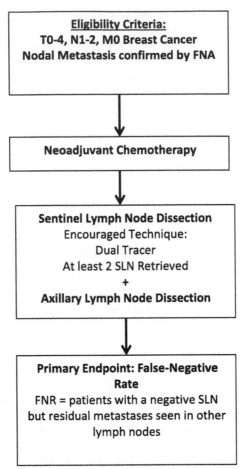

**Fig. 2.** ACOSOG Z1071 Trial.[43] The ACOSOG Z1071 trial was designed to test the reliability of SLND to restage the axillary lymph nodes after neoadjuvant chemotherapy in patients presenting with clinically positive lymph nodes. (*Data from* Boughey J, Suman V, Mittendorf E, et al. The role of sentinel lymph node surgery in patients presenting with node positive breast cancer (T0-T4), (N1-N2) who receive neoadjuvant chemotherapy - results from the ACOSOG Z1071. Cancer Res 2012;72(24):94s.)

patients should only undergo 1 SLN procedure for staging. The other arms focused on the possibility of accurately restaging the axillary nodes after NCT in clinically node-positive patients; however 1 important aspect of the trial to note is that the researchers did not require pathologic confirmation of lymph node involvement. In fact, only 149 of the 592 patients categorized as clinically node positive had an FNA to confirm metastases. The authors report an overall false-negative rate for SLND in these patients of 14.2%, with findings similar to the Z1071 trial in that the false-negative rate was lower when more SLNs were retrieved and dual tracers were used. Although the difference did not reach statistical significance, the false-negative rate of SLND in patients whose nodal disease was confirmed by FNA before NCT was 19%, compared with a false-negative rate of 12.3% in patients who were classified as node positive but did not have any pathologic confirmation of this status.

## ONGOING AND UPCOMING CLINICAL TRIALS ADDRESSING AXILLARY DISEASE MANAGEMENT

### Targeted Axillary Dissection

Further analysis of the trials such as ACOSOG Z1071 and the SENTINA trial will be necessary in order for clinicians to decide how to incorporate the findings into their clinical practice. One possibility being explored at MD Anderson Cancer Center is based on having radiologists place a clip in lymph nodes containing metastases when the initial biopsy is performed. This allows for the technique of targeted axillary dissection (TAD) after completion of NCT including the removal of the node known to harbor disease (with a clip in it) as well as the lymph nodes most likely to contain metastases (the SLNs) as a technique for reassessing the axillary nodes to confirm eradication of disease (www.clinicaltrials.gov, NCT1880645).[46]

### NSABP-51/RTOG 1304 Trial

With the acknowledgment that selected clinically node-positive patients who have a response to NCT may not undergo ALND in the future, cooperative groups are organizing trials to evaluate the optimal locoregional treatment for patients. One such trial, NSABP-51/RTOG 1304, will enroll clinically node-positive patients who undergo NCT and have no residual nodal disease (by SLND or ALND), and randomize them to axillary radiation versus no axillary radiation. The primary endpoints will be recurrence and survival, but information on toxicity, effect of radiation on cosmetic outcome, and quality of life will also be collected (www.clinicaltrials.gov, NCT01872975).

### ALLIANCE Trial A11202

Another cooperative group trial is being organized to look at those patients who do not have eradication of nodal disease after chemotherapy. The goal of the Alliance A11202 trial is to compare radiation plus ALND with radiation alone in clinically node-positive women who remain node positive (as demonstrated by a positive SLND) after NCT. The primary endpoints of the trial are locoregional recurrence and survival; however, there is a strong correlative component of the trial dedicated to lymphedema that should help delineate the differences in toxicity between axillary surgery and radiation together versus radiation alone. The trial should begin accruing patients within the next year (www.clinicaltrials.gov, NCT01901094).

## ADJUVANT RADIATION THERAPY

Locoregional management of patients with axillary nodal disease requires appropriate surgical resection as well as adjuvant radiation in selected patients. Understanding which patients will benefit from radiation is crucial to surgical planning, especially in cases requiring reconstruction, as well as for appropriate referrals. Surgeons and radiation oncologists should have open communication about shared patients in order to maximize locoregional control and to minimize morbidities.

### Breast Conservation Therapy

Whole breast radiation (WBRT) is standard after segmental mastectomy; however radiation fields are often designed based on nodal findings. The ACOSOG Z0011 trial led to a national conversation about how to tailor radiation fields in patients with small volume nodal metastases.[47] While regional nodal irradiation (RNI) was not allowed in the trial,[21] the tangential fields used in WBRT are known to treat the axillary nodal region. It has been estimated that standard tangential fields treat 80% of level 1 and 2 axillary lymph nodes.[48] Additionally, adjusting the superior border of the fields (with high tangents) can increase this coverage,[49] and has been recommended by some radiation oncologists in treating these patients.[47]

To provide more comprehensive coverage, regional nodal irradiation (RNI) is sometimes added to incorporate the draining nodal regions, including level 3 of the axilla as well as the supraclavicular region, and sometimes the internal mammary basin. This is a standard addition in patients with 4 or more involved lymph nodes, regardless of whether they undergo BCT or mastectomy. The possible benefit of RNI to WBRT in patients with less than 4 known positive lymph nodes, especially in the undissected axilla, is less clear. The NCIC-CTG MA.20 trial evaluated the addition of RNI (including internal mammary, supraclavicular, and high axillary nodal basins) to whole breast irradiation in high risk node-negative or node-positive patients following BCT.[50] After stratification based on number of positive nodes, number of axillary nodes removed, and systemic therapy, patients were randomized to WBRT (916 women) or WBRT plus RNI (916 women). The addition of RNI increased 5-year locoregional relapse-free survival (96.8% vs 94.5%), disease-free survival (89.7% vs 84%), and overall survival (92.3% and 90.7%). Eighty-five percent of the study population had 1 to 3 positive lymph nodes, which has brought consideration to the addition of RNI to these patients. These data will surely be the subject of much discussion once the full results are published.

### Postmastectomy Radiation Therapy

Landmark studies from Denmark[51,52] and British Columbia[53] first demonstrated benefits in overall survival and locoregional control in high-risk women who received Postmastectomy radiation therapy (PMRT) in addition to adjuvant tamoxifen or chemotherapy (cyclophosphamide, methotrexate, and fluorouracil), although the applicability of these data is unclear in contemporary patients with modern systemic therapy. A meta-analysis identified 25 trials of mastectomy and adjuvant chemotherapy that compared patients who received PMRT versus those did not have adjuvant radiotherapy. In node-positive patients, 5-year locoregional recurrences were seen in 5.8% of patients in the PMRT cohort compared with 22% in those without PMRT, translating to a 5% difference in 15-year disease-specific mortality. These benefits were not seen in node-negative patients.[54] ASCO guidelines recommending PMRT in patients with T3 or T4 tumors or at least 4 involved lymph nodes reflect evidence that these patients are at elevated risk for locoregional recurrence and thus benefit from PMRT.[55] Other candidates for PMRT are patients with pT4 tumors, extracapsular extension of lymphatic disease, and positive resection margins.

The decision to add PMRT in patients with 1 to 3 lymph nodes is more complex, and is often based on other variables. Although the addition of RNI to WBRT adds a small amount of toxicity,[50] the addition of PMRT based on nodal findings has a larger impact on patients undergoing mastectomy who would otherwise not receive radiation. In 1 study of patients with 1 to 3 positive lymph nodes who underwent mastectomy without adjuvant radiation, young age, tumor size greater than 3 cm, negative estrogen receptor status, and presence of lymphovascular invasion were used to define a group at high risk for locoregional relapse. The 4-year locoregional recurrence rate was 66.7% in patients with at least 3 of these factors compared with 7.8% in those with 0 to 2 of the factors.[56]

Another complication in adjuvant planning is the fact that patients with clinically positive lymph nodes often undergo neoadjuvant chemotherapy, further limiting the ability to accurately estimate the extent of nodal involvement. A retrospective review from MD Anderson evaluated the benefit of PMRT in patients who received NCT based on clinical staging as well as pathologic staging showing a decrease in 10-yr locoregional recurrence when PMRT was added in patients presenting with clinical N2-3 disease (40% vs 12%, $P = .0001$), or at least 4 lymph nodes were involved pathologically after chemotherapy (59% vs 16%, $P<.0001$).[57]

## SUMMARY

The evaluation and management of axillary lymph nodes is critical in breast cancer, with impact on locoregional as well as survival outcomes. Surgeons caring for breast cancer patients must be technically equipped to provide staging procedures such as SLND as well as understand the implications of these results. Although ALND has historically been the standard approach to patients with nodal metastases, emerging data have identified patients at low risk for regional recurrence who may be spared the morbidity of this procedure if other multidisciplinary teams are involved. It is important that clinicians keep the individual patient in mind, considering not only staging classifications but also tumor biology, evidence of response to therapy, and innate risk of recurrence when deciding on multidisciplinary care. This is an area of active investigation that is sure to lead to many changes in practice in the next few years.

## REFERENCES

1. Carter C, Allen C, Henson D. Relation of tumor size, lymph node status, and survival in 24,740 breast cancer cases. Cancer 1989;63(1):181–7.
2. Beenken S, Urist M, Zhang Y, et al. Axillary lymph node status, but not tumor size, predicts locoregional recurrence and overall survival after mastectomy for breast cancer. Ann Surg 2003;237(5):732–8.
3. Edge S, Byrd D, Compton C, et al, editors. AJCC cancer staging manual. 7th edition. New York: Springer; 2009.
4. Krag D, Anderson S, Julian T, et al. Sentinel lymph node resection compared with conventional axillary-lymph-node dissection in clinically node-negative patients with breast cancer: overall survival findings from the NSABP B-32 randomised phase 3 trial. Lancet Oncol 2010;11(10):927–33.
5. Sacre R. Clinical evaluation of axillar lymph nodes compared to surgical and pathological findings. Eur J Surg Oncol 1986;12(2):169–73.
6. Krishnamurthy S. Current applications and future prospects of fine-needle aspiration biopsy of locoregional lymph nodes in the management of breast cancer. Cancer 2009;117(6):451–62.
7. Krishnamurthy S, Sneige N, Bedi D, et al. Role of ultrasound-guided fine-needle aspiration of indeterminate and suspicious axillary lymph nodes in the initial staging of breast carcinoma. Cancer 2002;95(5):982–8.
8. Jain A, Haisfield-Wolfe M, Lange J, et al. The role of ultrasound-guided fine-needle aspiration of axillary nodes in the staging of breast cancer. Ann Surg Oncol 2008;15(2):462–71.
9. Cabanas R. An approach for the treatment of penile carcinoma. Cancer 1977; 39(2):456–66.
10. Morton D, Wen D, Wong J, et al. Technical details of intraoperative lymphatic mapping for early stage melanoma. Arch Surg 1992;127(4):392–9.
11. Krag D, Weaver D, Ashikaga T, et al. The sentinel node in breast cancer—a multicenter validation study. N Engl J Med 1998;339(14):941–6.
12. Veronesi U, Paganelli G, Viale G, et al. A randomized comparison of sentinel-node biopsy with routine axillary dissection in breast cancer. N Engl J Med 2003;349(6):546–53.

13. Giuliano A, Dale P, Turner R, et al. Improved axillary staging of breast cancer with sentinel lymphadenectomy. Ann Surg 1995;222(3):394–9.
14. Lucci A, McCall L, Beitsch P, et al. Surgical complications associated with sentinel lymph node dissection (SLND) plus axillary lymph node dissection compared with SLND alone in the American College of Surgeons Oncology Group Trial Z0011. J Clin Oncol 2007;25(24):3657–63.
15. National Comprehensive Cancer Network (NCCN) Clinical Practice Guidelines in Oncology: Breast, version 2.2008. 2008. Available at: www.nccn.org.
16. Lyman G, Giuliano A, Somerfield M, et al. American Society of Clinical Oncology guideline recommendations for sentinel lymph node biopsy in early-stage breast cancer. J Clin Oncol 2006;24(1):210–1.
17. Cserni G, Gregori D, Merletti F, et al. Meta-analysis of non-sentinel node metastases associated with micrometastatic sentinel nodes in breast cancer. Br J Surg 2004;91(10):1245–52.
18. van Deurzen C, de Boer M, Monninkhof E, et al. Non-sentinel lymph node metastases associated with isolated breast cancer cells in the sentinel node. J Natl Cancer Inst 2008;100(22):1574–80.
19. Yi M, Giordano S, Meric-Bernstam F, et al. Trends in and outcomes from sentinel lymph node biopsy (SLNB) alone vs. SLNB with axillary lymph node dissection for node-positive breast cancer patients: experience from the SEER database. Ann Surg Oncol 2010;17(Suppl 3):343–51.
20. Bilimoria K, Bentrem D, Hansen N, et al. Comparison of sentinel lymph node biopsy alone and completion axillary lymph node dissection for node-positive breast cancer. J Clin Oncol 2009;27(18):2946–53.
21. Giuliano A, Hunt K, Ballman K, et al. Axillary dissection vs no axillary dissection in women with invasive breast cancer and sentinel node metastasis: a randomized clinical trial. JAMA 2011;305(6):569–75.
22. Giuliano A, McCall L, Beitsch P, et al. Locoregional recurrence after sentinel lymph node dissection with or without axillary dissection in patients with sentinel lymph node metastases: the American College of Surgeons Oncology Group Z0011 randomized trial. Ann Surg 2010;252(3):426–32.
23. Galimberti V, Cole B, Zurrida S, et al. Axillary dissection versus no axillary dissection in patients with sentinel-node micrometastases (IBCSG 23-01): a phase 3 randomised controlled trial. Lancet Oncol 2013;14(4):297–305.
24. Caudle A, Hunt K, Kuerer H, et al. Multidisciplinary considerations concerning implementation of the findings from the American College of Surgeons Oncology Group (ACOSOG) Z0011 study: a practice-changing trial. Ann Surg Oncol 2011;18(9):2407–12.
25. Caudle A, Hunt K, Tucker S, et al. American College of Surgeons Oncology Group (ACOSOG) Z0011: impact on surgeon practice patterns. Ann Surg Oncol 2012;19(10):3144–51.
26. Camp M, Greenup R, Taghian A, et al. Application of ACOSOG Z0011 criteria reduces perioperative costs. Ann Surg Oncol 2013;20(3):836–41.
27. Gainer S, Hunt K, Beitsch P, et al. Changing behavior in clinical practice in response to the ACOSOG Z0011 trial: a survey of the American Society of Breast Surgeons. Ann Surg Oncol 2012;19(10):3152–8.
28. Giuliano A, Hawes D, Ballman K, et al. Association of occult metastases in sentinel lymph nodes and bone marrow with survival among women with early-stage invasive breast cancer. JAMA 2011;306(4):385–93.
29. Weaver D, Ashikaga T, Krag D, et al. Effect of occult metastases on survival in node-negative breast cancer. N Engl J Med 2011;364(5):412–21.

30. Mittendorf E, Sahin A, Tucker S, et al. Lymphovascular invasion and lobular histology are associated with increased incidence of isolated tumor cells in sentinel lymph nodes from early-stage breast cancer patients. Ann Surg Oncol 2008; 15(12):3369–77.
31. Cserni G, Bianchi S, Vezzosi V, et al. The value of cytokeratin immunohistochemistry in the evaluation of axillary sentinel lymph nodes in patients with lobular breast carcinoma. J Clin Pathol 2006;59(5):518–22.
32. Tan L, Giri D, Hummer A, et al. Occult axillary node metastases in breast cancer are prognostically significant: results in 368 node-negative patients with 20-year follow-up. J Clin Oncol 2008;26(11):1803–9.
33. Dominici L, Negron Gonzalez V, Buzdar A, et al. Cytologically proven axillary lymph node metastases are eradicated in patients receiving preoperative chemotherapy with concurrent trastuzumab for HER2-positive breast cancer. Cancer 2010;116(12):2884–9.
34. Fisher B, Brown A, Mamounas E, et al. Effect of preoperative chemotherapy on local-regional disease in women with operable breast cancer: findings from National Surgical Adjuvant Breast and Bowel Project B-18. J Clin Oncol 1997;15(7): 2479–82.
35. Kuerer H, Sahin A, Hunt K, et al. Incidence and impact of documented eradication of breast cancer axillary lymph node metastases before surgery in patients treated with neoadjuvant chemotherapy. Ann Surg 1999;230(1):72–8.
36. Jones J, Zabicki K, Christian R, et al. A comparison of sentinel node biopsy before and after neoadjuvant chemotherapy: timing is important. Am J Surg 2005;190(4):517–20.
37. Hunt K, Yi M, Mittendorf E, et al. Sentinel lymph node surgery after neoadjuvant chemotherapy is accurate and reduces the need for axillary dissection in breast cancer patients. Ann Surg 2009;250(4):558–66.
38. Rouzier R, Extra J, Klijanienko J, et al. Incidence and prognostic significance of complete axillary downstaging after primary chemotherapy in breast cancer patients with T1 to T3 tumors and cytologically proven axillary metastatic lymph nodes. J Clin Oncol 2002;20(5):1304–10.
39. Kakuda J, Stuntz M, Trivedi V, et al. Objective assessment of axillary morbidity in breast cancer treatment. Am Surg 1999;65(10):995–8.
40. Shen J, Gilcrease M, Babiera G, et al. Feasibility and accuracy of sentinel lymph node biopsy after preoperative chemotherapy in breast cancer patients with documented axillary metastases. Cancer 2007;109(7):1255–63.
41. Gimbergues P, Abrial C, Durando X, et al. Sentinel lymph node biopsy after neoadjuvant chemotherapy is accurate in breast cancer patients with a clinically negative axillary nodal status at presentation. Ann Surg Oncol 2008;15(5): 1316–21.
42. Classe J, Bordes V, Campion L, et al. Sentinel lymph node biopsy after neoadjuvant chemotherapy for advanced breast cancer: results of Ganglion Sentinelle et Chimiotherapie Neoadjuvante, a French prospective multicentric study. J Clin Oncol 2009;27(5):726–32.
43. Boughey J, Suman V, Mittendorf E, et al. The role of sentinel lymph node surgery in patients presenting with node positive breast cancer (T0-T4), (N1-N2) who receive neoadjuvant chemotherapy—results from the ACOSOG Z1071. Cancer Res 2012;72(24):94s.
44. Boughey JC, Suman VJ, Mittendorf EA, et al. Sentinel lymph node surgery after neoadjuvant chemotherapy in patients with node-positive breast cancer: the ACOSOG Z1071 (Alliance) clinical trial. JAMA 2013;310(14):1455–61.

45. Kuehn T, Bauerfeind I, Fehm T, et al. Sentinel-lymph-node biopsy in patients with breast cancer before and after neoadjuvant chemotherapy (SENTINA): a prospective, multicentre cohort study. Lancet Oncol 2013;14(7):609–18.
46. Matsuyama A, Kaneko M, Nagata C. Specific quenching of the fluorescence of benzo (a) pyrene by hepatic microsomes from 3-methylcholanthrene-treated rats. Biochem Biophys Res Commun 1977;77(3):918–24.
47. Haffty B, Hunt K, Harris J, et al. Positive sentinel nodes without axillary dissection: implications for the radiation oncologist. J Clin Oncol 2011;29(34):4479–81.
48. Schlembach P, Buccholz T, Ross M, et al. Relationship of sentinel and axillary level I-II lymph nodes to tangential fields used in breast irradiation. Int J Radiat Oncol Biol Phys 2001;51(3):671–8.
49. Reznik J, Cicchetti M, Degaspe B, et al. Analysis of axillary coverage during tangential radiation therapy to the breast. Int J Radiat Oncol Biol Phys 2005; 61(1):163–8.
50. Whelan T, Olivotto I, Ackerman I, et al. NCIC-CTG MA.20: an intergroup trial of regional nodal irradiation in early breast cancer. J Clin Oncol 2011;20(Suppl) [Abstr LBA 1003].
51. Overgaard M, Hansen P, Overgaard J, et al. Postoperative radiotherapy in high-risk premenopausal women with breast cancer who receive adjuvant chemotherapy. Danish Breast Cancer Cooperative Group 82b Trial. N Engl J Med 1997;337(14):949–55.
52. Overgaard M, Jensen M, Overgaard J, et al. Postoperative radiotherapy in high-risk postmenopausal breast-cancer patients given adjuvant tamoxifen: Danish Breast Cancer Cooperative Group DBCG 82c randomised trial. Lancet 1999; 353(9165):1641–8.
53. Ragaz J, Ilivotto I, Spinelli J, et al. Locoregional radiation therapy in patients with high-risk breast cancer receiving adjuvant chemotherapy: 20-year results of the British Columbia randomized trial. J Natl Cancer Inst 2005;97(2):116–26.
54. Clarke M, Collins R, Darby S, et al. Effects of radiotherapy and of differences in the extent of surgery for early breast cancer on local recurrence and 15-year survival: an overview of the randomised trials. Lancet 2005;366(9503): 2087–106.
55. Recht A, Edge S, Solin L, et al. Postmastectomy radiotherapy: clinical practice guidelines of the American Society of Clinical Oncology. J Clin Oncol 2001; 19(5):1539–69.
56. Cheng J, Chen C, Liu M, et al. Locoregional failure of postmastectomy patients with 1-3 positive axillary lymph nodes without adjuvant radiotherapy. Int J Radiat Oncol Biol Phys 2002;52(4):980–8.
57. Huang E, Tucker S, Strom E, et al. Postmastectomy radiation improves local-regional control and survival for selected patients with locally advanced breast cancer treated with neoadjuvant chemotherapy and mastectomy. J Clin Oncol 2004;22(23):4691–9.

# Lobular Neoplasia

Tari A. King, MD[a],*, Jorge S. Reis-Filho, MD, PhD, FRCPath[b]

## KEYWORDS

- Lobular carcinoma in situ • Atypical lobular hyperplasia • Lobular neoplasia
- E-cadherin • Breast cancer risk • Chemoprevention

## KEY POINTS

- Lobular carcinoma in situ (LCIS) and atypical lobular hyperplasia (ALH) are uncommon pathologic findings, representing part of a spectrum of epithelial proliferations referred to as lobular neoplasia (LN). LN can be considered both a nonobligate precursor of invasive breast cancer and a marker of increased risk.
- Loss of E-cadherin expression, caused by mutations, deletions, and methylation, is one of the defining features of LN; however, aberrant E-cadherin expression can be observed in a few lesions.
- A diagnosis of LCIS confers a long-term cumulative risk of a subsequent breast cancer that averages 1% to 2% per year and remains steady over time, resulting in relative risk of breast cancer that is 8-fold to 10-fold greater than the general population risk. ALH is associated with a relative risk of breast cancer 4-fold to 5-fold greater than the general population.
- A diagnosis of LN made by surgical excision does not require further surgical intervention; there is no indication to document margin status in specimens that contain only LN. The presence of LN in a lumpectomy specimen or at the margin is not a contraindication to breast conservation and does not require re-excision.
- Although routine surgical excision after a core biopsy diagnosis of LN is supported by National Comprehensive Cancer Network guidelines, the management of patients with this diagnosis requires a multidisciplinary approach. Excision is routinely recommended when there is radiologic-pathologic discordance and when the diagnosis indicates a less common histologic variant of LN.
- Patients with LN should be informed of their increased risk of breast cancer and counseled regarding both medical and surgical risk-reducing options.

The authors have nothing to disclose.
[a] Breast Service, Department of Surgery, Memorial Sloan-Kettering Cancer Center, 300 East 66th Street, New York, NY, 10065, USA; [b] Department of Pathology, Memorial Sloan-Kettering Cancer Center, 1275 York Avenue, New York, NY, 10065, USA
* Corresponding author.
*E-mail address:* kingt@mskcc.org

Surg Oncol Clin N Am 23 (2014) 487–503
http://dx.doi.org/10.1016/j.soc.2014.03.002
surgonc.theclinics.com

## INTRODUCTION

According to the current World Health Organization classification of breast lesions,[1] lobular neoplasia (LN) is defined as a term that encompasses the entire spectrum of atypical epithelial lesions that originate in the terminal duct-lobular unit (TDLU) of the breast and is characterized by a population of dyshesive cells, which expand the lobules and acini of the TDLUs, and may involve the terminal ducts in a pattern known as pagetoid spread. These lesions were traditionally described under the terms lobular carcinoma in situ (LCIS) and atypical lobular hyperplasia (ALH), which refer to the degree of involvement of the acinar structures of a given TDLU.

The first description of a lesion with features consistent with those currently used to define LCIS dates to 1919, when Ewing described an "atypical proliferation of acinar cells."[2] However, the main characteristics of LCIS were not thoroughly documented until the seminal study by Foote and Stewart in 1941,[3] in which the term LCIS was coined to refer to a spectrum of "noninfiltrative lesions of a definitely cancerous cytology." Based on the frequent identification of LCIS in association with invasive lobular carcinoma (ILC), and following the analogy of ductal carcinoma in situ (DCIS) and invasive ductal carcinoma (IDC), Foote and Stewart[3] hypothesized that the neoplastic cells of LCIS would still be contained within a basement membrane and that this lesion would constitute a precursor of breast cancer development, leading to the recommendation for mastectomy. Emerging data throughout the 1970s from Haagensen and colleagues[4] and others[5] showed that the risk of breast cancer development after a diagnosis of LCIS was lower than that expected for a direct precursor lesion (approximately 1% per year) and was conferred equally to both breasts, generating controversy regarding the significance of these lesions and leading to disparate recommendations for management, ranging from observation only to bilateral mastectomy.

The term ALH was coined in 1978 to refer to a less-prominent in situ proliferation composed of cells cytologically identical to those of LCIS, which were associated with a significantly lower risk of subsequent breast cancer development (approximately one-half of the risk associated with LCIS).[6] However, because the distinction between LCIS and ALH, which is based on quantitative rather than qualitative differences between the lesions (described later), often proves challenging in diagnostic specimens, Haagensen and colleagues[4] put forward the term LN to refer to the entire spectrum of these in situ lesions, including ALH and LCIS.[4]

In current practice, a diagnosis of LN is perceived as a risk factor for the subsequent development of breast cancer. However, observational data suggesting that the risk of breast cancer development after a diagnosis of LN is higher in the ipsilateral than in the contralateral breast, and compelling molecular data that show that ALH and LCIS are clonal neoplastic proliferations that commonly harbor the same genetic aberrations as those found in adjacent invasive cancers,[7-11] have reinstated the notion that ALH and LCIS are both nonobligate precursors and risk indicators of invasive breast cancer. In this article, the clinicopathologic and molecular characteristics of LN are revisited, and the impact of recent developments on the management of these lesions is discussed.

## ANATOMIC PATHOLOGY AND CLASSIFICATION
### ALH and Classic LCIS

Before introducing the histologic features of LN, it should be emphasized that the terms ALH, LCIS, and LN do not have histogenetic implications and do not imply that these lesions originate in the breast lobules. The term LCIS was chosen by Foote and Stewart to emphasize the histologic similarities between the cells of LCIS and those of frankly invasive lobular carcinoma, and it was acknowledged in their seminal study that LCIS would likely originate in the TDLUs and small ducts.[3]

From a histologic standpoint, LN encompasses a spectrum of noninvasive lesions that affect the TDLUs, which are characterized by a constellation of architectural and cytologic features. In its classic form, LN is characterized by variable enlargement and distention of the acinar structures by a neoplastic population of monomorphic, dyshesive, small, round, or polygonal cells, often with inconspicuous cytoplasm. However, the lobular architecture is largely maintained, and the neoplastic cells show the characteristic dyshesiveness and a regularly spaced distribution. Intracytoplasmic lumina and vacuoles, sometimes containing a central eosinophilic dot (known as magenta body), are usually found.[1,3,4,12] Mitotic figures and necrosis are not commonly found in classic LN. Pagetoid spread within the affected TDLU or to adjacent ducts, whereby the neoplastic cells extend between intact overlying epithelium and underlying myoepithelial layer and basement membrane, is frequently observed.

In the classic forms of LN, some degree of cytologic variation can be observed, and 2 cytologic subtypes have been described, namely type A cells, which are small, dyshesive cells, with scant cytoplasm and nuclei approximately 1.5 times the size of that of a lymphocyte, and type B cells, which show a slightly greater degree of variation, have more abundant and often clear cytoplasm, have nuclei that are slightly bigger than those of type A cells (ie, approximately 2 times the size of that of a lymphocyte), and show mild to moderate nuclear atypia; nucleoli, in type B cells, are also indistinct or absent (**Table 1**).[12,13] Although the subclassification of LN into these cytologic subtypes has not been shown to be of clinical usefulness and does not have a direct correlation with the risk of invasive breast cancer development, it is by no means a mere academic exercise. It serves as a reminder that some cytologic variation can be observed in bona fide cases of classic LN, and these features should not be overinterpreted as representing the pleomorphic variant of LCIS (described later).

LN has traditionally been subclassified into ALH and LCIS, based on quantitative rather than qualitative features of the lesions.[1] A diagnosis of LCIS requires more than half the acini in an involved lobular unit to be filled and distended by the characteristic LN cells, leaving no central lumina. In objective terms, lobular distention is defined as the presence of 8 or more cells in the cross-sectional diameter of an acinus. ALH is defined as a less well-developed and less-extensive lesion, in which the characteristic cells only partly fill the acini, less than half of the acini of the TDLU are involved, and there is minimal or no distention of the lobule.[1,10,14,15]

The arbitrary and subjective nature of this classification system, which is also dependent on the extent of sampling of a given lesion, frequently leads to high levels of inter-observer and intra-observer variability, creating difficulties in routine clinical practice. Yet, this classification system has been widely adopted given the lower risk of breast cancer development conferred by ALH than by LCIS (described later).

## Pleomorphic LCIS

In addition to the classic forms of LN, several variants of LN have also been described. Of potential clinical significance is the pleomorphic variant, first described in its pure form by Sneige and colleagues[13] under the name of pleomorphic LCIS (PLCIS). This variant is characterized by pleomorphic cells that are substantially bigger than those of classic LN,[16] and by more abundant, pink, and often finely granular cytoplasm. Features of apocrine differentiation are frequently found[16,17] but are not essential for a diagnosis of PLCIS. The pleomorphism observed in cells of PLCIS is greater than that found in type B cells; PLCIS nuclei are more than 4 times the size of a lymphocyte nucleus, show more overt pleomorphism and atypia, and the nucleoli are conspicuous

**Table 1**
Cytologic and histopathologic features of classic and pleomorphic lobular carcinomas

| Type of Carcinoma | Nuclear Characteristics | Cytoplasm | Cell Cohesiveness | Necrosis and Calcifications | Phenotype |
|---|---|---|---|---|---|
| LCIS type A | Small and bland nuclei (1.5× the size of a lymphocyte) Nuclear grade 1 (rarely 2) Inconspicuous nucleoli | Scant | Dyshesion present but often inconspicuous | Necrosis absent and infrequent calcifications | ER and PR positive (>95%) HER2 negative |
| LCIS type B | Slightly larger nuclei (2× the size of a lymphocyte) Nuclear grade 1 or 2 Small nucleoli may be present | Moderate | Conspicuous dyshesion | Necrosis absent and infrequent calcifications | ER and PR positive (>95%) HER2 negative |
| PLCIS | Large and pleomorphic nuclei (4× the size of a lymphocyte) Predominant nuclear grade 3 Nuclei present | Moderate to abundant | Conspicuous dyshesion | Necrosis and calcifications often found | ER and PR often positive, but often at lower levels than in type A/B HER2 occasionally amplified |
| Apocrine PLCIS | Large and pleomorphic nuclei (4× the size of a lymphocyte) Nuclear grade 3 Nuclei present Vesicular chromatin | Abundant with fine eosinophilic granules | Conspicuous dyshesion | Necrosis and calcifications often found | ER and PR often negative or low levels HER2 often amplified |

*Abbreviations:* ER, estrogen receptor; PR, progesterone receptor.

(**Fig. 1**, see **Table 1**). Although PLCIS also distends the acinar structures of TDLUs, it is not uncommon to find lesions with central, comedo-type necrosis and microcalcifications. However, necrosis and microcalcifications are not required for a diagnosis of PLCIS.

Recognition of the pleomorphic subtype of LCIS is important, given that its histologic features (namely, the combination of marked pleomorphism, comedo-type necrosis, and calcification) can lead to difficulty in differentiating between PLCIS and DCIS, and, potentially, overtreatment; however, data regarding the natural history of PLCIS are limited, and the management of these lesions is still largely based on empiricism. Although some advocate for a more aggressive approach in the management of patients with PLCIS, with treatment recommendations akin to those for DCIS, this approach is supported only by molecular studies, which have shown that PLCIS shares many similarities with pleomorphic ILC, not by long-term outcome studies showing the risk of subsequent cancer development. Other variants of LN, with a biological and clinical significance that also remains to be determined, include the apocrine, histiocytoid, rhabdoid, endocrine, and amphicrine variants of classic LCIS, and the apocrine variant of PLCIS.[1,12]

## Lobular Intraepithelial Neoplasia

The lobular intraepithelial neoplasia (LIN) classification system was proposed as a unifying terminology to encompass both classic and pleomorphic LN. In this system, LIN lesions are subclassified by morphologic criteria and clinical outcome into 3 grades (LIN 1, LIN 2, and LIN 3), with LIN 3 representing PLCIS and additional LN variants at the higher end of the spectrum, including those variants with extensive lobule involvement and necrosis, and lesions composed of signet ring cells.[18,19] This system

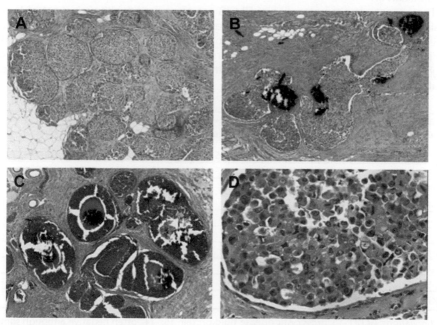

**Fig. 1.** PLCIS. Scanning magnification of a PLCIS. Note the distention of TDLUs by large, discohesive cells (*A, D*). Calcifications and comedo-type necrosis can often be observed (*B, C*). The neoplastic cells of PLCIS are characterized by atypical and pleomorphic nuclei, with conspicuous nucleoli; cytoplasm is abundant and often finely granular.

presupposes that the risk of invasive carcinoma development is related to increasing grade of LIN, a notion that is not supported by level I evidence. This classification system has the merit of sparing women from a diagnosis of carcinoma in the case of LCIS; however, it is supported by limited evidence and has not been endorsed in the latest edition of the World Health Organization classification.[1]

## MOLECULAR FEATURES AND PATHOPHYSIOLOGY

Genomic and transcriptomic analyses of invasive breast cancers and their precursors are leading to a better understanding of the molecular pathways involved in the evolution of breast cancers and their impact on the clinical behavior of these lesions.[1,9] It is accepted that estrogen receptor (ER)-positive and ER-negative breast cancers are fundamentally different diseases, with distinct patterns of gene expression changes[20] and, to an extent, different repertoires of genetic aberrations.[21] Classic invasive lobular lesions are low-grade ER-positive breast cancers, characterized by recurrent losses of 16q and gains of 1q and 16p. Molecular studies of LN, showing similar findings, provide evidence to suggest that ALH and LCIS are nonobligate precursors of invasive cancer and have also been instrumental in highlighting the role of E-cadherin inactivation in the development of lobular lesions.

### Phenotypic Characteristics of LN

LN, in its classic forms, is typically characterized by strong expression of ER-$\alpha$ (ER$\alpha$), ER-$\beta$ (ER$\beta$), and progesterone receptor (PR); low proliferation indices as defined by Ki-67, and lack of expression of HER2 and p53 (**Table 2**), features that are consistent with those of ER-positive breast cancers with a less aggressive clinical behavior (ie, luminal A).

The phenotypic characteristics of PLCIS are more varied; although most of these lesions do express ER and PR, their expression is usually at lower levels, and truly ER-negative cases of PLCIS have been documented. HER2 gene amplification and HER2 overexpression can also be found in a subset of PLCIS, and intermediate to high Ki-67 labeling indices, usually higher than those of classic LCIS, are a common feature of these lesions.

**Table 2**
**Summary of immunohistochemical marker status**

|  | LN Encompassing ALH and LCIS | PLCIS | Apocrine PLCIS |
|---|---|---|---|
| ER | + | +/– | –/+ |
| PR | + | +/– | –/+ |
| HER2 | Not amplified | Occasionally amplified | Often amplified |
| E-cadherin | Negative[a] | Negative[a] | Negative[a] |
| $\beta$-catenin | Negative[b] | Negative[b] | Negative[b] |
| p120 catenin | Cytoplasmic | Cytoplasmic | Cytoplasmic |
| GCDFP-15 | –/+ | +/– | + |
| p53 | –/+ | +/– | +/– |
| Ki-67 | Low | Intermediate to high | Often high |

Abbreviations: GCDFP-15, gross cystic disease fluid protein 15; –/+, often negative although sometimes positive; +/–, often positive although sometimes negative.
[a] Abnormal discontinuous or fragmented staining patterns or cytoplasmic dots can occasionally be observed.
[b] $\beta$-catenin nuclear expression is rare in LN and PLCIS.

The apocrine subtype of PLCIS, which is composed of cells with overt apocrine cytology and which express gross cystic disease fluid protein 15, a marker of apocrine differentiation,[1,12,17] are frequently found to have *HER2* gene amplification and high proliferation rates; however, the criteria to differentiate between PLCIS and apocrine PLCIS remain a matter of controversy.

## E-Cadherin and Related Proteins in LN

Both classic and pleomorphic forms of LN are characterized by a dysfunctional E-cadherin-catenin adhesion complex. E-cadherin is encoded by the *CDH1* gene, which maps to 16q22, a locus often lost in LN and ILCs. E-cadherin, a transmembrane adhesion molecule found in adherens junctions, mediates homophilic-homotypic adhesion between epithelial cells and interacts with p120 catenin and β-catenin through its intracytoplasmic domain. When E-cadherin is lost in breast epithelial cells, cytoplasmic, and occasionally nuclear, accumulation of p120 catenin is observed, as is loss of β-catenin membranous expression; however, nuclear accumulation of β-catenin or activation of the canonical Wnt pathway is not found.[22,23]

LN, both classic and pleomorphic, and ILCs lack or show marked downregulation of E-cadherin expression in more than 95% of cases (see **Table 2**). This molecular aberration is believed to be the cause of the characteristic dyshesiveness of LN and PLCIS cells.[1,9,12,17,24,25] LN, PLCIS, and ILCs have also been shown to have abnormal patterns of expression of the other components of the cadherin-catenin complex, including lack of β-catenin membranous expression and cytoplasmic expression of p120 catenin.[26] This knowledge has provided a wealth of ancillary markers for the differentiation of LN from its mimickers, in particular, for the distinction between LN and cases of solid low-grade DCIS. E-cadherin has been advocated for the classification of low-grade solid in situ proliferations with indeterminate features, such that lesions with positive E-cadherin staining should be considered as DCIS, those lacking E-cadherin expression should be classified as LCIS,[9,12,25,26] and lesions composed of populations of E-cadherin–positive and E-cadherin–negative cells should be classified as mixed.

Although E-cadherin has proved to be a useful ancillary marker in diagnostic breast pathology, its indiscriminate use has led to misconceptions about the diagnostic value of this marker, particularly when a detailed inspection of staining is not performed.[26] Aberrant expression patterns of E-cadherin, in the form of fragmented, focal, or beaded patterns, are not uncommonly observed.[1,12,26,27] Although the prevalence of E-cadherin positive classic LN is yet to be established, anecdotal cases of classic LN with strong and continuous E-cadherin expression have been reported.[28] In addition, approximately 10% to 16% of ILCs may be E-cadherin positive.[1,12,26,27] Hence, membranous expression of E-cadherin in a lesion with clear-cut histologic features of LN should not preclude a diagnosis of LN. In these cases, β-catenin and p120 catenin may provide additional evidence to differentiate between LN and DCIS.

One of the most frequent genetic aberrations in low-grade ER-positive breast lesions is 16q loss, which occurs in most cases and is believed to be an early event in the neoplastic development of LN and low-grade DCIS.[1,7,9,11,12] Although the target gene of 16q deletions in DCIS and IDC remains to be identified, in LN and ILC, the *CDH1* gene has been shown to be the target.[1,9,11,12] Loss of E-cadherin expression in LN, PLCIS, and ILCs stems from a combination of genetic, epigenetic, and transcriptional mechanisms affecting the *CDH1* gene. Loss of 16q is often accompanied by *CDH1* inactivating mutations, *CDH1* homozygous deletions, or *CDH1* gene promoter methylation, which result in biallelic silencing of the gene and loss of protein expression.[1,9,12]

The study of *CDH1* mutations has had a dramatic impact on our understanding of LN. First, the identification of identical *CDH1* gene mutations in LN and synchronous ILC components from individual patients has provided direct evidence to show that some LN and ILCs are clonally related[1,9,11,12] and that at least some LNs are precursors of ILC. In addition, conditional mouse models in which *CDH1* gene mutations and *p53* knockout were targeted in an epithelium-specific manner have provided strong circumstantial evidence to suggest that *CDH1* gene inactivation is a driver of the lobular phenotype.[29]

In addition to the genetic mechanisms reported to result in *CDH1* gene inactivation, transcriptional changes that result in E-cadherin dysfunction have been reported. Transforming growth factor β pathway activation, and upregulation of SNAIL, SLUG, and *ZEB1*, have been shown to result in downregulation of E-cadherin in lobular lesions.[1,27,30] In addition, transcriptomic and immunohistochemical analyses have shown that there is a stepwise decrease of the messenger RNA and proteins of the E-cadherin and catenin families from LCIS to ILC concurrent with upregulation of TWIST and SNAIL.[24]

Despite the clear role of loss of E-cadherin in the biology of LN, germline mutations of the *CDH1* gene do not seem to be a major cause of familial LN. Although *CDH1* germline gene mutations account for approximately 30% of cases of hereditary diffuse gastric carcinoma, which are also composed of dyshesive cells and have a growth pattern similar to that of lobular carcinomas,[1,31] germline truncating mutations of *CDH1* have been shown to play a limited role in familial LN and ILC. Although ILCs have been reported in the context of hereditary diffuse gastric cancer syndrome, patients with truncating *CDH1* germline gene mutations presenting solely with LN or ILCs are rare.[1,32]

### Genomics of LN

Comparative genomic hybridization (CGH) and single nucleotide polymorphism (SNP) array analyses of LN have shown that these lesions are clonal and neoplastic, that their most frequent copy number changes include loss of material from 16p, 16q, 17p, and 22q, and gain of material from 6q.[1,7,9,17,33,34]

Genomic studies have also corroborated the observations in regards to the potential precursor nature of LN made from *CDH1* gene sequencing. SNP array analyses of LN and invasive breast cancers have provided direct evidence that classic LCIS and many adjacent synchronous lesions, including ER-positive DCIS, ILC, and ER-positive IDC, are often clonally related.[7] Clonal patterns between LN and ILC have also been observed in CGH studies,[34] and in studies based on mitochondrial DNA heteroplasmy and mitochondrial gene mutation analyses.[8]

Genomic analyses of PLCIS and pleomorphic ILCs have established 2 important points. First, that PLCIS and pleomorphic ILCs are variants of classic LN and classic ILC, given that they harbor the hallmark genetic features of classic LN and ILCs, including loss of 16q, and gain of 1q and 16p. However, they do have more complex genomes[17,19,35,36] and amplification of genomic loci involving oncogenes associated with an aggressive phenotype, such as *MYC* (8q24) and HER2 (17q12).[17,35,36] One study[17] in which PLCIS was subclassified into those with and without apocrine features suggested that only apocrine, but not conventional PLCIS, would have more complex patterns of chromosomal copy number aberrations than classic LCIS. However, this observation requires further validation, given that the histologic features required to distinguish between PLCIS and apocrine PLCIS have yet to be fully defined. Second, these studies have shown that PLCIS and pleomorphic ILC are genetically related entities,[17,19,35,36] highlighting the potential precursor role of

PLCIS in the development of pleomorphic ILC akin to the relationship between LCIS and ILC.

## EPIDEMIOLOGY AND CLINICAL FEATURES

LCIS and ALH are uncommon noninvasive breast lesions, which are often incidental findings in breast biopsies performed for other reasons.[3,4] Both historical series from the pre-mammography era,[4,5,37] and more recent series of image-guided core needle biopsies,[38] suggest that LN, ALH, or LCIS are present in up to 5% of otherwise benign breast biopsies.

Population-based data reported to SEER (Surveillance, Epidemiology and End Results) from 1978 to 1998[39] show an incidence of 3.19 per 100,000 women for LCIS, with the highest incidence rate (11.47 per 100,000 person-years) in 1998 among women 50 to 59 years of age. During this period, there was an observed 4-fold increase in the number of LCIS cases reported among women older than 40 years. Possible explanations for this trend include increasing uptake of mammographic screening during this period,[39,40] the use of postmenopausal hormone replacement, and more accurate pathologic diagnosis of LN based on ancillary immunohistochemical markers, as described earlier.

Histologically, LCIS is often multifocal and bilateral, with more than 50% of patients diagnosed with LCIS showing multiple foci in the ipsilateral breast, and bilateral lesions are reported in approximately one-third of patients.[41,42] This pattern of presentation, combined with the lack of reliable radiographic or clinical features, has contributed to the uncertainty in defining optimal clinical management strategies for women with LCIS. Recent imaging series suggest that LCIS may be associated with microcalcifications,[38] and LCIS has been reported to enhance on magnetic resonance imaging (MRI)[43]; however, imaging criteria to differentiate LCIS from overt malignancy are lacking. Women with LCIS are frequently subject to multiple biopsies showing otherwise benign findings.

Compared with the general population, women with LCIS have an 8-fold to 10-fold increased risk of breast cancer.[14,15,44] The characteristics that support its role as a risk factor include the cumulative long-term risk of breast cancer development, which is conferred equally to both breasts, averaging 1% to 2% per year, and the observation that not all breast cancers developing after a diagnosis of LCIS are of lobular histology (reviewed in Ref.[45]). The incidence of invasive breast cancer after a diagnosis of LCIS is also steady over time. In the series with the longest follow-up,[46] the probability of developing DCIS or invasive cancer by 10 years after a diagnosis of LCIS was 13%, 26% after 20 years, and 35% by 35 years. Others have also reported the cumulative long-term risk, with one study[5] reporting that more than 50% of patients developed breast cancer between 15 and 30 years of follow-up.

ALH is also associated with an increased risk of subsequent breast cancer; however, this is of a lower magnitude than that conferred by LCIS. Patients diagnosed with ALH have a 4-fold to 5-fold higher risk than the general population (ie, women of comparable age who have had a breast biopsy performed with no atypical proliferative disease diagnosed). Hence, these observations suggest that the term LN, albeit helpful to describe this group of lesions collectively, may not suffice to guide the management of patients with lobular lesions, and specific classification of LN into ALH and LCIS, may still be justified. However, as noted earlier, the distinctions between ALH and LCIS are subjective, and the differences between these 2 categories of LN are often more easily expressed in words than in practice.[47]

Early observations that the risk of breast cancer development after a diagnosis of ALH or LCIS was bilateral, combined with the fact that not all subsequent cancers that developed in women with LN were of the lobular phenotype, led to the notion that these lesions should be considered as risk factors for breast cancer, as opposed to precursor lesions.[41,45,48] In contrast, more recent reports showing a higher rate of breast cancer development in the ipsilateral breast,[10,12,49] most of which are of lobular histology,[9,12,47] support a precursor role for LCIS. These clinical observations, in parallel with SEER data showing an increasing incidence of both LCIS and ILC from the late 1980s to the mid-1990s among women 50 years of age and older,[39,50] and molecular data showing the clonality between LN and synchronous invasive breast cancer (as described earlier), support the contention that LN is not only a risk indicator but also a nonobligate precursor of invasive breast cancer.

## CLINICAL MANAGEMENT

In current practice, a diagnosis of ALH or LCIS is typically perceived as a marker of increased risk, and conservative management remains the mainstay of treatment. However, the long-term cumulative risk associated with these lesions, and our inability to predict which women will develop breast cancer, generates uncertainty among both patients and providers.[51]

### Surgical Considerations

A diagnosis of classic LCIS or ALH made by surgical excision does not require further surgical intervention, and there is no indication to document margin status in a specimen that contains only classic LN.[12] Similarly, the finding of classic LCIS or ALH in the surrounding breast parenchyma of a lumpectomy specimen containing DCIS or invasive carcinoma does not alter surgical management of the breast primary and does not increase the rate of local recurrence in patients undergoing breast conservation.[52–54]

The importance of clear margins in the presence of an LCIS variant is largely unknown. Although there is considerable speculation that PLCIS represents a more aggressive subtype of LCIS, data regarding the natural history of this lesion are limited to 2 small retrospective reports describing recurrences of PLCIS after excision,[13,55] with one series specifically reporting on margin status.[55] At a mean follow-up of 46 months (range, 4–108 months), 1 of 6 patients whose original excision showed PLCIS at the margin developed recurrent PLCIS. Until additional data are available, it is reasonable to pursue margin-negative excision for PLCIS.

### Core Needle Biopsy

The term LN is preferred for diagnostic purposes in core needle biopsy specimens, because it removes the variability of the ALH/LCIS nomenclature.[12,56] In the guidelines of breast cancer screening programs (eg, the United Kingdom National Health Service Breast Screening Programme),[56] it is recommended that in core biopsy specimens, no attempts to distinguish ALH and LCIS should be made, and in the presence of lobular lesions, a diagnosis of LN should be rendered.

The National Comprehensive Cancer Network (NCCN) guidelines recommend surgical excision after a core biopsy diagnosis of LN to rule out an adjacent malignancy.[57] However, these guidelines are largely based on limited data from retrospective series, which report the upgrade rate at surgical excision for a core biopsy diagnosis of LN to range from 0% to 50%.[51,58–62] More recent series reporting upgrade rates of 3% to 4% after surgical excision of consecutive cases of LN[63,64] show that with a multidisciplinary approach, including careful pathologic review to exclude other high-risk lesions as well as an assessment of radiologic-pathologic concordance, not all patients with a core biopsy of LN require surgical excision. Rendi and colleagues[64] reported an upgrade rate of 4% after surgical excision of 68 cases of LN on core biopsy; similarly, Murray and colleagues[63] reported an upgrade rate of 3% after surgical excision of 72 cases of LN on core biopsy. In both these series, the cancers identified were small, low-grade malignancies. Additional reports focusing on upgrade rates after a core biopsy diagnosis of pure ALH also support observation for select cases.[65,66] In cases of ALH or LCIS that are not surgically excised, short-term mammographic follow-up is recommended.

As described earlier, diversity within the spectrum of LN has led to the diagnosis of several LCIS variants. Available data support routine excision when PLCIS is diagnosed on core biopsy, with upgrade rates consistently exceeding 25%.[67] Until additional information regarding the biological and clinical significance of other LCIS variants is available, excision of these lesions when diagnosed on core biopsy should also be pursued.

## Discussing Risk

Once a concurrent malignancy has been excluded, women with LCIS should be counseled regarding their increased risk of breast cancer. There are two different ways to describe risk for breast cancer: absolute risk, measured either over a patient's lifetime (usually up to 90 years of age) or within a given time interval (eg, 2.5% over the next 5 years); and relative risk (RR), measured as a comparison of the incidence of disease between a population with a risk factor and a second population without it. Information about risk for an individual patient is best provided in terms of absolute risk within a given period. For LN, it is important to stress that the risk remains steady over their lifetimes at ~1% to 2% per year; therefore, the absolute risk of breast cancer for an individual is affected by their age at LCIS diagnosis. However, most women with LCIS do not develop invasive breast cancer.

## Surveillance

The NCCN Breast Cancer Screening and Diagnosis Clinical Practice Guidelines for women with LCIS include annual mammography and clinical breast examination (CBE) every 6 to 12 months, with consideration of annual MRI.[68] However, the American Cancer Society (ACS) guidelines do not support routine use of MRI in this setting, stating that there is not enough evidence to recommend for or against MRI screening in women at increased risk from LCIS.[69] The ACS guidelines are based on the increased sensitivity of MRI in women at high risk because of an inherited predisposition or strong family history of breast cancer; however, the biology of the breast cancers that develop in women with LCIS differs from those that develop in women at risk from BRCA mutations, and a recent longitudinal cohort study of women in surveillance for a diagnosis of LCIS suggests that routine MRI screening is not warranted in these patients.[70]

Similarly, until additional information on the natural history of PLCIS is available, minimal surveillance strategies for this lesion should include biannual CBE and annual mammography, and the decision to incorporate MRI screening should be made on an individual basis after a full discussion of the potential risks and benefits of this approach.

## Chemoprevention

The potential preventive benefit of tamoxifen for women at increased risk of breast cancer, including those at increased risk because of LN, was first reported more than 10 years ago in the National Surgical Adjuvant Breast and Bowel Projected (NSABP) BCPT P-1 (Breast Cancer Prevention Trial),[71] and shortly thereafter for raloxifene in the NSABP STAR P-2 (Study of Tamoxifen and Raloxifene) trial.[72] Women with LCIS were well represented in both of these studies, comprising 6.2% of 13,338 participants in the P-1 trial and 9.2% of 19,747 participants in the STAR trial. In both subsets, chemoprevention reduced the risk of developing breast cancer by more than 50%. Despite these findings, these agents have not been commonly used for risk reduction among women at varying levels of hereditary risk or among those at increased risk because of LN.[51,73]

Clinical practice recommendations for the use of pharmacologic interventions for breast cancer were first published by the American Society of Clinical Oncology (ASCO) in 1999,[43,74] with updates in 2002[31,75] and 2009[49,76] stating that tamoxifen or raloxifene "may be offered" to reduce the risk of ER-positive invasive breast cancer in high-risk premenopausal and postmenopausal women, respectively. In the recent 2013 updated guidelines,[77] "may be offered" has been replaced with "should be discussed as an option," reflecting the increasing weight of evidence from randomized phase 3 trials showing a reduction in breast cancer risk for both tamoxifen and raloxifene. The MAP.3 (National Cancer Institute of Canada Clinical Trials Group Mammary Prevention.3) trial also showed that, compared with placebo, exemestane reduced the risk of invasive breast cancer by 65% in postmenopausal women, and appeared to be beneficial in women with a history of ADH, ALH, or LCIS.[78] Recommendations regarding exemestane for risk reduction are now also included in the ASCO guidelines.

These findings and others included in the updated ASCO guidelines strongly support the need to improve efforts to educate both high-risk patients and their health care providers about the benefits of chemoprevention in decreasing breast cancer risk.

### Risk-Reducing Surgery

When LCIS was first described, it was treated as a malignancy necessitating mastectomy, like all breast carcinomas at the time. Studies showing that the of risk of breast cancer was conferred equally to both breasts led to the recommendation for bilateral mastectomy, and, in parallel with the trend toward more conservative therapy for the treatment of invasive breast cancer, aggressive surgical therapy for LCIS fell out of favor. In the modern Memorial Sloan Kettering Cancer Center experience, only a few (5%) women with LCIS pursue bilateral prophylactic mastectomy (BPM).[51] Nevertheless, BPM may be a reasonable option for a subset of women with LCIS and other risk factors, such as a strong family history or extremely dense breasts.

The current standard of care for prophylactic mastectomy is total mastectomy (with or without reconstruction), with the goal of removing the entire mammary gland as would be performed during therapeutic mastectomy. Historically, BPM was reported to result in an ~90% risk reduction for the development of subsequent cancer.[79] However, this figure was based on a retrospective analysis of 639 women with a family history of breast cancer undergoing BPMs between 1960 and 1993. Although it is important to educate patients that prophylactic mastectomy does not completely eliminate cancer risk, many women in this series underwent subcutaneous mastectomy (an operation that has fallen out of favor because of the amount of breast tissue frequently left behind), and a more recent retrospective case-cohort study[80] evaluating the efficacy of BPM in a community practice setting reported a 95% risk reduction.

Patients considering surgery for risk reduction need to be fully aware of all the risks and benefits of this approach, and should be encouraged to consider the impact that prophylactic surgery may have on their quality of life with respect to body image and sexual functioning. If reconstruction is to be pursued, they should also have a reasonable expectation for the most likely cosmetic outcome. The decision to undergo BPM is highly individualized and should not be undertaken without ample time to consider all of the available options for risk management.

## REFERENCES

1. Lakhani SR, Ellis IO, Schnitt SJ, et al, editors. WHO classification of tumours of the breast. Lyon (France): IARC Press; 2012.
2. Ewing J. Neoplastic diseases: a textbook on tumors. Philadelphia: WB Saunders; 1919.
3. Foote FW, Stewart FW. Lobular carcinoma in situ: a rare form of mammary cancer. Am J Pathol 1941;17(4):491–6, 3.
4. Haagensen CD, Lane N, Lattes R, et al. Lobular neoplasia (so-called lobular carcinoma in situ) of the breast. Cancer 1978;42(2):737–69.
5. Rosen PP, Kosloff C, Lieberman PH, et al. Lobular carcinoma in situ of the breast. Detailed analysis of 99 patients with average follow-up of 24 years. Am J Surg Pathol 1978;2(3):225–51.
6. Page DL, Vander Zwaag R, Rogers LW, et al. Relation between component parts of fibrocystic disease complex and breast cancer. J Natl Cancer Inst 1978; 61(4):1055–63.
7. Andrade VP, Ostrovnaya I, Seshan VE, et al. Clonal relatedness between lobular carcinoma in situ and synchronous malignant lesions. Breast Cancer Res 2012; 14(4):R103.
8. Aulmann S, Penzel R, Longerich T, et al. Clonality of lobular carcinoma in situ (LCIS) and metachronous invasive breast cancer. Breast Cancer Res Treat 2008;107(3):331–5.
9. Lopez-Garcia MA, Geyer FC, Lacroix-Triki M, et al. Breast cancer precursors revisited: molecular features and progression pathways. Histopathology 2010; 57(2):171–92.
10. Page DL, Schuyler PA, Dupont WD, et al. Atypical lobular hyperplasia as a unilateral predictor of breast cancer risk: a retrospective cohort study. Lancet 2003; 361(9352):125–9.
11. Vos CB, Cleton-Jansen AM, Berx G, et al. E-cadherin inactivation in lobular carcinoma in situ of the breast: an early event in tumorigenesis. Br J Cancer 1997; 76(9):1131–3.
12. Reis-Filho JS, Pinder SE. Non-operative breast pathology: lobular neoplasia. J Clin Pathol 2007;60(12):1321–7.
13. Sneige N, Wang J, Baker BA, et al. Clinical, histopathologic, and biologic features of pleomorphic lobular (ductal-lobular) carcinoma in situ of the breast: a report of 24 cases. Mod Pathol 2002;15(10):1044–50.
14. Page DL. Atypical hyperplasia, narrowly and broadly defined. Hum Pathol 1991; 22(7):631–2.
15. Page DL, Dupont WD, Rogers LW, et al. Atypical hyperplastic lesions of the female breast. A long-term follow-up study. Cancer 1985;55(11):2698–708.
16. Eusebi V, Magalhaes F, Azzopardi JG. Pleomorphic lobular carcinoma of the breast: an aggressive tumor showing apocrine differentiation. Hum Pathol 1992;23(6):655–62.

17. Chen YY, Hwang ES, Roy R, et al. Genetic and phenotypic characteristics of pleomorphic lobular carcinoma in situ of the breast. Am J Surg Pathol 2009; 33(11):1683–94.
18. Bratthauer GL, Saenger JS, Strauss BL. Antibodies targeting p63 react specifically in the cytoplasm of breast epithelial cells exhibiting secretory differentiation. Histopathology 2005;47(6):611–6.
19. Boldt V, Stacher E, Halbwedl I, et al. Positioning of necrotic lobular intraepithelial neoplasias (LIN, grade 3) within the sequence of breast carcinoma progression. Genes Chromosomes Cancer 2010;49(5):463–70.
20. Reis-Filho JS, Pusztai L. Gene expression profiling in breast cancer: classification, prognostication, and prediction. Lancet 2011;378(9805):1812–23.
21. Cancer Genome Atlas Network. Comprehensive molecular portraits of human breast tumours. Nature 2012;490(7418):61–70.
22. Geyer FC, Lacroix-Triki M, Savage K, et al. beta-Catenin pathway activation in breast cancer is associated with triple-negative phenotype but not with CTNNB1 mutation. Mod Pathol 2011;24(2):209–31.
23. Dabbs DJ, Bhargava R, Chivukula M. Lobular versus ductal breast neoplasms: the diagnostic utility of p120 catenin. Am J Surg Pathol 2007;31(3):427–37.
24. Morrogh M, Andrade VP, Giri D, et al. Cadherin-catenin complex dissociation in lobular neoplasia of the breast. Breast Cancer Res Treat 2012;132(2):641–52.
25. Jacobs TW, Pliss N, Kouria G, et al. Carcinomas in situ of the breast with indeterminate features: role of E-cadherin staining in categorization. Am J Surg Pathol 2001;25(2):229–36.
26. Dabbs DJ, Schnitt SJ, Geyer FC, et al. Lobular neoplasia of the breast revisited with emphasis on the role of E-cadherin immunohistochemistry. Am J Surg Pathol 2013;37(7):e1–11.
27. Rakha EA, Patel A, Powe DG, et al. Clinical and biological significance of E-cadherin protein expression in invasive lobular carcinoma of the breast. Am J Surg Pathol 2010;34(10):1472–9.
28. Da Silva L, Parry S, Reid L, et al. Aberrant expression of E-cadherin in lobular carcinomas of the breast. Am J Surg Pathol 2008;32(5):773–83.
29. Derksen PW, Liu X, Saridin F, et al. Somatic inactivation of E-cadherin and p53 in mice leads to metastatic lobular mammary carcinoma through induction of anoikis resistance and angiogenesis. Cancer Cell 2006;10(5):437–49.
30. Aigner K, Dampier B, Descovich L, et al. The transcription factor ZEB1 (deltaEF1) promotes tumour cell dedifferentiation by repressing master regulators of epithelial polarity. Oncogene 2007;26(49):6979–88.
31. Guilford P, Hopkins J, Harraway J, et al. E-cadherin germline mutations in familial gastric cancer. Nature 1998;392(6674):402–5.
32. Schrader KA, Masciari S, Boyd N, et al. Germline mutations in CDH1 are infrequent in women with early-onset or familial lobular breast cancers. J Med Genet 2011;48(1):64–8.
33. Lu YJ, Osin P, Lakhani SR, et al. Comparative genomic hybridization analysis of lobular carcinoma in situ and atypical lobular hyperplasia and potential roles for gains and losses of genetic material in breast neoplasia. Cancer Res 1998; 58(20):4721–7.
34. Hwang ES, Nyante SJ, Yi Chen Y, et al. Clonality of lobular carcinoma in situ and synchronous invasive lobular carcinoma. Cancer 2004;100(12):2562–72.
35. Reis-Filho JS, Simpson PT, Jones C, et al. Pleomorphic lobular carcinoma of the breast: role of comprehensive molecular pathology in characterization of an entity. J Pathol 2005;207(1):1–13.

36. Simpson PT, Reis-Filho JS, Lambros MB, et al. Molecular profiling pleomorphic lobular carcinomas of the breast: evidence for a common molecular genetic pathway with classic lobular carcinomas. J Pathol 2008;215(3):231–44.

37. Wheeler JE, Enterline HT, Roseman JM, et al. Lobular carcinoma in situ of the breast. Long-term followup. Cancer 1974;34(3):554–63.

38. Hussain M, Cunnick GH. Management of lobular carcinoma in-situ and atypical lobular hyperplasia of the breast–a review. Eur J Surg Oncol 2011;37(4): 279–89.

39. Li CI, Anderson BO, Daling JR, et al. Changing incidence of lobular carcinoma in situ of the breast. Breast Cancer Res Treat 2002;75(3):259–68.

40. Li CI, Malone KE, Saltzman BS, et al. Risk of invasive breast carcinoma among women diagnosed with ductal carcinoma in situ and lobular carcinoma in situ, 1988-2001. Cancer 2006;106(10):2104–12.

41. Urban JA. Bilaterality of cancer of the breast. Biopsy of the opposite breast. Cancer 1967;20(11):1867–70.

42. Rosen PP, Senie R, Schottenfeld D, et al. Noninvasive breast carcinoma: frequency of unsuspected invasion and implications for treatment. Ann Surg 1979;189(3):377–82.

43. Liberman L, Holland AE, Marjan D, et al. Underestimation of atypical ductal hyperplasia at MRI-guided 9-gauge vacuum-assisted breast biopsy. AJR Am J Roentgenol 2007;188(3):684–90.

44. Dupont WD, Page DL. Risk factors for breast cancer in women with proliferative breast disease. N Engl J Med 1985;312(3):146–51.

45. Chuba PJ, Hamre MR, Yap J, et al. Bilateral risk for subsequent breast cancer after lobular carcinoma-in-situ: analysis of surveillance, epidemiology, and end results data. J Clin Oncol 2005;23(24):5534–41.

46. Bodian CA, Perzin KH, Lattes R. Lobular neoplasia. Long term risk of breast cancer and relation to other factors. Cancer 1996;78(5):1024–34.

47. Fisher ER, Land SR, Fisher B, et al. Pathologic findings from the National Surgical Adjuvant Breast and Bowel Project: twelve-year observations concerning lobular carcinoma in situ. Cancer 2004;100(2):238–44.

48. Andersen JA. Lobular carcinoma in situ of the breast. An approach to rational treatment. Cancer 1977;39(6):2597–602.

49. Collins LC, Baer HJ, Tamimi RM, et al. Magnitude and laterality of breast cancer risk according to histologic type of atypical hyperplasia: results from the Nurses' Health Study. Cancer 2007;109(2):180–7.

50. Li CI, Anderson BO, Porter P, et al. Changing incidence rate of invasive lobular breast carcinoma among older women. Cancer 2000;88(11):2561–9.

51. Oppong BA, King TA. Recommendations for women with lobular carcinoma in situ (LCIS). Oncology (Williston Park) 2011;25(11):1051–6, 8.

52. Abner AL, Connolly JL, Recht A, et al. The relation between the presence and extent of lobular carcinoma in situ and the risk of local recurrence for patients with infiltrating carcinoma of the breast treated with conservative surgery and radiation therapy. Cancer 2000;88(5):1072–7.

53. Ben-David MA, Kleer CG, Paramagul C, et al. Is lobular carcinoma in situ as a component of breast carcinoma a risk factor for local failure after breast-conserving therapy? Results of a matched pair analysis. Cancer 2006;106(1): 28–34.

54. Ciocca RM, Li T, Freedman GM, et al. Presence of lobular carcinoma in situ does not increase local recurrence in patients treated with breast-conserving therapy. Ann Surg Oncol 2008;15(8):2263–71.

55. Downs-Kelly E, Bell D, Perkins GH, et al. Clinical implications of margin involvement by pleomorphic lobular carcinoma in situ. Arch Pathol Lab Med 2011; 135(6):737–43.
56. Walker RA, Hanby A, Pinder SE, et al, National Coordinating Committee for Breast Pathology Research Subgroup. Current issues in diagnostic breast pathology. J Clin Pathol 2012;65(9):771–85.
57. National Comprehensive Cancer Network. Available at: http://www.nccn.org. Accessed September 20, 2013.
58. Georgian-Smith D, Lawton TJ. Calcifications of lobular carcinoma in situ of the breast: radiologic-pathologic correlation. AJR Am J Roentgenol 2001;176(5): 1255–9.
59. Kilbride KE, Newman LA. Lobular carcinoma in situ: clinical management. In: Harris JR, Lippman ME, Morrow M, et al, editors. Diseases of the breast. 4th edition. Philadelphia: Lippincott Williams & Wilkins; 2010. p. 341–8.
60. Lavoue V, Graesslin O, Classe JM, et al. Management of lobular neoplasia diagnosed by core needle biopsy: study of 52 biopsies with follow-up surgical excision. Breast 2007;16(5):533–9.
61. Mahoney MC, Robinson-Smith TM, Shaughnessy EA. Lobular neoplasia at 11-gauge vacuum-assisted stereotactic biopsy: correlation with surgical excisional biopsy and mammographic follow-up. AJR Am J Roentgenol 2006;187(4): 949–54.
62. Pacelli A, Rhodes DJ, Amrami KK, et al. Outcome of atypical lobular hyperplasia and lobular carcinoma in situ diagnosed by core needle biopsy: clinical and surgical follow-up of 30 cases. Am J Clin Pathol 2001;116(4):591–2.
63. Murray MP, Luedtke C, Liberman L, et al. Classic lobular carcinoma in situ and atypical lobular hyperplasia at percutaneous breast core biopsy: outcomes of prospective excision. Cancer 2013;119(5):1073–9.
64. Rendi MH, Dintzis SM, Lehman CD, et al. Lobular in-situ neoplasia on breast core needle biopsy: imaging indication and pathologic extent can identify which patients require excisional biopsy. Ann Surg Oncol 2012;19(3):914–21.
65. Shah-Khan MG, Geiger XJ, Reynolds C, et al. Long-term follow-up of lobular neoplasia (atypical lobular hyperplasia/lobular carcinoma in situ) diagnosed on core needle biopsy. Ann Surg Oncol 2012;19(10):3131–8.
66. Subhawong AP, Subhawong TK, Khouri N, et al. Incidental minimal atypical lobular hyperplasia on core needle biopsy: correlation with findings on follow-up excision. Am J Surg Pathol 2010;34(6):822–8.
67. King TA, Reis-Filho JS. Lobular carcinoma in situ: biology and management. In: Harris JR, Lippman ME, Morrow M, et al, editors. Diseases of the breast. 5th edition. Philadelphia: Lippincott Williams & Wilkins; in press.
68. Bevers TB, Anderson BO, Bonaccio E, et al. Breast cancer screening and diagnosis. J Natl Compr Canc Netw 2006;4(5):480–508.
69. Saslow D, Boetes C, Burke W, et al. American Cancer Society guidelines for breast screening with MRI as an adjunct to mammography. CA Cancer J Clin 2007;57(2):75–89.
70. King TA, Muhsen S, Patil S, et al. Is there a role for routine screening MRI in women with LCIS? Breast Cancer Res Treat 2013;142(2):445–53.
71. Fisher B, Costantino JP, Wickerham DL, et al. Tamoxifen for prevention of breast cancer: report of the National Surgical Adjuvant Breast and Bowel Project P-1 Study. J Natl Cancer Inst 1998;90(18):1371–88.
72. Vogel VG, Costantino JP, Wickerham DL, et al. Effects of tamoxifen vs raloxifene on the risk of developing invasive breast cancer and other disease outcomes: the

NSABP Study of Tamoxifen and Raloxifene (STAR) P-2 trial. JAMA 2006;295(23): 2727–41.

73. Ropka ME, Keim J, Philbrick JT. Patient decisions about breast cancer chemo-prevention: a systematic review and meta-analysis. J Clin Oncol 2010;28(18): 3090–5.

74. Chlebowski RT, Collyar DE, Somerfield MR, et al. American Society of Clinical Oncology technology assessment on breast cancer risk reduction strategies: tamoxifen and raloxifene. J Clin Oncol 1999;17(6):1939–55.

75. Chlebowski RT, Col N, Winer EP, et al. American Society of Clinical Oncology technology assessment of pharmacologic interventions for breast cancer risk reduction including tamoxifen, raloxifene, and aromatase inhibition. J Clin Oncol 2002;20(15):3328–43.

76. Visvanathan K, Chlebowski RT, Hurley P, et al. American Society of Clinical Oncology clinical practice guideline update on the use of pharmacologic inter-ventions including tamoxifen, raloxifene, and aromatase inhibition for breast cancer risk reduction. J Clin Oncol 2009;27(19):3235–58.

77. Visvanathan K, Hurley P, Bantug E, et al. Use of pharmacologic interventions for breast cancer risk reduction: American Society of Clinical Oncology clinical practice guideline. J Clin Oncol 2013;31(23):2942–62.

78. Goss PE, Ingle JN, Ales-Martinez JE, et al. Exemestane for breast-cancer pre-vention in postmenopausal women. N Engl J Med 2011;364(25):2381–91.

79. Hartmann LC, Schaid DJ, Woods JE, et al. Efficacy of bilateral prophylactic mastectomy in women with a family history of breast cancer. N Engl J Med 1999;340(2):77–84.

80. Geiger AM, Yu O, Herrinton LJ, et al. A population-based study of bilateral pro-phylactic mastectomy efficacy in women at elevated risk for breast cancer in community practices. Arch Intern Med 2005;165(5):516–20.

# Neoadjuvant Therapy in the Treatment of Breast Cancer

Mediget Teshome, MD, Kelly K. Hunt, MD*

## KEYWORDS

- Breast cancer • Neoadjuvant chemotherapy • Preoperative chemotherapy
- Pathologic complete response

## KEY POINTS

- Neoadjuvant chemotherapy in the treatment of breast cancer offers comparable survival benefit to adjuvant chemotherapy.
- Response to neoadjuvant systemic therapy and molecular subtype holds important implications for prognosis and individualized patient outcomes.
- The addition of trastuzumab to neoadjuvant chemotherapy improves pathologic complete response in patients with HER2-positive breast cancer.
- Neoadjuvant endocrine therapy with aromatase inhibitors in postmenopausal women with hormone receptor-positive tumors can significantly decrease tumor burden, thereby facilitating breast-conserving surgery.
- Neoadjuvant chemotherapy safely allows for a more limited operative approach with breast-conserving surgery and sentinel lymph node dissection without an increase in local-regional recurrence rates in selected patients.

## INTRODUCTION

The treatment of breast cancer has evolved from a primary surgical approach with a focus on local-regional control to multidisciplinary management with an emphasis on systemic therapy resulting in significantly improved survival. The optimal timing of systemic therapy relative to operative management has been studied for several decades with strong evidence supporting a neoadjuvant approach to systemic therapy in certain populations. Neoadjuvant therapy implies the initiation of systemic therapy

The authors have nothing to disclose.
Department of Surgical Oncology, The University of Texas MD Anderson Cancer Center, 1400 Pressler Street, Houston, TX 77030, USA
* Corresponding author. The University of Texas MD Anderson Cancer Center, 1400 Pressler Street, Unit 1484, Houston, TX 77030.
*E-mail address:* khunt@mdanderson.org

Surg Oncol Clin N Am 23 (2014) 505–523
http://dx.doi.org/10.1016/j.soc.2014.03.006
1055-3207/14/$ – see front matter © 2014 Elsevier Inc. All rights reserved.

before definitive local-regional management. It is also referred to as primary systemic therapy or preoperative chemotherapy. Although historically reserved for patients with inoperable disease, contemporary management of breast cancer involves a neoadjuvant approach for patients with inflammatory breast cancer, locally advanced disease, and selected patients with early-stage, operable breast cancer. Neoadjuvant chemotherapy has emerged as a powerful treatment modality with individualized prognostic significance based on response to therapy.

## RATIONALE FOR NEOADJUVANT CHEMOTHERAPY

The paradigm shift from adjuvant to neoadjuvant chemotherapy is rooted in observations of tumor kinetics and the hypothesis of micrometastatic disease present in the early stages of breast malignancy.[1] Fisher and colleagues[2] performed animal studies and observed a change in tumor kinetics with increased cellular proliferation at metastatic sites after resection of the primary tumor. Another concern was resistance to chemotherapy with increased tumor growth resulting in increased drug-resistant variants, suggesting the optimal time for chemotherapy administration was early after diagnosis.[3] These observations along with multiple clinical studies showing benefit in decreasing the primary tumor burden prompted randomized trials examining the potential survival benefit of neoadjuvant chemotherapy over adjuvant systemic therapy in treating disseminated micrometastatic disease. Although this survival advantage was not ultimately demonstrated, a decrease in the primary tumor burden converted some patients to operative candidates and facilitated breast conservation in at least 25%. In addition, insights into prognosis based on tumor response arose as significant clinical implications of neoadjuvant chemotherapy.

## COMPARISON OF NEOADJUVANT TO ADJUVANT SYSTEMIC THERAPY

Initiated in 1988, the National Surgical Adjuvant Breast and Bowel Project (NSABP) B-18 protocol was one of the earliest and largest randomized trials of neoadjuvant versus adjuvant chemotherapy for women with operable breast cancer. This study randomized 1523 women to surgery followed by 4 cycles of AC (doxorubicin 60 mg/$m^2$ and cyclophosphamide 600 mg/$m^2$) or preoperative AC followed by surgery. The planned surgical approach was determined before randomization. All women who were 50 years of age or older were treated with tamoxifen after the completion of chemotherapy and those treated with breast conservation received whole breast radiation therapy. The primary objective of the B-18 study was to determine if neoadjuvant chemotherapy resulted in improved overall survival (OS) and disease-free survival (DFS) as compared with delivery of the same chemotherapy in the adjuvant setting. Secondary aims were to evaluate the effect of neoadjuvant chemotherapy on response in the primary tumor, response in axillary lymph nodes, and facilitation of breast conservation.[4] The investigators found no difference in OS or DFS in women treated with preoperative chemotherapy as compared with those treated with adjuvant chemotherapy. This finding has persisted after 16 years of follow-up.[5] Patients in the preoperative AC group showed 79% objective clinical response, 43% clinical partial response, 36% clinical complete response, and 13% pathologic complete response (pCR) after treatment. This group also had increased incidence of pathologically negative axillary nodal disease and rates of breast conservation. There was a nonstatistically significant trend in increased ipsilateral breast tumor recurrence (IBTR) following preoperative chemotherapy. pCR and posttreatment pathologic negative nodal status emerged as strong predictors of both OS and DFS.

Similar to the NSABP B-18 trial, the European Organization Research and Treatment of Cancer Trial 10902 examined neoadjuvant chemotherapy in women with operable breast cancer as compared with adjuvant therapy.[6] This study randomized 698 women to 4 cycles of preoperative FEC (fluorouracil 600 mg/m$^2$, epirubicin 60 mg/m$^2$, and cyclophosphamide 600 mg/m$^2$) followed by surgery or the same regimen postoperatively. The investigators found no difference between the treatment groups in OS, progression-free survival, or time to local-regional recurrence. They observed an overall response rate of 49% in the preoperative chemotherapy group with 6.6% of patients experiencing complete clinical response and 3.7% with pCR. They also showed an increased survival advantage with pCR that was not demonstrated with complete clinical response. There was a significant down-sizing in clinical tumor size to less than 2 cm in the preoperative arm from 14% at diagnosis and 47% after treatment compared with 14% and 26% in the postoperative arm, respectively. In the preoperative group, 23% of patients initially planned for mastectomy underwent breast conservation.

A meta-analysis evaluating 9 randomized trials addressing outcomes after neoadjuvant and adjuvant chemotherapy in 3946 patients reached similar conclusions. Investigators reported no difference in OS, disease progression, and distant disease recurrence between the 2 groups. There was a 22% increased relative risk of local-regional recurrence with neoadjuvant chemotherapy. Although this was a statistically significant finding, it was attributed to 3 trials in which patients were not obligated to surgery after complete clinical response and received radiation therapy only. This finding underscores the importance of operative intervention in patients with complete clinical response for maintenance of local control. pCR varied from 4% to 29% reported in 5 studies. In addition, there was a higher rate of breast conservation in the preoperative chemotherapy group.[7] A more recent meta-analysis reviewing 14 trials randomizing a total of 5500 women to neoadjuvant chemotherapy or adjuvant chemotherapy confirmed these findings. Local-regional recurrence, after exclusion of the studies omitting surgical management, was similar among the neoadjuvant and adjuvant chemotherapy groups.[8]

Although these trials did not find increased survival rates following neoadjuvant chemotherapy as hypothesized, they asserted an equivalence of survival benefit with neoadjuvant treatment as compared with the adjuvant setting. In addition, they established the role for neoadjuvant chemotherapy in decreasing the primary tumor burden and facilitating breast conservation without increased risk of local recurrence. Importantly, they demonstrated tumor response as a strong predictor of outcome as evidenced by the association of pCR and survival.

## Introduction of Taxanes

The addition of taxanes to an anthracycline-based regimen in the preoperative setting was evaluated in the NSABP B-27 protocol. This study, initiated in 1995, randomized 2411 women with operable breast cancer to receive 4 cycles of preoperative AC followed by surgery, preoperative AC and docetaxel (100 mg/m$^2$) followed by surgery, and preoperative AC followed by surgery and postoperative docetaxel. The primary objective was to determine if the addition of docetaxel could increase OS and DFS. Additional objectives included the effect of preoperative docetaxel in local-regional control, pCR, pathologic axillary down-staging, and breast-conserving surgery.

The investigators found significantly increased rates of objective clinical response (86% vs 91%, $P<.001$) and pCR (13% vs 26%, $P<.001$) with the addition of neoadjuvant docetaxel to AC. Also observed were decreased rates of pathologically positive nodes and no further increase in the rates of breast conservation. Again, no difference in

OS and DFS was found with the addition of preoperative or postoperative docetaxel. However, patients who experienced a pCR and those who were found to have pathologically negative nodes after treatment continued to show an associated survival benefit.[5]

The above studies suggest that it is not the timing of chemotherapy but rather the chemosensitivity and responsiveness of the tumor influencing OS.

## PROGNOSTIC SIGNIFICANCE OF TUMOR RESPONSE

Perhaps the most intriguing implication of preoperative chemotherapy is the ability to observe in vivo tumor chemosensitivity and the prognostic impact of tumor response.

### Pathologic Complete Response (pCR)

Neoadjuvant chemotherapy trials have revealed the phenomenon of pCR, defined as no residual invasive tumor on pathologic assessment after therapy. Virtually every study examining the impact of pCR after neoadjuvant chemotherapy for breast cancer has demonstrated an associated survival benefit. Furthermore, neoadjuvant chemotherapy has the potential to decrease the axillary nodal disease burden significantly with 23% of patients converting from clinically node-positive to pathologically node-negative after treatment with anthracycline-based chemotherapy. Patients who achieve pCR in the primary tumor are more likely to have negative pathologic axillary nodal status and the degree of axillary nodal involvement after chemotherapy is highly predictive of outcome.[9]

Discrepancies exist in the literature in defining pCR with some studies reporting pCR in the breast only and others defining pCR as complete response in the breast and axillary nodes, the latter being the currently accepted definition. Importantly, it is only the residual invasive component and not the presence of carcinoma in situ that influences outcome.[10] Factors found to be associated with an increased likelihood of pCR include age less than 40, smaller tumors (<2.0 cm), ductal histology, high nuclear grade tumors, high rate of cellular proliferation (Ki-67), estrogen receptor negativity, triple negative subtype, and human epidermal growth factor receptor 2 (HER2)-positive disease.[11] Although associated with improved survival overall, a small percentage of patients who achieve pCR will develop disease recurrence and distant disease.[12] Significant factors associated with distant metastasis after pCR include clinical stage IIIB or higher, premenopausal status, and 10 or less lymph nodes examined.[13]

The presence of pCR has emerged as a powerful predictor of patient outcome and is used as a surrogate endpoint for prognosis in many clinical trials. As such, pCR has entered into contemporary policy with the recent adoption for use in accelerating drug approval by the Food and Drug Administration.[14]

### Prognosis After Neoadjuvant Chemotherapy

In patients who do not achieve pCR, the residual cancer burden (RCB) can be a useful tool to predict survival. This continuous value incorporates 4 parameters that hold prognostic significance after neoadjuvant chemotherapy: the primary tumor dimension, cellularity of the invasive cancer, size of largest nodal metastasis, and number of positive lymph nodes. Increasing RCB values after chemotherapy are associated with increased risk of 5-year distant relapse. When stratified by extent of residual disease, one study showed rates of distant relapse at 5 years were 2.4% in those with minimal residual disease (RCB-I) and 53.6% in those with extensive residual disease (RCB-III). Furthermore, in patients with minimal or no detectable residual disease (RCB-0 or RCB-I) at 5 years, the prognosis was similar to those with pCR. Conversely, patients with extensive residual disease (RCB-III) carried a poor prognosis independent of the type of chemotherapy, adjuvant hormonal therapy, or pathologic stage. In comparison with posttherapy American Joint Committee on Cancer (AJCC) stage group, the RCB was able to classify patients with stage II disease further into 3 distinct groups and stage III disease into 2 distinct groups with different prognoses.[15]

Traditionally, prognosis has been informed by pretreatment TNM (tumor-node-metastasis) clinical stage based on the AJCC system. In the neoadjuvant setting, prognosis is influenced by response to therapy and biologic markers that are not incorporated in traditional staging systems. To address this disparity, a system specifically incorporating the pretreatment clinical stage and posttreatment pathologic stage after neoadjuvant chemotherapy has been described. The Clinical-Pathologic Scoring (CPS) system stratifies patients into groups with increasing CPS scores associated with decreasing 5-year distant metastasis-free survival and disease-specific survival (DSS). A second system, CPS + EG, incorporating estrogen receptor (ER)-negative status and nuclear grade 3 tumors as independent risk factors for poor prognosis, was developed.[16] The CPS + EG system provided refinement of 5-year DSS from 23% to 99% compared with 61% to 92% by clinical stage and 58% to 95% by pathologic stage and recurrence-free survival (RFS) with 5-year RFS rates from 15% to 95% ($P<.001$). This system was subsequently validated in an independent cohort, suggesting generalizability among varying institutions with differing populations and practice patterns.[17]

The RCB index and CPS + EG staging system provide further refinement of prognosis by response beyond pCR status to stratify and predict patient outcomes after neoadjuvant chemotherapy. They are prospective tools for clinicians available online that can assist with decision-making and advising patients regarding individualized outcome.

## Impact of Molecular Subtype on pCR

Determining molecular tumor subtype (luminal, basal, HER2-positive, and normal-like)[18] and approximation of subtype by immunochemistry reveal consistently distinct behavior by subtype in response to neoadjuvant chemotherapy. Generally, more aggressive tumor biology is associated with higher pCR rates and these patients have improved outcomes. Patients with more favorable subtypes are less likely to achieve pCR with neoadjuvant chemotherapy. A meta-analysis of 30 studies examining pCR after neoadjuvant chemotherapy in 11,695 patients found an overall pooled estimate pCR of 19.2% when studies with unknown subtype were excluded. Tumor subtype was strongly associated with pCR% and odds of achieving pCR were 7 times higher for those with HER2-positive/hormone receptor (HR)-negative and 5 times higher for triple-negative subtypes in comparison with the HR-positive subtype. Estimates of pCR were 8.3% in the HR-positive/HER2-negative subtype, 18.7% in the HER2-positive/HR-positive subtype, 38.9% in the HER2-positive/HR-negative subtype, and 31.1% in the triple negative subtype ($P = .002$).[19]

Negative HR status has been associated with increased chemosensitivity and improved pCR as compared with HR-positive disease. However, regardless of HR status, pCR has been shown to result in improved progression-free survival and OS when compared with those who do not achieve pCR.[20] This finding is challenged by a pooled analysis of 6377 patients treated with anthracycline-taxane-based neoadjuvant chemotherapy demonstrating variation in the prognostic impact of pCR by tumor factors. In low proliferative subgroups, including lobular histology, grade 1 disease, and positive HR status, achieving pCR conferred no predictive power in DFS or OS. In contrast, in those with ductal histology, grade 2 or 3 tumors and negative HR status, pCR was associated with improved DFS and OS, suggesting that pCR may not be a suitable endpoint in luminal A and luminal B/HER2-negative subtypes.[21]

Some studies have documented a change in HR or HER2 receptor status when biopsy samples are compared with tissue samples obtained from the same patient after neoadjuvant chemotherapy. Change in HR status from positive to negative after neoadjuvant chemotherapy was evaluated in 259 patients from the Shanghai Cancer Center. This study found a positive to negative change in HR status in 15.2% of tumors. In the cases with a change in HR status, there was a higher proportion of tumors with increased Ki-67 index as compared with tumors showing no change in HR status. In addition, the 5-year DFS and OS rates were significantly lower in the group with change in HR status (43.2% and 60.4%, respectively) as compared with the group with no change (67.9% and 81.8%, respectively).[22] Similarly, loss of HER2 amplification after neoadjuvant chemotherapy with trastuzumab has been associated with decreased 3-year RFS as compared with patients who retain HER2 amplification (50.0% vs 87.5%, $P = .041$).[23]

### Neoadjuvant Therapy in Patients with HER2-positive Tumors

Trastuzumab, a humanized monoclonal antibody targeted against the extracellular domain of the HER2 receptor, has revolutionized the treatment of women with HER2-positive breast cancer with increased survival rates reported in the metastatic and adjuvant settings when used in combination with chemotherapy. In the neoadjuvant setting, significantly increased rates of pCR have been observed in patients treated with trastuzumab and chemotherapy versus chemotherapy alone. In a small trial conducted by Buzdar and colleagues,[24] the increased pCR when trastuzumab was combined with chemotherapy was so dramatic (65.2% vs 26.3%, $P = .016$) that after review by the data and safety monitoring board, the control arm of this phase III, randomized study was terminated prematurely.

Several groups have investigated the use of anti-HER2 therapies in the neoadjuvant setting (Table 1).[24–28] In the NeOAdjuvant Herceptin (NOAH) trial, women with locally

**Table 1**
Phase II and III trials evaluating the addition of trastuzumab to chemotherapy for HER2-positive tumors in the neoadjuvant setting

| Study | Clinical Stage | Neoadjuvant Regimen | n | pCR (%) | DFS (%) | OS (%) |
|---|---|---|---|---|---|---|
| Buzdar et al,[24,25] 2005, 2007 | II and IIIA | P → FEC [P → FEC] + H | 19 23 | 26.3 65.2 $P = .016$ | 85.3 100 $P = .041$ | NR |
| GeparQuattro,[26] 2010 | III | [EC → T or EC → TX or EC → T → X] + H | 445 | 40 | NR | NR |
| NOAH,[27] 2010 | III | AP → P → CMF [AP → P → CMF] + H | 113 115 | 19 38 $P = .004$ | 56 71 $P = .013$ | 79 87 $P = .114$ |
| TECHNO,[28] 2011 | II and III | EC → [P + H] | 217 | 38.7 | 77.9 | 89.4 |

*Abbreviations:* AP, doxorubicin paclitaxel; CMF, cyclophosphamide methotrexate fluorouracil; EC, epirubicin cyclophosphamide; H, trastuzumab; n, number; NR, not reported; P, paclitaxel; T, docetaxel; TX, docetaxel capecitabine; X, capecitabine.

advanced breast cancer were randomized to trastuzumab (loading dose of 8 mg/m$^2$ followed by 10 cycles of 6 mg/m$^2$) in addition to neoadjuvant chemotherapy (3 cycles of doxorubicin 60 mg/m$^2$ plus paclitaxel 150 mg/m$^2$ followed by 4 cycles of paclitaxel 175 mg/m$^2$ followed by 3 cycles of cyclophosphamide 600 mg/m$^2$, methotrexate 40 mg/m$^2$, and fluorouracil 600 mg/m$^2$) versus neoadjuvant chemotherapy alone. Trastuzumab was given for 1 year postoperatively. Patients receiving neoadjuvant trastuzumab experienced an increased pCR in the breast and axillary lymph nodes as compared with those treated with chemotherapy alone (38% vs 19%, $P$ = .001). The investigators reported an improved 3-year event-free survival (71% vs 56%, $P$ = .013) with low cardiac toxicity in those patients receiving concurrent trastuzumab with chemotherapy.[27] The use of neoadjuvant trastuzumab was also associated with a trend toward increased breast-conserving surgery (23% vs 13%, $P$ = .07) without an increase in local recurrence, particularly in patients with noninflammatory breast cancer and HR-negative disease.[29]

To address the need for concurrent administration of trastuzumab in combination with anthracyclines to achieve high pCR rates, the American College of Surgeons Oncology Group (ACOSOG) Z1041 trial compared pCR rates in the breast for 280 women with operable or locally advanced breast cancer randomized to FEC-75 (fluorouracil 500 mg/m$^2$, epirubicin 75 mg/m$^2$, and cyclophosphamide 500 mg/m$^2$) followed by paclitaxel (80 mg/m$^2$) with trastuzumab (4 mg/kg first dose, 2 mg/kg subsequent doses) [sequential group] to women treated with paclitaxel with trastuzumab followed by FEC-75 with trastuzumab [concurrent group]. There was no difference in the breast pCR rates between the 2 groups (56.5% vs 54.2%), suggesting that trastuzumab does not need to be delivered concurrently with anthracyclines to achieve high pCR rates. Although cardiac toxicities were low in both arms, further follow-up is needed to assess the cardiac safety of these regimens.

More recently, other HER2-targeted therapies have also been examined in the neoadjuvant setting with and without chemotherapy. The HER2-positive arm of the GeparQuinto trial compared trastuzumab plus chemotherapy with lapatinib plus chemotherapy in the neoadjuvant setting. This trial randomized 620 women with HER2-positive breast cancer and found pCR rates of 30.3% in the trastuzumab arm and 22.7% in the lapatinib arm (odds ratio [OR] 0.68, 95% confidence interval [CI] 0.47–0.97, $P$ = .04), concluding that trastuzumab was superior to lapatinib as HER2-directed monotherapy in the neoadjuvant setting.[30]

Other trials have investigated dual HER2 targeting in the neoadjuvant setting with lapatinib, pertuzumab, and trastuzumab, all of which have differing mechanisms of action (**Table 2**) and toxicity (**Table 3**).[31–35] The NeoALTTO trial, a multicenter phase III trial randomized 455 women to receive either lapatinib, trastuzumab, or the combination in addition to paclitaxel. The investigators found significantly increased breast pCR rates (51.3% vs 29.5%, OR 2.6, 97.5% CI 1.50–4.58, $P$ = .0001), breast and axilla pCR rates (46.8% vs 27.6%, OR 2.39, 97.5% CI 1.36–4.26, $P$ = .0007), and an increased proportion of patients with pathologically negative axillary lymph nodes after surgery (73% vs 58.6%, $P$ = .0115) in the lapatinib plus trastuzumab arm as compared with the trastuzumab-only arm. There was no difference between the lapatinib-only and the trastuzumab-only arms. Toxicity was highest in the lapatinib-treated groups with diarrhea and hepatic toxicity limiting therapy or prompting dose adjustments.[31] Similarly, the NeoSphere study, a randomized multicenter phase II trial investigating the addition of pertuzumab to trastuzumab with or without docetaxel, found a doubling of pCR rates in women treated with dual HER2 therapy in comparison with trastuzumab and chemotherapy alone (45.8% vs 29%, $P$ = .0141). Of note, in the treatment arm whereby patients received dual HER2-targeted therapy without any

**Table 2**
**Phase II and III trials evaluating dual anti-HER2-directed therapy in the neoadjuvant setting**

| Study | Clinical Stage | Neoadjuvant Regimen | n | pCR (Breast) (%) | pCR (Breast & Axilla) (%) |
|---|---|---|---|---|---|
| NeoALTTO,[31] 2012 | II and IIIA | Lapatinib → lapatinib + P | 154 | 24.7 | 20 |
| | | H → H + P | 149 | 29.5* | 27.6* |
| | | Lapatinib + H → lapatinib + H + P | 152 | 51.3* | 46.8* |
| | | | | *P = .0001 | *P = .0007 |
| NeoSphere,[32] 2012 | II and III | H + T | 107 | 29* | 21.5 |
| | | Pertuzumab + H + T | 107 | 45.8* | 39.3 |
| | | Pertuzumab + H | 107 | 16.8 | 11.2 |
| | | Pertuzumab + T | 96 | 24 | 17.7 |
| | | | | *P = .0140 | |
| CHER-LOB,[33] 2012 | II and IIIA | [P → FEC] + H | 36 | NR | 25 |
| | | [P → FEC] + lapatinib | 39 | | 26.3 |
| | | [P → FEC] + H + lapatinib | 46 | | 46.7 |
| | | | | | P = .019 |
| TBCRC 006,[34] 2013 | II and IIIA | Lapatinib + H | 113 | 27 | NR |
| TRYPHAENA,[35] 2013 | II and III | [FEC → T] + H + pertuzumab | 72 | 61.6 | 50.7 |
| | | FEC → [T + H + pertuzumab] | 75 | 57.3 | 45.3 |
| | | Carboplatin + H + pertuzumab | 76 | 66.2 | 51.9 |

*Abbreviations:* H, trastuzumab; n, number; NR, not reported; P, paclitaxel; T, docetaxel.

chemotherapy, the pCR rate was 16.8%, suggesting some patients may benefit from HER2-directed therapy alone without chemotherapy.[32]

### Neoadjuvant Therapy in Patients with Triple Receptor-negative Breast Cancer

Triple receptor-negative breast cancer (TNBC) is distinguished by the lack of expression of estrogen, progesterone, and HER2 receptors and uniformly carries a poor prognosis. Following neoadjuvant chemotherapy, investigators have shown increased pCR rates in patients with TNBC as compared with non-TNBC subtypes (22% vs 11% OR = 1.53, 95% CI 1.03–2.26, P = .034). In addition, those patients with TNBC achieving a pCR were found to have comparable OS rates to non-TNBC patients. Unfortunately, patients with TNBC who have residual disease after neoadjuvant chemotherapy have a particularly poor prognosis.[36,37]

The lack of specific targets in patients with TNBC has prompted investigators to examine alternative chemotherapeutic regimens in this population. Several studies have shown improved pCR rates with sequential anthracycline-taxane–based neoadjuvant chemotherapy in TNBC.[38] Given the similarities between TNBC and BRCA1-associated cancers, use of platinum-containing drug regimens has been of particular interest. These agents promote interstrand DNA cross-linking triggering apoptosis. Another area of investigation has been the use of PARP (poly-ADP-ribose polymerase) inhibitors. These agents compromise DNA repair leading to selective cell death and have shown mixed results in TNBC.[39] The use of these agents in combination with chemotherapy is the subject of ongoing clinical trials in patients with TNBC.

### Neoadjuvant Therapy in Patients with HR-positive Breast Cancer

Numerous studies have documented that patients with ER-positive tumors have decreased clinical and pathologic response rates to neoadjuvant chemotherapy

**Table 3**
Reported toxicity associated with dual anti-HER2 therapy in the neoadjuvant setting

| Study | Neoadjuvant Regimen | n | LVEF <50% & >10% Points from Baseline | CHF | Diarrhea (Grade ≥3) | Hepatic (Grade ≥3)[a] | Neutropenia (Grade ≥3) | Skin (Grade ≥3) | Death |
|---|---|---|---|---|---|---|---|---|---|
| NeoALTTO,[31] 2012 | Lapatinib → lapatinib + P | 154 | 1 (0.6%) | 0 (0%) | 36 (23.4%) | 28 (18.2%) | 24 (15.6%) | 10 (6.5%) | 0 (0%) |
| | H → H + P | 149 | 1 (0.7%) | 0 (0%) | 3 (2%) | 11 (7.4%) | 4 (2.7%) | 4 (2.7%) | 0 (0%) |
| | Lapatinib + H → Lapatinib + H + P | 152 | 1 (0.6%) | 1 (0.6%) | 32 (21.1%) | 16 (10.5%) | 13 (8.6%) | 10 (6.6%) | 1 (0.6%)[b] |
| NeoSphere,[32] 2012 | H + T | 107 | 1 (1%) | 0 (0%) | 4 (4%) | 3 (3%) | 61 (57%) | 2 (2%) | 0 (0%) |
| | Pertuzumab + H + T | 107 | 3 (3%) | 0 (0%) | 6 (6%) | 1 (1%) | 48 (45%) | 2 (2%) | 1 (1%)[c] |
| | Pertuzumab + H | 107 | 1 (1%) | 1 (1%) | 0 (0%) | 0 (0%) | 1 (1%) | 0 (0%) | 0 (0%) |
| | Pertuzumab + T | 96 | 1 (1%) | 0 (0%) | 4 (4%) | 1 (1%) | 52 (55%) | 1 (1%) | 1 (1%)[d] |
| CHER-LOB,[33] 2012 | [P → FEC] + H | 36 | 1 (2.7%) | 0 (0%) | 1 (2.7%) | 2 (5.5%) | 14 (39%) | 2 (5.5%) | NR |
| | [P → FEC] + lapatinib | 39 | 0 (0%) | 0 (0%) | 14 (35.9%) | 5 (12.8%) | 14 (36%) | 6 (15.4%) | NR |
| | [P → FEC] + H + lapatinib | 46 | 0 (0%) | 0 (0%) | 16 (34.8%) | 4 (8.7%) | 19 (41%) | 5 (10.8%) | NR |
| TBCRC 006,[34] 2013 | Lapatinib + H | 113 | NR | NR | 2 (3%) | 3 (5%) | NR | 1 (2%) | NR |
| TRYPHAENA,[35] 2013 | [FEC → T] + H + pertuzumab | 72 | 4 (5.6%) | 0 (0%) | 3 (4.2%) | 0 (0%) | 34 (47.2%) | NR | 0 (0%) |
| | FEC → [T + H + pertuzumab] | 75 | 4 (5.3%) | 2 (2.7%) | 4 (5.3%) | 0 (0%) | 32 (42.7%) | NR | 0 (0%) |
| | Carboplatin + H + pertuzumab | 76 | 3 (3.9%) | 0 (0%) | 9 (11.8%) | 3 (3.9%) | 35 (46.1%) | NR | 0 (0%) |

*Abbreviations:* CHF, congestive heart failure; H, trastuzumab; LVEF, left ventricle ejection fraction; n, number; NR, not reported; P, paclitaxel; T, docetaxel.
[a] Hepatic toxicity reported based on elevation of ALT.
[b] Death secondary to hypoglycemia in patient with diabetes.
[c] Death secondary to fulminant hepatitis.
[d] Death secondary to lung metastasis/progressive disease.

compared with other subtypes. Because the major impact on recurrence and survival in patients with HR-positive tumors is attributed to endocrine therapies, there has been an interest in using this approach in the neoadjuvant setting. Although neoadjuvant endocrine therapies have not been associated with significant pCR rates, a significant clinical impact has been demonstrated in down-staging tumors and increasing rates of breast-conservation therapy (BCT) in this population. Expression of the proliferation marker, Ki-67, after short-term exposure to endocrine therapy has also been shown to be a useful tool for assessing clinical benefit.[40]

Patients best suited for neoadjuvant endocrine therapy are postmenopausal women with large or locally advanced ER-positive tumors and elderly women who are unable to tolerate toxicities associated with chemotherapy or are not surgical candidates secondary to significant comorbidities. To date, a role for neoadjuvant endocrine therapy has not been established in the treatment of premenopausal women with breast cancer. Early trials with endocrine therapy primarily used tamoxifen, a competitive inhibitor of estradiol that binds to the estrogen receptor. Aromatase inhibitors, which inactivate the aromatase enzyme thereby inhibiting the conversion of adrenal androgens to estrogen, have also been investigated in the neoadjuvant setting.

Several trials have compared the efficacy of tamoxifen and aromatase inhibitors in the neoadjuvant setting (**Table 4**).[41–43] A multicenter study evaluating 324 postmenopausal women with ER and/or PR-positive breast cancer randomized participants to tamoxifen 20 mg daily or letrozole 2.5 mg daily for 4 months followed by surgery. No women were considered BCT candidates at baseline. The investigators found a superior overall response (both complete and partial response) in the letrozole group (55% vs 36%, $P<.001$). Also significant was an increased conversion to BCT in the letrozole group (45% vs 35%, $P = .022$).[41]

Similar findings were noted in the Immediate Preoperative Anastrozole, Tamoxifen, or Combined with Tamoxifen (IMPACT) trial, which examined the efficacy of anastrozole versus tamoxifen and a combination of anastrozole and tamoxifen in the neoadjuvant setting. Three hundred thirty postmenopausal women with ER-positive, operable, or locally advanced breast cancer were randomized to 1 of 3 treatment arms (tamoxifen 20 mg daily, anastrozole 1 mg daily, or both tamoxifen 20 mg and anastrozole 1 mg daily) and treated for 3 months before surgery. There was no difference in overall response rates (by clinical examination and ultrasound) or conversion

**Table 4**
Phase II and III trials evaluating neoadjuvant endocrine therapy with tamoxifen versus aromatase inhibitors in postmenopausal women with ER-positive breast cancer

| Study | Neoadjuvant Regimen | Duration | n | Overall Clinical Response (%) | Overall Response by US (%) | Feasibility of BCT (%) |
|---|---|---|---|---|---|---|
| Letrozole P024,[41] 2001 | Letrozole | 16 wk | 154 | 55 | 35 | 45 |
| | Tamoxifen | | 170 | 36 | 25 | 35 |
| | | | | $P<.001$ | $P = .042$ | $P = .022$ |
| IMPACT,[42] 2005 | Anastrozole + placebo | 12 wk | 113 | 37 | 24 | 46* |
| | Tamoxifen + placebo | | 108 | 36 | 20 | 22* |
| | Tamoxifen + anastrozole | | 109 | 39 | 28* | 26 |
| | | | | $P = NS$ | $P = NS$ | $*P = .03$ |
| PROACT,[43] 2006 | Anastrozole + placebo | 12 wk | 142 | 48.6 | 36.6 | 43 |
| | Tamoxifen + placebo | | 120 | 35.8 | 24.2 | 30.8 |
| | | | | $P = .04$ | $P = .03$ | $P = .04$ |

*Abbreviations:* n, number; US, ultrasound.

to breast-conservation rates among the groups. However, when tamoxifen was compared with anastrozole, there was an improvement in breast conservation eligibility from 22% to 46%, respectively (OR 2.94, CI 1.11–7.81, $P = .03$). No difference was observed when comparing tamoxifen with the combination of anastrozole and tamoxifen. The investigators also found an increased response to therapy with increased ER levels.[42]

These studies demonstrated the superiority of aromatase inhibitors over tamoxifen as primary endocrine therapy for postmenopausal women with ER-positive breast cancer in down-staging tumors and allowing for breast conservation.

The ACOSOG Z1031 phase II trial directly compared all 3 aromatase inhibitors (exemestane, letrozole, and anastrozole) in the neoadjuvant setting. This study analyzed 374 postmenopausal women with stage II or III ER-positive breast cancer randomized to receive one of the aromatase inhibitors for 16 weeks. The investigators found similar clinical response rates among the 3 agents with the highest response observed with letrozole treatment (74.8% compared with 62.9% with exemestane and 69.1% with anastrozole). There were similar rates of BCT in each group. The 3 treatments were also similar in biologic effect as evidenced by mean percentage decrease in Ki-67 from baseline to that measured after therapy.[44]

There are limited data comparing neoadjuvant endocrine therapy with neoadjuvant chemotherapy. Semiglazov and colleagues[45] reported results from a randomized phase II trial comparing 239 postmenopausal women with ER-positive stage IIA to stage IIIB breast cancer randomized to endocrine therapy (exemestane 25 mg daily or anastrozole 1 mg daily) or chemotherapy (4 cycles of doxorubicin 60 mg/m$^2$ and paclitaxel 200 mg/m$^2$) for 3 months before surgery. The investigators found no statistically significant difference in overall objective response between the neoadjuvant chemotherapy and neoadjuvant endocrine groups. The pCR rate was 6% and 3%, respectively. There was also no difference in breast conservation or local recurrence at 36 months. A higher rate of adverse events was noted in the neoadjuvant chemotherapy group. This study suggests that neoadjuvant aromatase inhibitor therapy is similar to neoadjuvant chemotherapy in postmenopausal women with ER-positive tumors in terms of clinical and pathologic response rates and confers less toxicity.

## Poor Response to Neoadjuvant Chemotherapy

Unfortunately, most patients do not achieve pCR with neoadjuvant therapy and studies have consistently demonstrated reduced survival outcomes in those patients with residual disease. Those with disease progression on therapy have an unfavorable prognosis and present a clinical challenge with limited therapeutic options to improve outcome. Early identification of poor response or disease progression is important to spare patients the toxicity of ineffective therapy. Once identified, this typically prompts surgical intervention or a change in chemotherapeutic regimen.

The benefit of switching to a non-cross-resistant regimen has not been demonstrated in clinical trials. The GeparTrio trial studied the impact of changing chemotherapeutic regimens in patients who showed poor response early in the neoadjuvant course. This phase III study enrolled 2072 women, 67.1% of which demonstrated response to therapy. The remaining 622 women whose tumors did not respond to 2 initial cycles of TAC (doxorubicin 50 mg/m$^2$, cyclophosphamide 500 mg/m$^2$, and docetaxel 75 mg/m$^2$) were randomized to 4 additional cycles of TAC or 4 cycles of NX (vinorelbine 25 mg/m$^2$ and capecitabine 1000 mg/m$^2$). Similar efficacy between the 2 treatment arms was observed with pCR rates of 5.3% in the TAC group and 6.0% in the NX group.[46] These patients, classified as nonresponders, show decreased responsiveness to neoadjuvant chemotherapy likely secondary to a lack of inherent chemosensitivity conferring a worse outcome. By comparison, responders achieved a pCR rate of 21.0% after 6 additional cycles of TAC and 23.5% after 8 additional cycles of TAC.[47]

There are currently efforts underway to determine genetic changes that may identify resistant tumors at diagnosis so that these patients might be targeted for novel agents. In addition, biomarkers are being investigated that can be used to direct therapies in patients with significant residual disease after neoadjuvant therapy.

## MONITORING OF RESPONSE TO NEOADJUVANT THERAPY

During the neoadjuvant treatment course, patients are monitored with physical examination to assess changes in the primary tumor and regional lymph nodes. There are currently no established recommendations for imaging surveillance during therapy.[11] The pretreatment placement of radiopaque clips in the primary tumor for patients planning to pursue breast conservation is important for tumor localization in the setting of a complete radiographic response and has been associated with improved local control.[48] On completion of neoadjuvant therapy, the residual tumor burden is typically estimated by clinical and radiographic methods to assess response.

The combination of mammography and ultrasound has been shown to correlate with pCR better than physical examination alone with a sensitivity and specificity in predicting pCR of 78.6% and 92.5%, respectively. However, pathologic residual may vary with underlying tumor biology and specifically may be underestimated with invasive lobular histology and overestimated with poorly differentiated tumors.[49]

Contrast-enhanced breast magnetic resonance imaging (MRI) has shown promise in predicting response after neoadjuvant chemotherapy. In the American College of Radiology Imaging Network (ACRIN) 6657/I-SPY (investigation of serial studies to predict your therapeutic response with imaging and molecular analysis) trial, investigators were able to demonstrate superiority of MRI as compared with physical examination in predicting response to therapy, with the greatest predictive ability in change in tumor volume occurring early in the treatment course.[50] MRI has also been studied with respect to its predictive power in detecting patients with pCR. Evaluation of radiographic complete response (rCR) by MRI and pCR in the Translational Breast Cancer Research Consortium (TBCRC) Trial 017 found an overall accuracy of 74% for MRI in predicting pCR in 746 patients after neoadjuvant chemotherapy for breast cancer. Triple-negative subtype, HER2-positive tumors, and lower T classification at presentation were found to be independently associated with increased rCR. Similarly, these variables were found to be associated with achieving pCR with the addition of African American race.[51]

The impact of breast imaging in measuring early response to neoadjuvant therapy and predicting pCR may be a powerful tool informing a change in systemic therapy for poor responders or possibly identifying a subset of patients in association with tumor subtype who will not ultimately require surgical intervention.

## IMPACT OF NEOADJUVANT CHEMOTHERAPY ON LOCAL-REGIONAL THERAPIES
### Breast Conserving Therapy

An established benefit of neoadjuvant systemic therapy is a decrease in tumor burden such that patients with large tumors become candidates for breast conservation. This benefit is contingent on the patient's desire for breast conservation, candidacy for adjuvant radiotherapy, and consideration of cosmesis. Factors associated with decreased feasibility for BCT include lobular histology, multicentricity, and diffuse calcifications on mammography.[52]

The primary concern in breast conservation after neoadjuvant chemotherapy is the risk of local-regional recurrence (LRR). The NSABP B-18 trial suggested a slight increase in IBTR in the neoadjuvant group; however, this difference was not statistically significant.[4] Increased local recurrence after neoadjuvant chemotherapy has been described however, primarily in the setting of radiotherapy alone without surgical intervention in patients with complete clinical response,[7] highlighting the distinction that complete clinical response does not confer pCR and the critical role for operative intervention in achieving local control. When breast-conserving surgery is followed with whole breast radiation therapy, several studies have shown no significant increase in local recurrence after neoadjuvant chemotherapy. Furthermore, prior treatment with neoadjuvant chemotherapy does not compromise salvage after LRR in these patients.[53]

To identify selection criteria for BCT better after neoadjuvant chemotherapy, 4 statistically significant predictors of IBTR and LRR were used to develop the MD Anderson prognostic index. These predictors were clinical N2 or N3 disease, residual pathologic tumor size greater than 2 cm, a multifocal pattern of residual disease, and lymphovascular space invasion. Each variable, if present, is assigned a score of 1 and calculated into an overall score. Stratification by low risk (score 0–1), intermediate risk (score 2), and high risk (score 3–4) resulted in a 5-year IBTR-free survival of 97%, 88%, and 82%, respectively ($P = .0001$) and 5-year LRR-free survival of 94%, 83%, and 58%, respectively ($P = .0001$).[54,55]

In addition, LRR after neoadjuvant chemotherapy is influenced by tumor subtype following BCT or mastectomy. Specifically, the basal subtype (ER/PR-negative/HER2-negative) seems to be associated with increased LRR as compared with luminal A (ER/PR-positive/HER2-negative), luminal B (ER/PR-positive/HER2-positive), and HER2-enriched (ER/PR-negative/HER2-positive) subtypes ($P = .03$).[56]

### Nodal Assessment After Chemotherapy

In addition to the primary tumor, neoadjuvant chemotherapy also has an impact on down-staging or eradicating disease in the axillary lymph nodes. Pathologically negative axillary nodes after neoadjuvant chemotherapy remain a strong predictor of prognosis.[5] In this setting, concerns initially arose over the identification and accuracy of sentinel lymph node (SLN) dissection in staging the axilla following neoadjuvant chemotherapy. Reports from many single-institution studies have shown the utility and safety of SLN dissection after neoadjuvant chemotherapy in clinically node-negative patients with comparable identification and false-negative rates to those undergoing surgery first, thus, decreasing the role for completion axillary lymph node dissection and sparing the potential associated morbidity in these patients.[57,58]

In patients with clinically node-positive disease at presentation, the role of SLN dissection is more controversial. These patients present a clinical challenge, because approximately 42% will achieve a pCR with pathologically negative disease at the time of axillary lymph node dissection.[59] The ACOSOG Z1071 trial specifically addressed this question, evaluating 756 women with clinically positive lymph nodes before neoadjuvant chemotherapy. All patients underwent SLN dissection and subsequent axillary lymph node dissection. Identification of at least one sentinel lymph node was achieved in 92.7% of patients with a false-negative rate of 12.6%. Although this false-negative rate was higher than the preset false-negative rate defined by the study, the investigators reported that improved accuracy was obtained with use of both blue dye and radioactive tracer and removal of 2 or more SLNs.[60] Furthermore, when the SLN correlated with the radiographically suspicious lymph node evidenced by inclusion of a clip marker placed before treatment, the false-negative rate was reduced to 7.4%.

### Reconstructive Surgery

Although neoadjuvant chemotherapy improves rates of breast conservation, many women still require mastectomy for optimal local-regional control. In this population, postmastectomy breast reconstruction is an important multidisciplinary consideration. This consideration is particularly true given that after neoadjuvant chemotherapy women are less likely to undergo immediate reconstruction.[61] One contributing concern limiting immediate reconstruction is the delay of adjuvant therapy; however, a single-institution retrospective review from the Institut of Gustave-Roussy found no difference in interval from surgery to adjuvant chemotherapy or radiotherapy based on receipt of neoadjuvant chemotherapy or type of reconstruction (implant versus autologous tissue flap). This study also found no difference in 5-year local relapse-free survival with respect to timing of reconstruction. The 5- and 10-year distant DFS rates were improved in the group with delayed reconstruction, which is postulated to be secondary to the exclusion of patients with metastatic disease from delayed reconstruction.[62]

An additional concern is the potential for increased postoperative complications with reconstruction following chemotherapy and radiation. A study from the Dana-Farber Cancer Institute found no association between neoadjuvant chemotherapy and increased postoperative complications after immediate or delayed reconstruction.[61] Similarly, an investigation using the American College of Surgeons National Surgical Quality Improvement Program (ACS-NSQIP) database found that neoadjuvant chemotherapy did not increase wound complications following breast conservation or mastectomy. They did observe a nonsignificant trend toward increased wound complications in patients who underwent neoadjuvant chemotherapy and immediate reconstruction after mastectomy.[63]

### Radiation Therapy

Although the role of whole breast radiation therapy in BCT is undisputed, postmastectomy radiation therapy (PMRT) after neoadjuvant chemotherapy is not as well studied. There seems to be a benefit of radiation therapy in patients with stage III disease treated with neoadjuvant chemotherapy followed by mastectomy in improving local-regional control even after achieving pCR. In one study, the 10-year LRR rate was 7.3% after PMRT compared with 33.3% in those who did not receive radiation ($P = .040$). In addition, there was a significant difference in OS, distant metastasis-free survival, and cause-specific survival in this population when treated with PMRT.[64]

The NSABP B-51/RTOG 1304 (NRG 9353) study is a phase III trial planned to investigate the role of radiation therapy after neoadjuvant chemotherapy in women with T1-3 N1 disease and pathologically negative axillary nodal disease after treatment. Patients will be randomized to regional lymph node radiation after whole breast radiation for BCT and radiation to the chest wall and regional lymphatics after mastectomy versus no additional radiation.

### SUMMARY

The use of neoadjuvant chemotherapy has evolved from its role in inoperable and locally advanced breast cancer to the treatment of selected patients with early-stage, operable disease. Survival is comparable with treatment with adjuvant systemic therapy; however, the neoadjuvant approach carries the benefit of decreasing tumor burden thus facilitating breast-conserving surgery, and tumor response to therapy holds individualized prognostic value by tumor subtype. Neoadjuvant endocrine therapy with aromatase inhibitors in postmenopausal women with HR-positive tumors has a role in tumor down-staging, particularly in patients who are not acceptable candidates for chemotherapy or surgery. Neoadjuvant chemotherapy also decreases the incidence of positive axillary lymph nodes resulting in a reduction in the number of patients requiring axillary lymph node dissection on completion of chemotherapy.

Future directions include further refinement of predictors of response to therapy, development of targeted treatments, and optimization of chemotherapeutic regimen by subtype. Clinical trials are now addressing the role of additional treatment in patients with residual disease and high-risk subtypes and determination of patients who may not require surgical management after neoadjuvant chemotherapy.

## REFERENCES

1. Mamounas EP, Fisher B. Preoperative (neoadjuvant) chemotherapy in patients wlth breast cancer. Semin Oncol 2001;28:389–99.
2. Fisher B, Gunduz N, Saffer EA. Influence of the interval between primary tumor removal and chemotherapy on kinetics and growth of metastases. Cancer Res 1983;43:1488–92.
3. Ragaz J, Baird R, Rebbeck P, et al. Neoadjuvant (preoperative) chemotherapy for breast cancer. Cancer 1985;56:719–24.
4. Fisher B, Bryant J, Wolmark N, et al. Effect of preoperative chemotherapy on the outcome of women with operable breast cancer. J Clin Oncol 1998;16:2672–85.
5. Rastogi P, Anderson SJ, Bear HD, et al. Preoperative chemotherapy: updates of National Surgical Adjuvant Breast and Bowel project protocols B-18 and B-27. J Clin Oncol 2008;26:778–85.
6. van der Hage JA, van de Velde CJ, Julien JP, et al. Preoperative chemotherapy in primary operable breast cancer: results from the European Organization for Research and Treatment of Cancer trial 10902. J Clin Oncol 2001;19: 4224–37.
7. Mauri D, Pavlidis N, Ioannidis JP. Neoadjuvant versus adjuvant systemic treatment in breast cancer: a meta-analysis. J Natl Cancer Inst 2005;97:188–94.
8. Mieog JS, van der Hage JA, van de Velde CJ. Neoadjuvant chemotherapy for operable breast cancer. Br J Surg 2007;94:1189–200.
9. Kuerer HM, Newman LA, Smith TL, et al. Clinical course of breast cancer patients with complete pathologic primary tumor and axillary lymph node response to doxorubicin-based neoadjuvant chemotherapy. J Clin Oncol 1999;17:460–9.
10. Mazouni C, Peintinger F, Wan-Kau S, et al. Residual ductal carcinoma in situ in patients with complete eradication of invasive breast cancer after neoadjuvant chemotherapy does not adversely affect patient outcome. J Clin Oncol 2007; 25:2650–5.
11. Kaufmann M, von Minckwitz G, Mamounas EP, et al. Recommendations from an international consensus conference on the current status and future of neoadjuvant systemic therapy in primary breast cancer. Ann Surg Oncol 2012;19: 1508–16.
12. Ju NR, Jeffe DB, Keune J, et al. Patient and tumor characteristics associated with breast cancer recurrence after complete pathological response to neoadjuvant chemotherapy. Breast Cancer Res Treat 2013;137:195–201.

13. Gonzalez-Angulo AM, McGuire SE, Buchholz TA, et al. Factors predictive of distant metastases in patients with breast cancer who have a pathologic complete response after neoadjuvant chemotherapy. J Clin Oncol 2005;23:7098–104.

14. Prowell TM, Pazdur R. Pathological complete response and accelerated drug approval in early breast cancer. N Engl J Med 2012;366:2438–41.

15. Symmans WF, Peintinger F, Hatzis C, et al. Measurement of residual breast cancer burden to predict survival after neoadjuvant chemotherapy. J Clin Oncol 2007;25:4414–22.

16. Jeruss JS, Mittendorf EA, Tucker SL, et al. Combined use of clinical and pathologic staging variables to define outcomes for breast cancer patients treated with neoadjuvant therapy. J Clin Oncol 2008;26:246–52.

17. Mittendorf EA, Jeruss JS, Tucker SL, et al. Validation of a novel staging system for disease-specific survival in patients with breast cancer treated with neoadjuvant chemotherapy. J Clin Oncol 2011;29:1956–62.

18. Perou CM, Sorlie T, Eisen MB, et al. Molecular portraits of human breast tumours. Nature 2000;406:747–52.

19. Houssami N, Macaskill P, von Minckwitz G, et al. Meta-analysis of the association of breast cancer subtype and pathologic complete response to neoadjuvant chemotherapy. Eur J Cancer 2012;48:3342–54.

20. Guarneri V, Broglio K, Kau SW, et al. Prognostic value of pathologic complete response after primary chemotherapy in relation to hormone receptor status and other factors. J Clin Oncol 2006;24:1037–44.

21. von Minckwitz G, Untch M, Blohmer JU, et al. Definition and impact of pathologic complete response on prognosis after neoadjuvant chemotherapy in various intrinsic breast cancer subtypes. J Clin Oncol 2012;30: 1796–804.

22. Chen S, Chen CM, Yu KD, et al. Prognostic value of a positive-to-negative change in hormone receptor status after neoadjuvant chemotherapy in patients with hormone receptor-positive breast cancer. Ann Surg Oncol 2012;19:3002–11.

23. Mittendorf EA, Wu Y, Scaltriti M, et al. Loss of HER2 amplification following trastuzumab-based neoadjuvant systemic therapy and survival outcomes. Clin Cancer Res 2009;15:7381–8.

24. Buzdar AU, Ibrahim NK, Francis D, et al. Significantly higher pathologic complete remission rate after neoadjuvant therapy with trastuzumab, paclitaxel, and epirubicin chemotherapy: results of a randomized trial in human epidermal growth factor receptor 2-positive operable breast cancer. J Clin Oncol 2005;23: 3676–85.

25. Buzdar AU, Valero V, Ibrahim NK, et al. Neoadjuvant therapy with paclitaxel followed by 5-fluorouracil, epirubicin, and cyclophosphamide chemotherapy and concurrent trastuzumab in human epidermal growth factor receptor 2-positive operable breast cancer: an update of the initial randomized study population and data of additional patients treated with the same regimen. Clin Cancer Res 2007;13:228–33.

26. Untch M, Rezai M, Loibl S, et al. Neoadjuvant treatment with trastuzumab in HER2-positive breast cancer: results from the GeparQuattro study. J Clin Oncol 2010;28:2024–31.

27. Gianni L, Eiermann W, Semiglazov V, et al. Neoadjuvant chemotherapy with trastuzumab followed by adjuvant trastuzumab versus neoadjuvant chemotherapy alone, in patients with HER2-positive locally advanced breast cancer (the NOAH trial): a randomised controlled superiority trial with a parallel HER2-negative cohort. Lancet 2010;375:377–84.

28. Untch M, Fasching PA, Konecny GE, et al. Pathologic complete response after neoadjuvant chemotherapy plus trastuzumab predicts favorable survival in human epidermal growth factor receptor 2-overexpressing breast cancer: results from the TECHNO trial of the AGO and GBG study groups. J Clin Oncol 2011;29:3351–7.

29. Semiglazov V, Eiermann W, Zambetti M, et al. Surgery following neoadjuvant therapy in patients with HER2-positive locally advanced or inflammatory breast cancer participating in the NeOAdjuvant Herceptin (NOAH) study. Eur J Surg Oncol 2011;37:856–63.

30. Untch M, Loibl S, Bischoff J, et al. Lapatinib versus trastuzumab in combination with neoadjuvant anthracycline-taxane-based chemotherapy (GeparQuinto, GBG 44): a randomised phase 3 trial. Lancet Oncol 2012;13:135–44.

31. Baselga J, Bradbury I, Eidtmann H, et al. Lapatinib with trastuzumab for HER2-positive early breast cancer (NeoALTTO): a randomised, open-label, multicentre, phase 3 trial. Lancet 2012;379:633–40.

32. Gianni L, Pienkowski T, Im YH, et al. Efficacy and safety of neoadjuvant pertuzumab and trastuzumab in women with locally advanced, inflammatory, or early HER2-positive breast cancer (NeoSphere): a randomised multicentre, open-label, phase 2 trial. Lancet Oncol 2012;13:25–32.

33. Guarneri V, Frassoldati A, Bottini A, et al. Preoperative chemotherapy plus trastuzumab, lapatinib, or both in human epidermal growth factor receptor 2-positive operable breast cancer: results of the randomized phase II CHER-LOB study. J Clin Oncol 2012;30:1989–95.

34. Rimawi MF, Mayer IA, Forero A, et al. Multicenter phase II study of neoadjuvant lapatinib and trastuzumab with hormonal therapy and without chemotherapy in patients with human epidermal growth factor receptor 2-overexpressing breast cancer: TBCRC 006. J Clin Oncol 2013;31:1726–31.

35. Schneeweiss A, Chia S, Hickish T, et al. Pertuzumab plus trastuzumab in combination with standard neoadjuvant anthracycline-containing and anthracycline-free chemotherapy regimens in patients with HER2-positive early breast cancer: a randomized phase II cardiac safety study (TRYPHAENA). Ann Oncol 2013;24:2278–84.

36. Liedtke C, Mazouni C, Hess KR, et al. Response to neoadjuvant therapy and long-term survival in patients with triple-negative breast cancer. J Clin Oncol 2008;26:1275–81.

37. Carey LA, Dees EC, Sawyer L, et al. The triple negative paradox: primary tumor chemosensitivity of breast cancer subtypes. Clin Cancer Res 2007;13:2329–34.

38. Nahleh Z. Neoadjuvant chemotherapy for "triple negative" breast cancer: a review of current practice and future outlook. Med Oncol 2010;27:531–9.

39. Chang HR, Glaspy J, Allison MA, et al. Differential response of triple-negative breast cancer to a docetaxel and carboplatin-based neoadjuvant treatment. Cancer 2010;116:4227–37.

40. Dowsett M, Smith IE, Ebbs SR, et al. Prognostic value of Ki67 expression after short-term presurgical endocrine therapy for primary breast cancer. J Natl Cancer Inst 2007;99:167–70.

41. Eiermann W, Paepke S, Appfelstaedt J, et al. Preoperative treatment of postmenopausal breast cancer patients with letrozole: a randomized double-blind multicenter study. Ann Oncol 2001;12:1527–32.

42. Smith IE, Dowsett M, Ebbs SR, et al. Neoadjuvant treatment of postmenopausal breast cancer with anastrozole, tamoxifen, or both in combination: the

Immediate Preoperative Anastrozole, Tamoxifen, or Combined with Tamoxifen (IMPACT) multicenter double-blind randomized trial. J Clin Oncol 2005;23: 5108–16.

43. Cataliotti L, Buzdar AU, Noguchi S, et al. Comparison of anastrozole versus tamoxifen as preoperative therapy in postmenopausal women with hormone receptor-positive breast cancer: the Pre-Operative "Arimidex" Compared to Tamoxifen (PROACT) trial. Cancer 2006;106:2095–103.

44. Ellis MJ, Suman VJ, Hoog J, et al. Randomized phase II neoadjuvant comparison between letrozole, anastrozole, and exemestane for postmenopausal women with estrogen receptor-rich stage 2 to 3 breast cancer: clinical and biomarker outcomes and predictive value of the baseline PAM50-based intrinsic subtype–ACOSOG Z1031. J Clin Oncol 2011;29:2342–9.

45. Semiglazov VF, Semiglazov VV, Dashyan GA, et al. Phase 2 randomized trial of primary endocrine therapy versus chemotherapy in postmenopausal patients with estrogen receptor-positive breast cancer. Cancer 2007;110:244–54.

46. von Minckwitz G, Kummel S, Vogel P, et al. Neoadjuvant vinorelbine-capecitabine versus docetaxel-doxorubicin-cyclophosphamide in early nonresponsive breast cancer: phase III randomized GeparTrio trial. J Natl Cancer Inst 2008;100: 542–51.

47. von Minckwitz G, Kummel S, Vogel P, et al. Intensified neoadjuvant chemotherapy in early-responding breast cancer: phase III randomized GeparTrio study. J Natl Cancer Inst 2008;100:552–62.

48. Oh JL, Nguyen G, Whitman GJ, et al. Placement of radiopaque clips for tumor localization in patients undergoing neoadjuvant chemotherapy and breast conservation therapy. Cancer 2007;110:2420–7.

49. Peintinger F, Kuerer HM, Anderson K, et al. Accuracy of the combination of mammography and sonography in predicting tumor response in breast cancer patients after neoadjuvant chemotherapy. Ann Surg Oncol 2006;13:1443–9.

50. Hylton NM, Blume JD, Bernreuter WK, et al. Locally advanced breast cancer: MR imaging for prediction of response to neoadjuvant chemotherapy–results from ACRIN 6657/I-SPY TRIAL. Radiology 2012;263:663–72.

51. De Los Santos JF, Cantor A, Amos KD, et al. Magnetic resonance imaging as a predictor of pathologic response in patients treated with neoadjuvant systemic treatment for operable breast cancer. Translational Breast Cancer Research Consortium trial 017. Cancer 2013;119:1776–83.

52. Newman LA, Buzdar AU, Singletary SE, et al. A prospective trial of preoperative chemotherapy in resectable breast cancer: predictors of breast-conservation therapy feasibility. Ann Surg Oncol 2002;9:228–34.

53. Weksberg DC, Allen PK, Hoffman KE, et al. Outcomes and predictive factors for salvage therapy after local-regional recurrence following neoadjuvant chemotherapy and breast conserving therapy. Ann Surg Oncol 2013;20:3430–7.

54. Chen AM, Meric-Bernstam F, Hunt KK, et al. Breast conservation after neoadjuvant chemotherapy. Cancer 2005;103:689–95.

55. Akay CL, Meric-Bernstam F, Hunt KK, et al. Evaluation of the MD Anderson prognostic index for local-regional recurrence after breast conserving therapy in patients receiving neoadjuvant chemotherapy. Ann Surg Oncol 2012;19: 901–7.

56. Meyers MO, Klauber-Demore N, Ollila DW, et al. Impact of breast cancer molecular subtypes on locoregional recurrence in patients treated with neoadjuvant chemotherapy for locally advanced breast cancer. Ann Surg Oncol 2011;18: 2851–7.

57. Hunt KK, Yi M, Mittendorf EA, et al. Sentinel lymph node surgery after neoadjuvant chemotherapy is accurate and reduces the need for axillary dissection in breast cancer patients. Ann Surg 2009;250:558–66.

58. Tan VK, Goh BK, Fook-Chong S, et al. The feasibility and accuracy of sentinel lymph node biopsy in clinically node-negative patients after neoadjuvant chemotherapy for breast cancer–a systematic review and meta-analysis. J Surg Oncol 2011;104:97–103.

59. Alvarado R, Yi M, Le-Petross H, et al. The role for sentinel lymph node dissection after neoadjuvant chemotherapy in patients who present with node-positive breast cancer. Ann Surg Oncol 2012;19:3177–84.

60. Boughey JC, Suman VJ, Mittendorf EA, et al. Sentinel lymph node surgery after neoadjuvant chemotherapy in patients with node-positive breast cancer: the ACOSOG Z1071 (alliance) clinical trial. JAMA 2013;310:1455–61.

61. Hu YY, Weeks CM, In H, et al. Impact of neoadjuvant chemotherapy on breast reconstruction. Cancer 2011;117:2833–41.

62. Gouy S, Rouzier R, Missana MC, et al. Immediate reconstruction after neoadjuvant chemotherapy: effect on adjuvant treatment starting and survival. Ann Surg Oncol 2005;12:161–6.

63. Decker MR, Greenblatt DY, Havlena J, et al. Impact of neoadjuvant chemotherapy on wound complications after breast surgery. Surgery 2012;152:382–8.

64. McGuire SE, Gonzalez-Angulo AM, Huang EH, et al. Postmastectomy radiation improves the outcome of patients with locally advanced breast cancer who achieve a pathologic complete response to neoadjuvant chemotherapy. Int J Radiat Oncol Biol Phys 2007;68:1004–9.

# Advances in Breast Reconstruction of Mastectomy and Lumpectomy Defects

Tiffany Nicole S. Ballard, MD, Adeyiza O. Momoh, MD*

## KEYWORDS

- Breast reconstruction • Tissue expander • Implant • Autologous flap
- Tissue transfer • Acellular dermal matrix • Autologous fat grafting • Radiation

## KEY POINTS

- Breast reconstruction efforts complement oncologic interventions in breast cancer patients, with the ultimate goal of restoration of breast form and function.
- Use of acellular dermal matrices in tissue expander/implant–based breast reconstruction represents one of the most significant advances in implant reconstruction in the past decade.
- Free flap and perforator flap options expand patients' choices for reconstruction and result in breasts that are natural in both appearance and feel. These techniques are also better suited than implants for reconstruction of obese patients.
- Partial breast reconstruction options should be considered in all patients who opt for breast conservation therapy.
- Improvements in fat grafting techniques have the potential to improve on all existing forms of breast reconstruction and revolutionize the approach to breast reconstruction as a whole.

 Videos of intraoperative perfusion mapping of mastectomy flaps and an abdominal flap after an intravenous injection of indocyanine green dye accompany this article at http://www.surgonc.theclinics.com/

## INTRODUCTION

Breast reconstruction is achieved through various reconstructive techniques that attempt to restore the breast to near-normal shape, appearance, and size after oncologic surgical resection in the form of lumpectomy or mastectomy. Several factors, including earlier detection of breast cancer and advances in radiation therapy and

The authors have nothing to disclose.

Section of Plastic Surgery, Department of General Surgery, University of Michigan Health System, 1500 East Medical Center Drive, 2130 Taubman Center, SPC 5340, Ann Arbor, MI 48109-5340, USA

* Corresponding author.

E-mail address: amomoh@umich.edu

Surg Oncol Clin N Am 23 (2014) 525–548

http://dx.doi.org/10.1016/j.soc.2014.03.012

1055-3207/14/$ – see front matter © 2014 Elsevier Inc. All rights reserved.

surgonc.theclinics.com

systemic treatments, have contributed to increased use of breast preservation and skin-sparing surgical techniques in the management of breast cancer patients. As a complement to these changes in management, breast reconstruction has evolved from procedures aimed at simply creating a breast with a satisfactory appearance when clothed to a series of procedures aimed at creating a breast that meets high aesthetic standards when bare. The psychological, social, emotional, and functional benefits of breast reconstruction have been well documented over the past 30 years. Previous studies have demonstrated the positive effects of postmastectomy reconstruction on psychological health, self-esteem, sexuality, and body image.[1] These benefits will likely be enhanced as implant technology and surgical techniques evolve, with an improvement in the quality of the reconstructed breast. Today the surgical repertoire for breast reconstruction includes several autologous tissue flaps and prosthetic techniques using tissue expanders and implants. The most recent advances in breast reconstruction are presented.

## RECONSTRUCTION OF MASTECTOMY DEFECTS

Factors ranging from oncologic treatment plans to patient-specific factors are taken into consideration when planning a reconstructive strategy. A team-based approach with open communication between medical oncologists, radiation oncologists, oncologic surgeons, and reconstructive surgeons helps simplify planning. Key decisions that need to be made with a perspective of the treatment plan include the type and timing of reconstruction.

### Decisions on Type of Reconstruction

Several options are available to women who choose breast reconstruction after mastectomy. The 2 broad categories available to patients include techniques using prosthetic implants and those involving autologous tissue flaps.

Some women have an inherent preference with regards to the technique, whereas others' medical history or lifestyle may steer them toward a particular option. Although it is important that patients have a choice in the type of reconstruction performed, not all reconstructive options are available to every patient. **Fig. 1** provides an algorithm highlighting some factors that affect the choice of reconstructive technique offered. It is the responsibility of the reconstructive surgeon to provide information to the patient about all potential options and provide guidance that allows her to make a decision that results in the safest and most aesthetically pleasing outcome.

### Decisions on Timing of Reconstruction

The decision on immediate or delayed reconstruction in general is influenced by cancer staging, with delayed reconstruction favored in advanced-stage cancers that require postmastectomy radiation therapy (PMRT) or close surveillance. Most patients tend to prefer immediate reconstruction, which takes advantage of skin preservation while minimizing the length of time spent without a breast. Patients may also opt to wait on reconstruction if the combined process of oncologic treatment and reconstruction seems overwhelming. The need for PMRT tends to be the predominant reason influencing the choice for delayed reconstruction. Delayed reconstruction, for patients requiring radiation therapy, is typically advocated for several reasons, including the avoidance of untoward effects of radiation on the results of an immediate reconstruction and the potential for delaying oncologic treatment as a result of complications from reconstruction. In an attempt to take advantage of the skin preserved in a skin-sparing mastectomy in patients who require radiation, several plastic

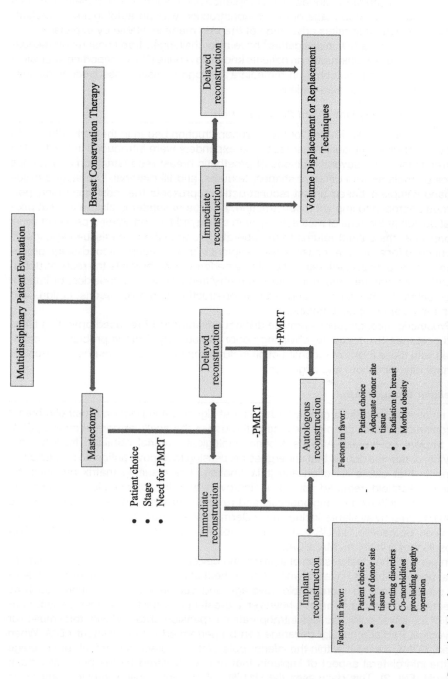

**Fig. 1.** Basic algorithm for decisions on reconstructive options following mastectomy or breast conservation therapy.

surgeons[2,3] have suggested the immediate placement of tissue expanders. The skin is initially expanded and then, prior to radiation therapy, the expander is deflated temporarily if needed and re-expanded after completion of radiation. These patients can then proceed to the second stage of their reconstruction with an autologous or implant-based technique that takes advantage of the skin made available by expansion.

In recent years, a few investigators[4] have also challenged traditional recommendations for delayed reconstruction in patients known to require PMRT, reporting equivalent clinical and aesthetic outcomes in immediate autologous tissue–based reconstructions in radiated and nonradiated patients.

### Tissue Expander/Implant–Based Reconstruction

The use of prosthetic devices for breast reconstruction began in the early 1960s with silicone gel–filled implants, whereas tissue expanders were introduced in the 1970s.[5] Currently there are several methods of prosthetic breast reconstruction and various types of implants with different shapes, textures, and fill material. The staged tissue expander/implant–based breast reconstruction represents the most commonly performed approach to implant reconstruction. A tissue expander is placed in a subpectoral pocket at the time of mastectomy or in a delayed fashion. After a period of serial expansions, the patient returns to the operating room, where the tissue expander is exchanged for a silicone- or saline-filled implant in an outpatient second-stage procedure. Subsequent procedures that could be performed to complete the reconstruction include contralateral procedures for symmetry (reductions, mastopexies, or implant augmentations in cases of unilateral reconstructions), nipple reconstruction, and nipple-areolar complex tattooing.

Prosthetic reconstructions provide distinct advantages of reduced operating times and postoperative recovery, obviating donor site surgery. Unique problems encountered with these forms of reconstruction include implant infection, exposure, capsular contracture, deflation, and migration.

### Acellular Dermal Matrix

An innovation that has arguably had the most significant impact on prosthetic breast reconstruction over the past decade is the use of the acellular dermal matrix (ADM) for implant coverage.[6] ADM is a biotechnological material obtained from human, bovine, or porcine dermis that undergoes processing to remove antigenic cellular components that cause rejection and inflammation. The resulting matrix provides the biologic scaffold required for tissue ingrowth and the biochemical components required for initiation of angiogenesis and revascularization. There are several types of ADM currently available, including AlloDerm (LifeCell, Branchburg, NJ, USA), FlexHD (Ethicon, Somerville, NJ, USA), Allomax (Davol, Warwick, RI, USA), and SurgiMend (TEI Biosciences, Waltham, MA, USA).

In general, the ideal position of a prosthetic device after mastectomy is in a subpectoral pocket. Studies have shown that placement of the implant in a purely submuscular position leads to more stable coverage and decreased complications, such as infection and seroma.[7] There is, however, a greater potential for malposition, less control of the lower pole, and less intraoperative expansion obtained with total muscular coverage. Partial muscular coverage can be performed with or without ADM. When used, ADMs are inset within the inferior pole of the mastectomy defect for coverage of the inferolateral aspect of implants that are not covered by the pectoralis major muscle (**Fig. 2**). This decreases the visibility of implant rippling, provides improved control of the inframammary fold, and allows for increased intraoperative fill (**Fig. 3**). During the expansion process, use of an ADM results in easier lower pole expansion,

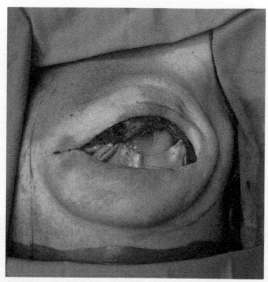

**Fig. 2.** Coverage of the inferior pole of a tissue expander with ADM during an immediate reconstruction after mastectomy. The superior pole of the tissue expander is covered with the pectoralis major muscle.

with increased lower pole projection and the potential for an improved final aesthetic result (**Fig. 4**).

ADMs can be used in most patients who are candidates for prosthetic reconstruction. It is less effective or relatively contraindicated in patients in whom prosthetic reconstruction may need to be delayed or avoided, including those who are morbidly obese, who are smokers, who have a history of radiation, or whose mastectomy skin flaps have questionable viability.

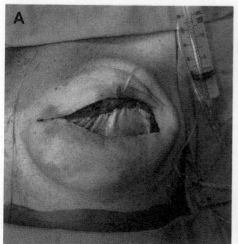
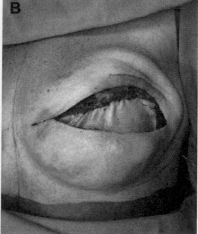

**Fig. 3.** Intraoperative filling of a tissue expander with saline after partial muscle coverage of the expander. The pectoralis major muscle is sutured to ADM (*A*). Final appearance following initial filling (*B*).

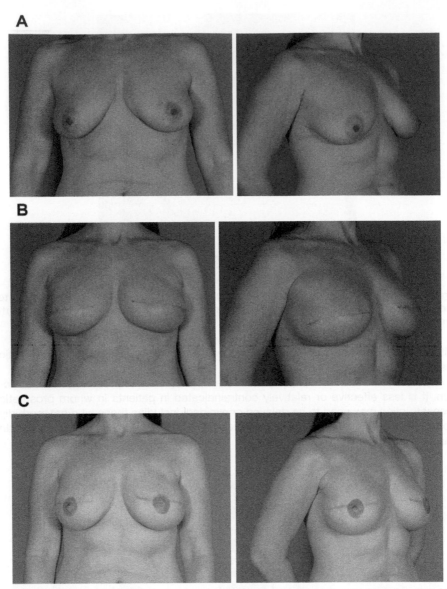

**Fig. 4.** A patient with right breast cancer prior to bilateral mastectomies (*A, left and right*), after completion of tissue expansion with ADM in place (*B, left and right*), and after exchange for implants, bilateral nipple reconstructions and nipple areola complex tattooing (*C, left and right*).

### Single-Stage Implant Breast Reconstruction

The improvement in the ability to achieve greater intraoperative fill volumes with ADMs has enabled the development of single-stage implant techniques. Fully filled saline implants or silicone implants are placed at the time of a skin- or nipple-sparing mastectomy (**Fig. 5**). This approach overcomes many of the disadvantages of tissue expander placement, including the need for multiple clinic

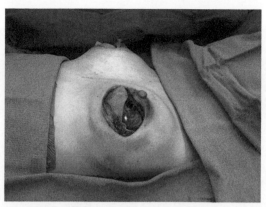

**Fig. 5.** Intraoperative placement of a silicone gel breast implants immediately after bilateral nipple-sparing mastectomies.

visits for expansions and a subsequent operation to exchange the expander for an implant. Caution must be used, however, when counseling patients to advise them that they may require an additional operation for revisions to achieve symmetry.

Ideal candidates for single-stage implant reconstruction include those with small to medium-sized breasts with mild to moderate ptosis who are undergoing skin- or nipple-sparing mastectomies (**Fig. 6**). Patients also have to be willing to be the same size or slightly smaller after reconstruction because the skin cannot be stretched at the time of the mastectomy without compromising flap perfusion. A moderate degree of preoperative ptosis is beneficial because expansions are not performed to increase the available skin envelope. Mastectomy flap viability is critical because the flaps must tolerate the additional weight and tension of an implant as opposed to a gradual increase in volume with a tissue expander.

The risks associated with single-stage implant reconstruction include infection, seroma, hematoma, skin necrosis, and capsular contracture. There is also a steep learning curve for surgeons. In a recent series of 439 patients undergoing this technique, the rate of reoperation was 11%, including a 3% rate of revision surgeries to deal with implant size changes, scar revisions, and inframammary fold revisions.[8] Overall, clinical experience over the past 10 years has demonstrated the effectiveness, safety, and long-term aesthetic benefits of this approach.

### Innovation in Prosthetic Devices

Since the development of breast implants as a medical technology device in the 1960s, significant improvements in safety and composition have been made. The first saline implants had shells created through high-temperature vulcanization and were prone to shell breakage, leakage, and spontaneous deflation. Contemporary saline implants are now made with stronger shells of a silicone elastomer manufactured with thicker, room-temperature vulcanized shells.

Five generations of silicone gel implants have been introduced since their development by American plastic surgeons, Thomas Cronin and Frank Gerow, and the Dow Corning Corporation in the 1960s (**Table 1**).[9] Key changes in implants over the years have centered on providing softer, more natural-appearing implants with a decreased risk of leakage of silicone gel.

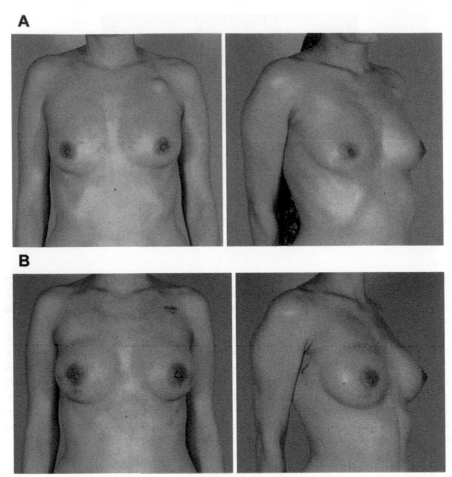

**Fig. 6.** Preoperative (*A, left and right*) and early postoperative results at 4 weeks (*B, left and right*) of a bilateral single-stage breast reconstruction with immediate placement of silicone implants after nipple-sparing mastectomies.

| Table 1 | | |
|---|---|---|
| **Generations of silicone gel breast implants** | | |
| **Generation** | **Time Period** | **Silicone Implant Characteristics** |
| First | 1960s | Thick shell<br>Thick, viscous gel<br>Dacron patch |
| Second | 1970s | Thin shell<br>Less viscous gel<br>No patch |
| Third | 1980s–1992 | Thick, silica-reinforced barrier coat shells |
| Fourth | 1992–present | Stricter manufacturing standards<br>Refined version of 3rd-generation implants |
| Fifth | 1993–present | Cohesive silicone gel–filled devices<br>Form stable devices, with textured outer shell |

On June 14, 2013, the Food and Drug Administration (FDA) approved the MemoryShape breast implant (Mentor Worldwide, Santa Barbara, CA, USA), making it 1 of 3 approved cohesive gel implants in the United States. The implant was known as the "gummy bear" implant to the general public as it was going through the testing and approval process. Unlike past round gel implants, the MemoryShape implant has a teardrop shape intended to provide a natural-shaped breast with preferential fullness of the lower pole (**Fig. 7**). The gel is highly cohesive secondary to increased cross-linking, leading to enhanced firmness and shape retention. Other similar implants with slight variations are made by Sientra and Allergan for use in the United States.

Early experience with these implants suggests that they provide a few advantages relative to round gel implants, including a more natural shape and less rippling. These implants, however, are firmer to the touch, require larger incisions for insertion, and occasionally rotate within the breast pocket resulting in an abnormal contour of the reconstructed breast. Implant malrotation may occur despite external shell texturing and precise pocket creation, 2 measures intended to limit implant movement.

### Breast Implants and Anaplastic Large Cell Lymphoma

The relationship between implants and breast surgery has been somewhat tumultuous with the moratorium on silicone gel implants in the 1990s and more recently a possible association with a type of lymphoma. In January 2011, the FDA released a medical device safety communication regarding the possible association between breast implants and the development of anaplastic large cell lymphoma (ALCL), a rare type of non-Hodgkin lymphoma. The FDA reported that women with breast implants may have a very low but increased risk of developing ALCL adjacent to the breast implant compared with women without implants. According to the Surveillance, Epidemiology, and End Results Program of the National Cancer Institute, an estimated 1 in 500,000 women per year in the United States is diagnosed with ALCL, with only 3 in 100 million women diagnosed with the disease in the breast. Globally, there have been approximately 60 cases of ALCL identified in women with breast implants, whereas 5 to 10 million women have received implants worldwide. Currently, additional data is required to fully evaluate the possible relationship between ALCL and breast implants. All cases of ALCL reported in women with breast implants are now tracked in the FDA MedWatch Program.

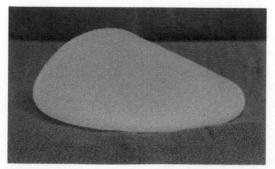

**Fig. 7.** The Memory-Shape breast implant (Mentor Worldwide, Santa Barbara, CA, USA) is a teardrop-shaped implant that maintains its contour as a result of the cohesive gel.

## Autologous Breast Reconstruction

Since Tansini first described the use of a pedicled latissimus dorsi flap in 1906 to reconstruct an anterior chest wall defect, the use of autologous flaps for breast reconstruction has evolved significantly.[10] Today's arsenal of possible autologous flaps includes pedicled flaps, such as the latissimus dorsi and transverse rectus abdominis myocutaneous (TRAM) flaps, and free flaps, which can be harvested from the abdomen, buttocks, or thighs (**Box 1**). The trend toward perforator flaps over the past 20 years has also expanded the options for patients desiring reconstruction using their own tissue.

Like expander/implant-based reconstruction, autologous reconstruction can be performed in an immediate fashion at the time of mastectomy or in delayed fashion months to years after a mastectomy.

Autologous reconstruction creates a more natural-appearing reconstructed breast by "replacing like with like." The results are durable and some of the complications encountered with implants, including infection, implant exposure, and implant failure, are avoided. The aesthetic benefits of autologous reconstruction in providing symmetry are especially evident in women undergoing unilateral mastectomies with reconstruction.

## Pedicled Flaps

The primary pedicled flaps used in breast reconstruction are the latissimus dorsi and the TRAM flaps. Both flaps are well established and take advantage of the regional vascular anatomy of the trunk, which makes it possible to transfer skin, adipose tissue, and muscles without completely disrupting their blood supply.

---

**Box 1**
**Autologous flaps for breast reconstruction**

Abdomen

  Pedicled TRAM

  Free TRAM

  Muscle-sparing free TRAM

  DIEP

  SIEA

Back

  Pedicled latissimus dorsi

  TDAP

Buttocks

  SGAP

  IGAP

  Septocutaneous gluteal artery perforator

Thigh

  TUG

  Anterolateral thigh

  Profunda artery perforator

The pedicled latissimus dorsi flap gained popularity in the 1970s and remains a workhorse flap in breast reconstruction due to its reliability, size, and location. It can be harvested as a muscle alone or as a myocutaneous flap with a skin paddle. Today the latissimus dorsi myocutaneous flap is typically used in combination with an implant to reconstruct the radiated breast. Reconstruction of the radiated breast with implants alone has been plagued with significantly higher rates of complications relative to similar reconstructions in nonradiated patients. Use of the lastissimus dorsi decreases postoperative morbidity in radiated patients.[11]

The pedicled TRAM flap, introduced by Hartrampf in 1982,[12] takes advantage of the superiorly based epigastric perfusion of the lower abdominal soft tissue adiposity that is present in many patients. Use of the pedicled TRAM flap requires the harvest of at least one rectus muscle (in unilateral reconstructions) and some overlying fascia, with the possibility of harvesting both rectus muscles with segments of fascia in bilateral breast reconstructions. Although effective for breast reconstruction, the pedicled TRAM flap, especially in bilateral reconstructions, places patients at risk for donor site complications related to abdominal wall integrity and function.[13–16] To avoid some of these potential donor site complications and with the growth of free tissue transfer techniques, there has been an evolution of procedures for harvest of similar volumes of skin and adipose tissue, without use of muscle and fascia.

### Abdominal-Based Perforator Flaps

The deep inferior epigastric perforator (DIEP) flap is an abdominal-based perforator flap that has increased in popularity over the past decade. Described by Koshima and Soeda[16] and first applied to reconstruction of the postmastectomy breast in 1994 by Allen and Treece,[17] the flap uses lower abdominal skin and adipose tissue while sparing the rectus abdominis muscle and fascia. Most patients who in the past were considered candidates for the TRAM flap are good candidates for DIEP flap breast reconstruction. Intramuscular perforators that run from the inferior epigastric vessels are identified, a few are selected based on their ability to adequately perfuse the flap, and these perforators are harvested along with the flap without the surrounding muscle and fascia (**Fig. 8**). Using microsurgical techniques, the flap is then transferred to the mastectomy defect where recipient vessels, typically the internal mammary or thoracodorsal vessels, are anastomosed to the flap vessels. Patients receive the dual benefit of restoration of the breast form and an improvement in contour of their lower abdomen (**Fig. 9**).

In comparison with implant-based reconstruction, studies have demonstrated superior symmetry, a better overall appearance, natural contour, and higher satisfaction with autologous reconstruction. Some controversy, however, exists as to the benefits of abdominal perforator flap reconstruction relative to TRAM flap reconstruction. Because the aesthetic results of all abdominal-based flaps are essentially similar, the differences between these procedures can be subtle and are often centered on complication profiles, abdominal wall function, and patients' experiences with the procedures. Several studies suggest an increase in abdominal wall functional morbidity with techniques that harvest greater amounts of muscle.[14,15,18,19] The pedicled TRAM is also associated with higher rates of abdominal wall hernias and bulges,[13,20,21] likely secondary to the magnitude of mechanical damage that results from muscle and fascia harvest. This mechanical damage to the muscle and fascia is of greater significance in bilateral flap harvests.

Aesthetic satisfaction for both pedicled TRAM flap patients and DIEP flap patients is similar.[13] Patients who have undergone DIEP flap reconstruction report higher general

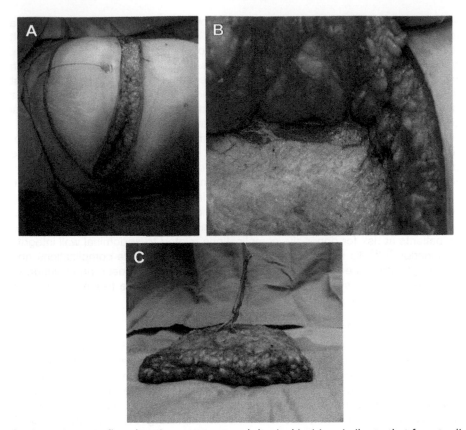

**Fig. 8.** During DIEP flap elevation a transverse abdominal incision similar to that for a traditional abdominoplasty is made (*A*). Selected intramuscular perforators from the inferior epigastric vessels to be included in the flap are exposed (*B*). The flap is harvested without the surrounding muscle (*C*).

satisfaction with reconstruction,[13] likely due to a shortened hospital stay and recovery, which are the secondary benefits of less muscle destruction.

Complications unique to abdominal perforator flap reconstruction stem from flap perfusion being dependent on a few selected perforators. As a result, fat necrosis occurs in approximately 14%[22] of flap reconstructions, with necrosis occurring in segments of adipose tissue with poor perfusion. Perforator selection is typically performed based on intraoperative clinical assessment and can be complemented with preoperative CT angiographic studies or intraoperative perfusion studies. The technical challenges involved in microsurgical breast reconstruction lend it to additional unique complications of microvascular thrombosis with the potential for flap loss. With greater experience this complication seldom occurs and is reported at a rate of less than 2% in high-volume centers.[13]

Representing the best possible abdominal flap option is the superficial inferior epigastric artery (SIEA) flap, which technically is not a perforator flap. The superficial inferior epigastric vessels are a branch of the femoral vessels and run superficial to the abdominal wall fascia and muscles. Harvest of this flap avoids incisions in the abdominal wall fascia and dissection through the rectus muscle that are required with harvest of a DIEP flap (**Fig. 10**). Abdominal wall morbidity is consequently avoided

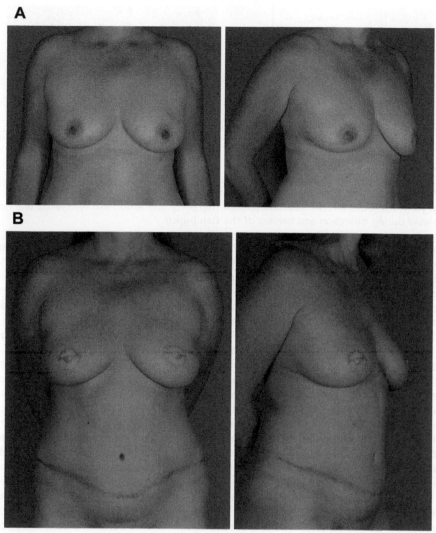

**Fig. 9.** A patient with left breast cancer prior to bilateral skin-sparing mastectomies (*A, left and right*) and after bilateral DIEP flap breast reconstruction (*B, left and right*). The patient also underwent a minor post-operative revision procedure and bilateral nipple reconstruction.

with this technique. The flap is transferred to the breast and microsurgical techniques similar to other free flaps are used. Unfortunately, not all patients have adequate-sized vessels or both an artery and vein present (sometimes due to previous incisions, such as the Pfannenstiel incision). Some investigators have reported that adequate-sized vessels are present in approximately 30% of potential candidates.[23] Flap perfusion tends to be unreliable across the midline with this vascular pedicle, making it better suited for hemiabdominal flaps, which limits the possible size of the reconstructed breast.

### Reconstruction of the Obese Patient

As the rates of obesity in America continue to rise, plastic surgeons will increasingly encounter obese patients who desire postmastectomy reconstruction. Studies

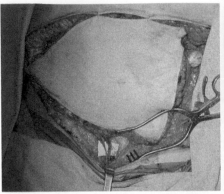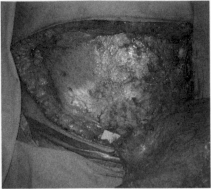

**Fig. 10.** A harvested left hemiabdominal SIEA flap (*left*). The abdominal wall fascia was not violated during dissection and harvest of the flap (*right*).

suggest that the rates of complications in both prosthetic and autologous reconstruction are higher in obese patients. An analysis of the American College of Surgeons National Surgery Quality Improvement Program database of more than 15,000 breast reconstructions revealed that obese patients have higher rates of comorbidities, require longer operative times, and have increased anesthetic risk. Obesity was also found to be a predictor for wound complications.[24]

In the past, a body mass index over 30 was considered a relative contraindication to abdominal-based autologous reconstruction. Kroll and Netscher[25] reported a weight-dependent increase in complication rates after pedicled TRAMs in a series of 82 patients. Increased use of free flaps for reconstruction has prompted a reassessment of this position on abdominal-based reconstruction in obese patients. Garvey and colleagues[26] studied outcomes of abdominal-based flap and implant reconstruction in obese patients and found that obese patients have higher reconstruction failure rates with implants for immediate reconstruction. Support for autologous microsurgical reconstruction in this patient population was again provided in a recent study by Momeni and colleagues,[27] which showed that the most common complications encountered in obese patients are minor and can be managed on an outpatient basis.

Currently, the largest gel implant available for reconstruction has an 800 mL volume. This volume is often insufficient to fill out the breast envelope of many obese patients. As the rates of obesity rise, the limits of autologous reconstruction will continue to be pushed to provide satisfactory reconstructive results and meet the needs of this patient population.

### Alternative Flaps

In select patients who are not good candidates for implant reconstruction or abdominal-based flap reconstruction, other forms of autologous flap reconstruction are available. The transverse upper gracilis (TUG) flap or transverse myocutaneous gracilis flap is a medial thigh flap that has increased in popularity as a second-line autologous flap option. Based on the medial circumflex branch of the profunda femoris artery, skin from the upper medial thigh is harvested along with the gracilis muscle and transferred to the chest as a free flap (**Fig. 11**). Given the limited volume of tissue in the medial thigh, it is best suited for reconstructing small to moderate-sized breasts (**Fig. 12**).

Also used as a second- or third-line flap option are gluteal perforator flaps. The superior gluteal artery perforator (SGAP) and inferior gluteal artery perforator (IGAP) flap tend to be options in patients with a gynecoid body habitus associated with ample

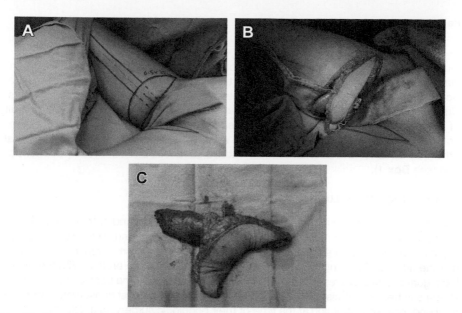

**Fig. 11.** Preoperative marking for a TUG flap along the medial right thigh (*A*), intraoperative elevation of the flap (*B*), and the flap following harvest (*C*).

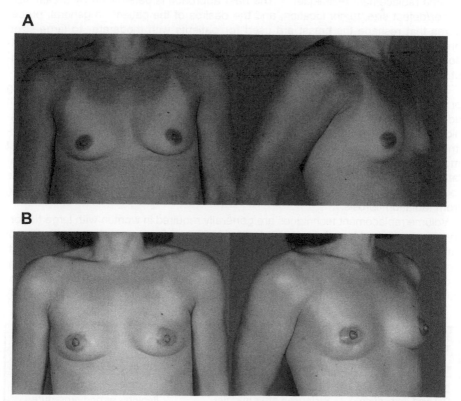

**Fig. 12.** A patient with left breast cancer prior to bilateral skin-sparing mastectomies (*A, left and right*) and a few months after immediate bilateral TUG flap reconstruction (*B, left and right*). The patient also underwent bilateral autologous fat grafting and nipple reconstruction in the postoperative period.

gluteal adiposity. Bilateral breast reconstruction in patients who lack sufficient abdominal tissue is especially made possible due to the availability of bilateral gluteal tissue. Scars tend to be well hidden with modest-sized undergarments or bathing suits. Compared with abdominal-based tissue transfers, gluteal flaps are firmer as a result of a difference in the quality of adipose tissue present in the buttocks, and these reconstructions present a greater challenge with higher rates of flap failure.[28] Several other flap options have been described but are used less often in breast reconstruction (see **Box 1**).

## RECONSTRUCTION OF LUMPECTOMY DEFECTS

Breast conservation therapy in the form of lumpectomy or quandrantectomy followed by adjuvant radiation is a popular treatment option for women with breast cancer. Coupled with equivalent survival rates compared with mastectomy, breast conservation has the additional advantage to patients of avoiding loss of the breast. With the oncologic goal of adequate resection of all local disease, however, the postoperative breast shape can be compromised. Women choosing to undergo breast conservation therapy may undergo reconstruction at the time of their oncologic surgery, in a delayed fashion after negative margins are confirmed, or after adjuvant radiation therapy (**Table 2**).

Reconstruction methods can be divided into volume displacement techniques and volume replacement techniques.[29] The best approach is determined by breast size, tumor/defect size, tumor location, and the desires of the patient. In general, procedures that reshape the breast are used for patients with moderate- to large-sized breasts with sufficient parenchyma remaining after resection. In contrast, when additional tissue and/or skin is required after resection, as in women with smaller or nonptotic breasts, then a volume replacement procedure is indicated (**Table 3**).

The breast reshaping, or volume displacement, techniques may involve advancing or rotating an adjacent area of breast parenchmya into the defect in women with adequate breast volume remaining after resection. Mastopexy and reduction techniques can be used to resect the tumor within the expected breast reduction specimen. The incisions are designed to preserve nipple viability, reshape the breast mound, and close the dead space. A similar technique can be performed in the contralateral breast for symmetry if necessary. Consideration should be given to keep the reconstructed breast slightly larger to account for the anticipated shrinkage resulting from radiation fibrosis.

Volume replacement techniques are generally required in women with large tumor-to-breast ratios and small to moderate-sized breasts. Such patients typically do not have sufficient breast parenchyma remaining after resection to reshape the breast. Therefore, reconstruction must be performed using regional or distant flaps. Often, a contralateral breast symmetry procedure is not required. The latissimus dorsi myocutaneous flap is a workhorse flap for defects for lateral and central, and occasionally

| Table 2 Timing of partial breast reconstruction | | |
|---|---|---|
| **Timing** | **Advantages** | **Disadvantages** |
| Immediate | Single surgery | Potential for positive margins |
| Delayed immediate | Performed after margins confirmed negative | Requires second procedure |
| Delayed | Know final breast shape after radiation | Operating on radiated, scarred breast |

| Table 3 | |
|---|---|
| **Reconstruction techniques after lumpectomy or quadrantectomy** | |
| **Volume Displacement Techniques** | **Volume Replacement Techniques** |
| Primary closure | Regional flaps |
| Local tissue rearrangement/advancement | Regional pedicled flaps |
| Mastopexy | Free flaps |
| Nipple-areola centralization | Implant augmentation |
| Reduction/mastopexy | Fat grafting |

even medial, defects (**Fig. 13**). It is a reliable flap with excellent blood supply that provides both muscle bulk for filling defects and skin for cutaneous deficiencies. Lateral defects can also be reconstructed with skin and adipose tissue from the lateral chest wall or back without harvest of muscle in the form of a pedicled thoracodorsal artery perforator (TDAP) flap or intercostal artery perforator (ICAP) flap. Significant medial or superomedial defects are more difficult to reconstruct and can result in poor cosmetic results as placement of scars on the superomedial aspect of the breast is less than ideal. Options still include regional flaps, but free flaps can be considered in addition to entertaining the alternative of a completion mastectomy with total breast reconstruction for both cosmetic and oncological reasons. Zaha and colleagues[30] have described the use of an endoscopically harvested free omental flap, citing its long pedicle, resistance to radiation, and soft and pliable characteristics as beneficial for reconstruction of a variety of partial defects. Breast augmentation with saline or silicone implants for restoration of volume is a possibility that obviates a donor site. Implants, however, do not address the cutaneous deficiencies or scar contractures that typically exist in these radiated breasts. These contractures can be released at the time of augmentation but can recur in the early postoperative period.

The ever-expanding use of autologous fat grafting has provided surgeons with another means of reconstructing partial defects. The fat can be used for core volume replacement and obviates musculocutaneous transposition required for many of the volume replacement techniques. The safety and efficacy of fat grafting are discussed below.

### Fat Grafting for Contour Deformities/Augmentation

Autologous fat grafting, described for a variety of applications as early as the 1980s,[31,32] was met with skepticism when considered for use in breast surgery based on concerns over calcifications associated with this procedure that might be problematic for tumor detection. In recent years there has been a resurgence of interest in this technique, with growing evidence of its efficacy and an improved ability to distinguish between calcifications from fat grafting and those suspicious for malignancy.[33–35] This technique has become a mainstay in breast reconstruction. Fat grafting is primarily used to address volume and contour deformities of the reconstructed breast[36,37] as well as lumpectomy defects. Adipose tissue is harvested using liposuction techniques and processed prior to injecting the grafts into the breast.[38,39] A commonly used technique for fat graft processing involves centrifugation of the lipoaspirate to allow for separation of its components (**Fig. 14**). The oily supernatant is wicked off and fluid at the dependent portion is decanted, leaving behind adipose tissue that can be injected. Small aliquots of the graft are then injected in different soft tissue layers to improve on adipocyte viability (**Fig. 15**). Because only a fraction of the grafted fat survives, multiple sessions of fat grafting are typically required to achieve desired results. The evidence to date, although limited, suggests that fat grafting does not increase the risk of breast cancer recurrence.[40] Questions persist regarding optimal harvest and grafting techniques and the long-term safety and efficacy of fat grafts.

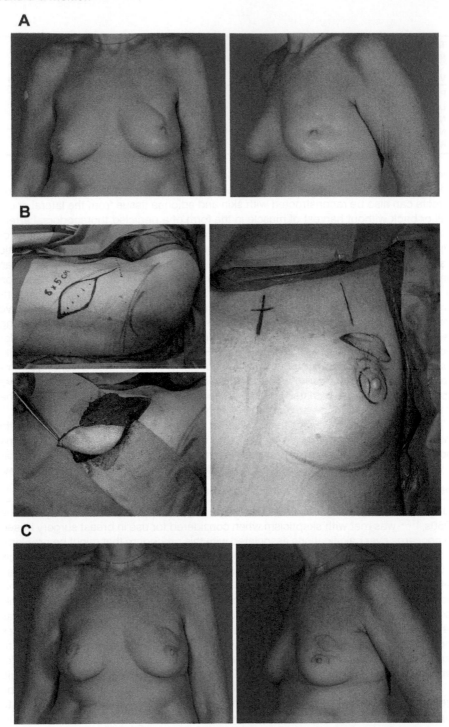

**Fig. 13.** A patient with a left breast superolateral contour deformity with superior retraction of the nipple after breast conservation therapy (*A, left and right*). Intraoperative markings (*B, top left*), harvest (*B, bottom left*), and inset (*B, right*) of a left muscle-sparing latissimus dorsi flap to reconstruct the contour deformity and address the skin deficiency. Postoperative result after flap reconstruction and a minor revision with autologous fat grafting (*C, left and right*).

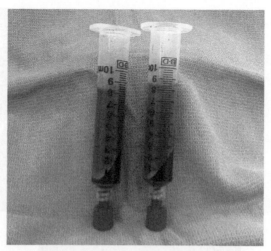

**Fig. 14.** Layering of lipoaspirate components after centrifugation.

## TECHNOLOGICAL AIDS IN BREAST RECONSTRUCTION
### Preoperative CT Angiography

Advances in CT with 3-D mapping capabilities have made this technology a useful tool in preoperative planning for perforator flap breast reconstruction (**Fig. 16**). It has been shown to be superior to duplex ultrasounds at identifying clinically important perforators.[41] By identifying perforators that most likely will be used for the reconstruction, it has the potential to decrease operative time and simplify some of the decision making. These scans provide a road map of the vascular anatomy from the larger pedicle all the way to the perforators, showing their course within the flap soft tissue. CT scans, however, do not give direct information on the perfusion expected with selected perforators.

### Intraoperative Evaluation of Mastectomy Skin Flap Perfusion

Perfusion based on selected perforators is better assessed using intraoperative mapping technology. The SPY Elite intraoperative perfusion assessment system (LifeCell Corporation, Branchburg, NJ, USA) is one such device that provides real-time

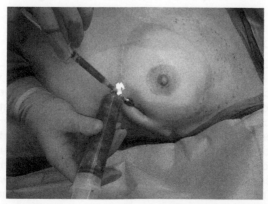

**Fig. 15.** Injection of autologous fat grafts into a reconstructed breast to address a contour deformity.

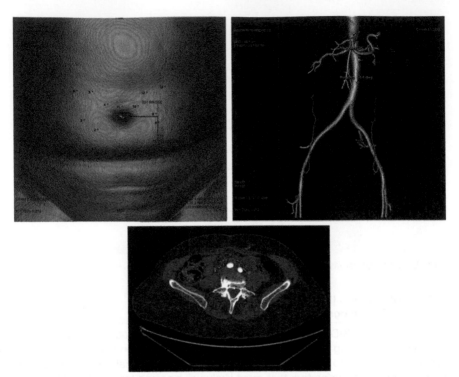

**Fig. 16.** CT angiogram of the abdomen for preoperative planning for harvest of a perforator free flap. The preoperative microvascular protocol with reformatting produces images including an external reconstructed image with mapping of perforator location (*top left*), a 3-D reconstruction of the aorta and its branches (*top right*), and a cross-sectional axial image (*bottom*).

information on flow within flap soft tissues. It is used as an adjunct to clinical assessment and can be used to assess the perfusion of mastectomy skin flaps in addition to perfusion of autologous flaps intraoperatively.[42] Patients are administered a dose of intravenous indocyanine green dye and perfusion is assessed with use of an infrared laser from the device, which stimulates fluorescent properties of the dye (Videos 1 and 2). Based on the information provided, intraoperative changes can be made to the planned operation.

## POSSIBLE DIRECTIONS IN THE FUTURE
### Patient-Performed Expansion

A disadvantage of tissue expander/implant–based reconstruction is the often uncomfortable and time-consuming process of tissue expansion that women must undergo. An ideal system would convert the intermittent delivery of volume into a more continuous, gradual process.

A potentially promising system recently developed was presented in 2011 by Connell,[43] who described a fully implantable device that provided tissue expansion in a controlled and guided manner without the need for percutaneous injections. The device contains a reservoir of compressed carbon dioxide and a wireless handheld dosage controller that a surgeon and/or patient uses to release carbon dioxide into the expander up to 3 times a day. Patients in this feasibility study reported that they were satisfied with their results and that the system was easy to use. Furthermore, the study found that the time to achieve the full volume was one-third the usual time, because patients were able to optimize their own rates of expansion. Potential drawbacks of the device relate to the use of carbon dioxide as an expansion medium, because permeation of the gas through the walls of the expander may necessitate intermittent dosing during the rest phase and patients may experience fluctuations in volume during air travel, necessitating a change-in-altitude restriction. Whether or not such patient-controlled tissue expanders become the standard of care is yet to be determined, but these new technologies are evidence of a continually evolving field.

## Total Reconstruction with Autologous Fat Grafting

Although use of autologous fat grafting for breast reconstruction revisions and for contouring of segmental breast defects has gained recent acceptance, fat grafting alone for total breast reconstruction remains a subject of interest in the early stages of investigation. A critical problem with autologous fat grafting has to do with resorption of the transferred volume because not all adipocytes survive.[44] Consequently, fat grafting is typically performed in multiple sessions over time to achieve a final result. With an understanding of the volumes of fat required to fully reconstruct a moderate- to large-sized breast, fat grafting alone in its present form would be problematic. A few studies in the aesthetic plastic surgery literature have described a technique of soft tissue pre-expansion that allows for large-volume fat transfer.[45] Proponents of this technique perform breast pre-expansion using an external expansion device known as BRAVA (BRAVA, Miami, Florida) for a few weeks before fat transfer and a few weeks afterward. This technique is thought to allow for larger-volume (>300 g) transfers with an increase in breast size ranging from 60% to 200% after 6 months of follow-up. Drawbacks to use of this technique are related to patient compliance with the external expansion process because it can be painful, noisy, and irritating to the skin. It also requires patient motivation to keep the device on for many hours of the day for an extended period of time. The applicability of this technology alongside fat transfer for total breast reconstruction is a subject that requires further investigation.

## SUPPLEMENTARY DATA

Videos related to this article can be found online at http://dx.doi.org/10.1016/j.soc. 2014.03.012.

## REFERENCES

1. Wilkins EG, Cederna PS, Lowery JC, et al. Prospective anlaysis of psychosocial outcomes in breast reconstruction: one-year postoperative results from the Michigan breast reconstruction outcomes study. Plast Reconstr Surg 2000;106(5): 1014–25.
2. Kronowitz SJ, Lam C, Terefe W, et al. A multidisciplinary protocol for planned skin-preserving delayed breast reconstruction for patients with locally advanced breast cancer requiring postmastectomy radiation therapy: 3-year follow up. Plast Reconstr Surg 2001;127(6):2154–66.
3. Fine NA, Hirsch EM. Keeping options open for patients with anticipated postmastectomy chest wall irradiation: immediate tissue expansion followed by reconstruction of choice. Plast Reconstr Surg 2009;123(1):25–9.
4. Chang EI, Liu TS, Festekjian JH, et al. Effects of radiation therapy for breast cancer based on type of free flap reconstruction. Plast Reconstr Surg 2013;131(1): 1e–8e.

5. Radovan C. Breast reconstruction after mastectomy using the temporary expander. Plast Reconstr Surg 1982;69(2):195–208.
6. Breuing K, Warren S. Immediate bilateral breast reconstruction with implants and inferolateral alloderm slings. Ann Plast Surg 2005;55(3):232–9.
7. Kim JY, Davila AA, Persing S, et al. A meta-analysis of human acellular dermis and submuscular tissue expander breast reconstruction. Plast Reconstr Surg 2012;129(1):28–41.
8. Salzberg C. Focus on technique: one-stage implant-based breast reconstruction. Plast Reconstr Surg 2012;130(5 Suppl 2):95S–103S.
9. Cronin TD, Gerow FJ. Augmentation mammoplasty: a new "natural feel" prosthesis. Transactions of the Third International Congress of Plastic and Reconstructive Surgery. Amsterdam: Excerpta Medica Foundation; 1964. p. 41–9.
10. Maxwell GP. Iginio Tansini and the origin of the latissimus dorsi musculocutaneous flap. Plast Reconstr Surg 1980;65(5):686–92.
11. Spear SL, Boehmler JH, Bogue DP, et al. Options in reconstructing the irradiated breast. Plast Reconstr Surg 2008;122(2):379–88.
12. Hartrampf CR, Scheflan M, Black PW. Breast reconstruction with a transverse abdominal island flap. Plast Reconstr Surg 1982;69(2):216–25.
13. Momoh AO, Colakoglu S, Westvik TS, et al. Analysis of complications and patient satisfaction in pedicled transverse rectus abdominis myocutaneous and deep inferior epigastric perforator flap breast reconstruction. Ann Plast Surg 2012; 69(1):19–23.
14. Selber JC, Nelson J, Fosnot J, et al. A prospective study comparing the functional impact of SIEA, DIEP and muscle-sparing free TRAM flaps on the abdominal wall: part I. Unilateral reconstruction. Plast Reconstr Surg 2010;126(4):1142–53.
15. Selber JC, Fosnot J, Nelson J, et al. A prospective study comparing the functional impact of SIEA, DIEP, and muscle-sparing free TRAM flaps on the abdominal wall: part II. Bilateral reconstruction. Plast Reconstr Surg 2010;126(5):1438–53.
16. Koshima I, Soeda S. Inferior epigastric artery skin flaps without rectus abdominis muscle. Br J Plast Surg 1989;42(6):645–8.
17. Allen RJ, Treece P. Deep inferior epigastric perforator flap for breast reconstruction. Ann Plast Surg 1994;32(1):32–8.
18. Man L, Selber JC, Serletti JM. Abdominal wall following free TRAM or DIEP flap reconstruction: a meta-analysis and critical review. Plast Reconstr Surg 2009; 124(3):752–64.
19. Alderman AK, Kuzon WM, Wilkins EG. A two-year prospective analysis of trunk function in TRAM breast reconstructions. Plast Reconstr Surg 2006;117(7):2131–8.
20. Blondeel N, Vanderstraeten GG, Monstrey SJ, et al. The donor site morbidity of free DIEP flaps and free TRAM flaps for breast reconstruction. Br J Plast Surg 1997;50(5):322–30.
21. Nahabedian MY, Dooley W, Singh N, et al. Contour abnormalities of the abdomen after breast reconstruction with abdominal flaps: the role of muscle preservation. Plast Reconstr Surg 2002;109(1):91–101.
22. Khansa I, Momoh AO, Patel PP, et al. Fat necrosis in autologous abdomen-based breast reconstruction: a systematic review. Plast Reconstr Surg 2013;131(3): 443–52.
23. Spiegel AJ, Khan FN. An intraoperative algorithm for use of the SIEA flap for breast reconstruction. Plast Reconstr Surg 2007;120(6):1450–9.
24. Fischer JP, Nelson JA, Kovach SJ, et al. Impact of obesity on outcomes in breast reconstruction: analysis of 15,937 patients from ACS-NSQIP datasets. J Am Coll Surg 2013;217(4):656–64.

25. Kroll SS, Netscher DT. Complications of TRAM flap breast reconstruction in obese patients. Plast Reconstr Surg 1989;84(6):886–92.
26. Garvey PB, Villa MT, Rozanski AT, et al. The advantages of free abdominal-based flaps over implants for breast reconstruction in obese patients. Plast Reconstr Surg 2012;130(5):991–1000.
27. Momeni A, Ahdoot M, Kim R, et al. Should we continue to consider obesity a relative contraindication for autologous microsurgical breast reconstruction? J Plast Reconstr Aesthet Surg 2012;65(4):420–5.
28. Mirzabeigi MN, Au A, Jandali S, et al. Trials and tribulations with the inferior gluteal artery perforator flap in autologous breast reconstruction. Plast Reconstr Surg 2011;128(6):614e–24e.
29. Losken A, Hamdi M. Partial breast reconstruction: current perspectives. Plast Reconstr Surg 2009;124(3):722–36.
30. Zaha H, Onomura M, Nomura H, et al. Free omental flap for partial breast reconstruction after breast-conserving surgery. Plast Reconstr Surg 2012;129(3):583–7.
31. Chajchir A, Benzaquen I. Liposuction fat grafts in face wrinkles and hemifacial atrophy. Aesthetic Plast Surg 1986;10(2):115–7.
32. Chajchir A, Benzaquen I. Fat-grafting injection for soft-tissue augmentation. Plast Reconstr Surg 1989;84(6):921–34 [discussion: 935].
33. Chala LF, de Barros N, de Camargo Morales P, et al. Fat necrosis of the breast: mammographic, sonographic, computed tomography, and magnetic resonance imaging findings. Curr Probl Diagn Radiol 2004;33(3):106–26.
34. Kneeshaw PJ, Lowry M, Manton D, et al. Differentiation of benign from malignant breast disease associated with screening detected microcalcifications using dynamic contrast enhanced magnetic resonance imaging. Breast 2006;15(1): 29–38.
35. Mizuno H, Hyakusoku H. Fat grafting to the breast and adipose-derived stem cells: recent scientific consensus and controversy. Aesthet Surg J 2010;30(3): 381–7.
36. Kannchwala SK, Glatt BS, Conant EF, et al. Autologous fat grafting to the reconstructed breast: the management of acquired contour deformities. Plast Reconstr Surg 2009;124(2):409–18.
37. De Blacam C, Momoh AO, Colakoglu S, et al. Evaluation of clinical outcomes and aesthetic results after autologous fat grafting for contour deformities of the reconstructed breast. Plast Reconstr Surg 2011;128(5):411e–8e.
38. Coleman SR. Structural fat grafting. St Louis (MO): Quality Medical; 2004. p. 30–175.
39. Coleman SR. Structural fat grafting: more than a permanent filler. Plast Reconstr Surg 2006;118(Suppl 3):108S–20S.
40. Seth AK, Hirsch EM, Kim JY, et al. Long-term outcomes following fat grafting in prosthetic breast reconstruction: a comparative analysis. Plast Reconstr Surg 2012;130(5):984–90.
41. Scott JR, Liu D, Said H, et al. Computed tomographic angiography in planning abdomen-based microsurgical breast reconstruction: a comparison with color duplex ultrasound. Plast Reconstr Surg 2010;125(2):446–53.
42. Komorowska-Timek E, Gurtner G. Intraoperative perfusion mapping with laser-assisted indocyanine green imaging can predict and prevent complications in immediate breast reconstruction. Plast Reconstr Surg 2010;125(4):1065–73.
43. Connell A. Patient-activated controlled expansion for breast reconstruction with controlled carbon dioxide inflation: a feasibility study. Plast Reconstr Surg 2011; 128(4):848–52.

44. Nguyen A, Pasyk KA, Bouvier TN, et al. Comparative study of survival of autologous adipose tissue taken and transplanted by different techniques. Plast Reconstr Surg 1990;85(3):378–86 [discussion: 387–9].
45. Del Vecchio DA, Bucky LP. Breast augmentation using preexpansion and autologous fat transplantation: a clinical radiographic study. Plast Reconstr Surg 2011; 127(6):2441–50.

# Nipple-Sparing Mastectomy
## An Oncologic and Cosmetic Perspective

Christine Laronga, MD[a,b,*], Paul Smith, MD[b]

## KEYWORDS

- Nipple-sparing mastectomy • Oncologic safety • Cosmesis

## KEY POINTS

- All new surgical techniques need to first be evaluated for safety and efficacy.
- Nipple-sparing mastectomy is technically feasible but challenging.
- On short-term follow-up, nipple-sparing mastectomy is oncologically safe.
- Impact on sensation, body image, and quality of life are yet to be fully determined.

 Video of bilateral nipple-sparing mastectomy with tissue expander/silicone implant reconstruction accompanies this article at http://www.surgonc. theclinics.com/

## HISTORICAL PERSPECTIVE

The surgical management of breast cancer has changed dramatically over the years.

- 1600 BC: oldest recorded history (a scroll) comes from ancient Egypt and stated that there was no treatment of breast cancer.[1]
- ~400 BC: Hippocrates also recommended no surgical management for breast cancer, because it would certainly only hasten the patient's death.
- First century AD: Greek physician, Leonides, performed the first operative management of breast cancer, called the escharotomy method.
  - A hot poker made repeated incisions, burning the entire breast off the chest wall. Most women died of surgical infection.

The authors have nothing to disclose.
[a] Comprehensive Breast Program, Department of Women's Oncology, Moffitt Cancer Center, 12902 Magnolia Drive, MCC BR-PROG, Tampa, FL 33612, USA; [b] Department of Surgery, University of South Florida, 13220 USF Laurel Drive, Tampa, FL 33612, USA
* Corresponding author. Comprehensive Breast Program, Moffitt Cancer Center, 12902 Magnolia Drive, MCC BR-PROG, Tampa, FL 33612.
E-mail address: Christine.laronga@moffitt.org

- 100 years later: Galen is credited with the first surgical cure for breast cancer.
- Renaissance era: new surgical instruments were being created. Without anesthesia or antisepsis, the goal was to remove the breast swiftly.
  - The Guillotine method: amputation of the breast with a large sharp knife without reapproximating the skin. Most women died of exsanguination or subsequent infection.
- Eighteenth century: birth of the nipple-sparing mastectomy.
  - A surgeon, Jean Louis Petit, advocated leaving all the skin not involved with tumor including the nipple-areola disk during the procedure and, in essence, described the concept of the nipple-sparing mastectomy.[2]
  - His beliefs and methods were not adopted.
- Late nineteenth century to mid-twentieth century: the Halsted era
  - Halsted described the exact technique to perform a radical mastectomy. Operative mortality decreased but the operation was disfiguring (**Fig. 1**).
  - He had 2 advantages: the advent of anesthesia and antisepsis.
  - The initial operation: complete removal of the breast with all the overlying skin (a skin graft for coverage of the chest wall) and removal of level I to III axillary lymph nodes and the pectoralis major and minor muscles.
  - Later operation: the additional removal of the latissimus dorsi, supscapularis, teres minor, and serratus muscles.
  - The Halsted radical mastectomy became the primary treatment of breast cancer for the next 70 years. During that era, a surgeon-pathologist (Hagensen) at Columbia University noted that the more radical the operation became, the survival rates from breast cancer did not likewise increase.[3]
  - This observation was also noted by European colleagues (Veronesi); this opened the door to consideration of a less radical operation.[4]
  - In 1948, Patey and Dyson[5] introduced the concept of the modified radical mastectomy; a modified radical mastectomy includes removal of the entire breast, level I to III lymph nodes, and the necessary skin (including nipple-areola disk) to allow primary closure flat against the chest wall, with minimal redundancy of skin. No muscles would be removed.

## BIRTH OF BREAST RECONSTRUCTION AND SUBCUTANEOUS MASTECTOMY

In the 1950s, silicone gel implants came on the scene. Women with breast cancer were not offered immediate reconstruction for 2 reasons:

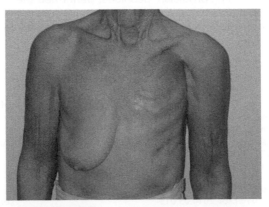

**Fig. 1.** The Halsted radical mastectomy.

- Development of a recurrence or distant disease, mostly likely within 3 years of a woman's cancer diagnosis. The woman would be declared a survivor before any breast reconstruction was performed.
- The techniques of immediate reconstruction after mastectomy were still in their infancy. If the woman lived with all the imperfections of a mastectomy without reconstruction for a significant period, she would be more appreciative of any reconstructive outcome.

Early experience with immediate breast reconstruction came from women having subcutaneous mastectomies for benign disease.[6,7] A subcutaneous mastectomy was performed using, most commonly, an inframammary incision, with removal of most of the breast tissue, leaving a rim of normal breast tissue on the undersurface of the native breast skin, especially subareolar. No skin was removed, including the nipple areolar disk, akin to a nipple-sparing mastectomy. Thick mastectomy flaps (>10 mm) were raised, leaving a cushion of tissue anterior to the implant and beneath the skin. This cushion maintained skin viability and created a more natural feel to the reconstruction. Because this operation was for benign disease, the oncologic safety was not questioned.

By the 1970s, the modified radical mastectomy was gaining traction and women demanded immediate reconstruction. Plastic surgeons had some native breast skin, albeit thinner than a subcutaneous mastectomy, to provide coverage over the implant. However, it was quickly learned that there was a high risk of implant exposure from wound dehiscence. The implant was too heavy for the delicate mastectomy skin. As a result, tissue expanders were developed (**Fig. 2**).

Tissue expanders are placed beneath the pectoralis major muscles at the time of mastectomy. They are slowly inflated with saline over time, stretching the pectoralis major muscle until the intended breast size is achieved. The rate of expansion is adjusted per patient based on skin integrity and patient tolerance. The expanders are subsequently exchanged for a permanent, more natural appearing, implant a few months later as an outpatient. The nipple can be reconstructed at a third operation a minimum of 6 weeks later.

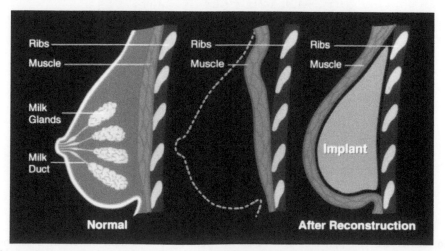

**Fig. 2.** Tissue expander/implant placement beneath the pectoralis muscle.

## COSMETIC IMPORTANCE OF THE NIPPLE-AREOLA COMPLEX

Plastic surgeons recognized that the nipple-areola complex defines a breast as a breast and therefore defined a reconstructed breast mound. Reconstruction is performed using skin from the local area or donated from the groin area. Alternatively, the nipple-areola disk could be harvested at the time of mastectomy, with banking of the nipple in the patient's groin as a full-thickness skin graft and later replacing it on the reconstructed breast (**Fig. 3**). Attempts to maintain the nipple in a tissue bank for future reimplantation resulted in poor viability of the preserved nipple-areola disk. However, whether banking in the groin or the biorepository, concerns about transplanting cancer contained within the preserved nipple started to appear in the literature[8–10]; thus, this practice fell out of favor. Focus shifted back to improving the techniques of nipple reconstruction and investigating the psychological importance of having recreation of a nipple on a reconstructed breast mound.[11]

## AUTOLOGOUS TISSUE FLAP RECONSTRUCTION AND SKIN-SPARING MASTECTOMY

In the 1980s, new methods of breast reconstruction were being developed, namely autologous tissue transfers. These modalities (latissimus dorsi and transverse rectus abdominus myocutaneous flaps) offered an alternative to expander/implant reconstruction and provided the ability to create a larger breast mound size, with ptosis if needed (**Figs. 4** and **5**).

In 1984, Toth and Lappert[12] introduced the concept of the skin-sparing mastectomy.

- A skin-sparing mastectomy removes the entire breast and provides access to the axilla for lymph node removal, but preserves a minimum of 80% of the native breast skin, but always removes the nipple-areola complex. By preserving the maximal amount of breast skin, the breast surgeon provides the patient with an envelope that is the same size, color, contour, and ptosis as her original breast. These investigators also recommended avoiding incisions in the upper part of the breast, which could affect cosmesis (**Fig. 6**).[12]

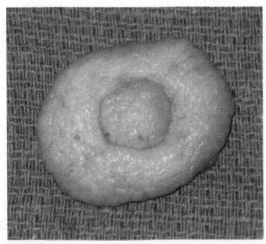

**Fig. 3.** Harvest of nipple-areola complex for banking and reimplantation at a second surgery.

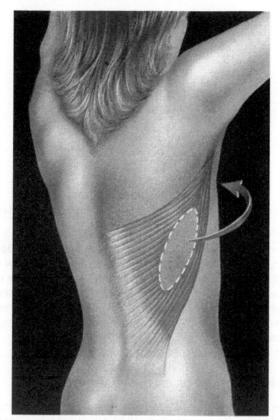

**Fig. 4.** Latissimus dorsi myocutaneous flap harvest site.

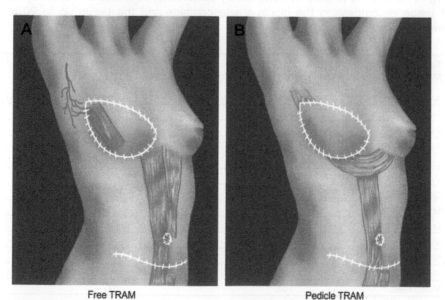

Free TRAM                                         Pedicle TRAM

**Fig. 5.** Transverse abdominus myocutaneous flap: (*A*) free flap; (*B*) pedicle flap.

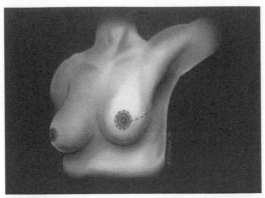

**Fig. 6.** Common incision used for a skin-sparing mastectomy with immediate reconstruction.

- Initial concerns regarding the oncologic safety of preserving additional skin were quelled by studies[13–18] proving the technical feasibility and low local recurrence rate. With all types of mastectomy, if the undersurface of the remaining native breast skin and the anterior surface of the pectoralis major muscles is scraped, approximately 1 g of normal breast epithelial cells could be identified.[19] Thus, the local recurrence rates were no different between skin-sparing and non–skin-sparing mastectomy.[13,14,17,18]
- Skin-sparing mastectomies are standard of practice.

## NIPPLE AREOLAR PRESERVATION OR RECONSTRUCTION

Aside from Petit in the eighteenth century, preserving the nipple-areola complex went against surgical dogma. Several studies (1970–1990) reported unsuspected nipple involvement in 6% to 58% of mastectomy specimens.[20] All studies took a cylinder of tissue encompassing the nipple-areola complex and the tissue up to 20 mm deep to it (**Table 1**).

| Table 1<br>Mastectomy specimens with occult cancer found in the nipples | | |
|---|---|---|
| **Author, Year** | **Number of Specimens** | **Nipple Involvement (%)** |
| Smith,[23] 1976 | 541 | 12 |
| Parry, 1977 | 200 | 8 |
| Andersen, 1979 | 40 | 50 |
| Lagios,[22] 1979 | 149 | 30 |
| Wertheim, 1980 | 1000 | 23 |
| Quinn, 1981 | 45 | 25 |
| Morimoto, 1985 | 141 | 31 |
| Luttges, 1987 | 166 | 38 |
| Santini, 1989 | 1291 | 12 |
| Menon, 1989 | 33 | 58 |
| Verma, 1997 | 26 | 0 |
| Vyas, 1998 | 140 | 16 |
| Laronga,[20] 1999 | 286 | 6 |

In current practice, 20 mm of tissue is not left on the nipple flap during a nipple-sparing mastectomy, but rather, it is the same as the rest of the flap (ie, 3–5 mm). Using a 5-mm zone behind the nipple-areola complex as the definition for involvement of the nipple with a true occult second cancer, the incidence would be lower (<5%).[20] Despite this knowledge, many surgeons still were not comfortable with the prospect of sparing the nipple and thus relied on the plastic surgeon to create a nipple.

Although there are many techniques to recreate a nipple, they all fall into 1 of 3 groups.

- The first method is called composite grafting, which entails borrowing tissue from a distant source (contralateral normal nipple, cartilage graft from the ear, skin from the groin area), use of various acellular dermal matrices, or use of fillers that can be injected/placed under the breast skin.
- The second approach uses local in situ breast skin flaps to recreate a projecting nipple with primary closure of the donor site.
- The final option, referred to as a skate flap, is a similar recreation of the nipple with local breast skin but rather than closing the donor site primarily, it uses a skin graft to cover the area that was borrowed from. Typically, this procedure manifests itself as a round graft mimicking an areolar disk.

Despite numerous advances in nipple reconstruction, loss of projection, diminished color variation, and asymmetry continued to plague the plastic surgeon.

## BIRTH OF THE AREOLA-SPARING MASTECTOMY

In the late 1990s, surgeons began exploring the option of areola-sparing mastectomy. The areola disk is a skin appendage and not breast tissue. Therefore, it cannot make a de novo breast cancer. Akin to skin-sparing mastectomy, the technique needed to be defined and more specifically, what the areola disk would be used for. The 2 options were:

- Leave the areola disk in situ and create a nipple using donor skin from the autologous tissue transfer
- Use the areola disk to create a nipple, and then later, tattoo the areola disk around the newly created nipple

The areola made a natural appearing nipple and did a better job maintaining its projection than recreating a nipple using the donor skin, especially if the donor skin was used at the initial reconstruction operation (**Fig. 7**A, B). On the down side, the color tones and pigmentation within the areola are typically variegated and highly individual, defying exact match by even the most skillful tattoo artist (see **Fig. 7**C).

It was also learned that areola-sparing mastectomy was not only technically feasible but oncologically safe. There have been no reports of a de novo breast cancer arising from the preserved areola disk, regardless of whether it is maintained as an areola disk or used to create the nipple.[21]

## REBIRTH OF THE NIPPLE-SPARING MASTECTOMY

The time had come to reexplore the option of nipple-sparing mastectomy.

Factors that predict occult nipple involvement formed the basis for initial eligibility criteria:

- Poorly differentiated primary tumors larger than 2 cm and centrally located[20,22,23]

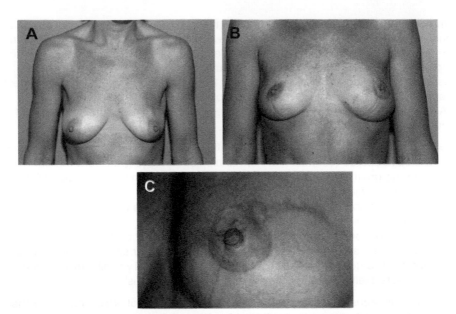

**Fig. 7.** (*A*) Before and (*B*) after an areola-sparing mastectomy using the areolar disk to make the nipple. (*C*) Close-up of the areolar disk as a nipple.

- Multicentric tumors
- Presence of lymphovascular invasion and lymph node involvement

## TECHNICAL DEVELOPMENT

- The incision must allow for complete removal of the breast and access to the axilla for staging.
- Ability to easily obtain tissue from the base of the nipple for assessment of atypia or occult cancer was an absolute requirement (**Fig. 8**).
- The base of the nipple could be examined by imprint cytology or frozen section. If any atypical or cancerous cells were identified or if the vascular viability was concerning by the end of the procedure, the nipple would be sacrificed.

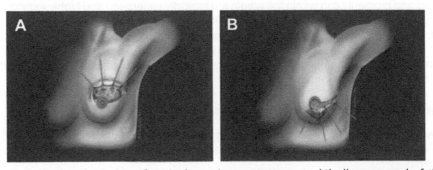

**Fig. 8.** Designing the incision for nipple-sparing mastectomy to (*A*) allow removal of the entire breast with access to axilla and (*B*) allow access to easily sample the base of the nipple.

## TIMELINE

- 1999: first case report presented at the Southwestern Surgical Congress.
- 2000: editorial describing the technique in *Annals of Surgical Oncology*.[24]
- 2003: the first reported series came from separate institutions.[25,26]
  - The Petit group (Milan, Italy) described a subcutaneous mastectomy and use of 20 Gy of intraoperative radiation (ELIOT [ELectron Bean Intra_Operative Radiation Therapy]) to the nipple-areola complex and remaining breast tissue.[25] This technique uses a radial incision in the upper outer quadrant of the breast from areola border to axilla, and an intraoperative frozen section of the base of the nipple is always obtained. At 6 months of follow-up in 25 patients, no local recurrences were reported.
  - The study by Gerber and colleagues[26] looked at 61 patients having nipple-sparing mastectomy and compared them with women having skin-sparing or non–skin-sparing mastectomy. The local recurrence rate at a mean follow-up of 4.9 years was the same (5%) in all 3 cohorts.
- 2004: Crowe and colleagues[27] reported on 44 patients having nipple-sparing mastectomy for breast cancer treatment or prophylaxis with no local recurrences at a short 6 weeks mean follow-up.

Initially, many nipple-sparing mastectomies were performed as prophylactic mastectomies in high-risk women not for the treatment of breast cancer. In these women, many of whom were later confirmed to be BRCA mutation carriers, the nipple-sparing mastectomy was performed as a subcutaneous mastectomy. However, the development of a primary breast cancer in the residual breast tissue was higher than anticipated (1.9% at median follow-up of 6.4 years in the Rebbeck study) and begs the question of oncologic safety of a subcutaneous mastectomy in this high-risk population.[28,29]

By 2008 to 2009, a plethora of reports surfaced in the literature[30–32] spouting technical feasibility but with small numbers of patients and short-term follow-up (**Table 2**). Some articles focused on generating an algorithm for eligibility, without providing much information about their own institutional experience or outcomes from a cosmesis standpoint.[33,34]

**Table 2**
Early experience of many centers after the initial reporting of nipple-sparing mastectomy in 2003–2004

| Author, Year | Number of Cases | Indication for Surgery | Follow-Up (mo) | LR or New (%) |
|---|---|---|---|---|
| Sookhan,[30] 2008 | 18 NSM 2 ASM | Treatment Prevention | 10.8 | 0 |
| Voltura,[31] 2008 | 51 NSM (NAC+ 6%) | Treatment Prevention | 18 | 5.9 |
| Kiluk, 2008 | 87 NSM | Treatment Prevention | 6.5 | 0 |
| Petit,[39] 2009 | 579 NSM + ELIOT | Treatment | 19 | 0.9/y |
| Garwood,[32] 2009 | 170 NSM | Treatment Prevention | 13 | 0.6 |
| Gerber,[38] 2009 | 60 NSM | Treatment | 101 | 11.7 |
| Petit,[39] 2009 | 1001 NSM + ELIOT | Treatment | 20 | 1.4 |

*Abbreviations:* LR, local recurrence; New, new primary breast cancer; NSM, nipple-sparing mastectomy.

- Memorial Sloan Kettering early experience:
  - ○ 25 women had 42 nipple-sparing mastectomies, of which 81% were prophylactic.[34]
  - ○ All of these women had tissue expander/implant reconstruction.
  - ○ Partial nipple loss was seen in 5% of mastectomies, and complete nipple loss happened in 2% of women. In addition, at 2 weeks after the operation, 48% had nipple discoloration or ischemia. Ischemia was most common with a lateral incision (curvilinear at the edge of the breast in the lower outer quadrant).
- De Alcantara and colleagues[35] have updated the Memorial Sloan Kettering Cancer Center experience, reflecting a change in eligibility criteria, including more women with breast cancer. Still, only 4% of all their mastectomies are nipple sparing, showing continued careful selection criteria, resulting in no local recurrences on short-term follow-up and only 1 patient with distant metastasis. None of these investigators' nipple-sparing mastectomies was performed using an inframammary approach.

Incision choice affects cosmesis, technical ease of performing the operation, and vascular viability of the nipple.

- In a study by Kiluk and colleagues,[36] all the patients had an inframammary incision akin to that used in breast augmentation or subcutaneous mastectomies, but this was a true nipple-sparing mastectomy (**Fig. 9**). No counterincision was made in the axilla for sentinel lymph node biopsy. Showing technical feasibility of this incision to accomplish all the goals (complete removal of the breast, access to the axilla for staging, and ease of obtaining pathologic assessment of the base of the nipple) set the bar high for nipple-sparing mastectomies in the future.

## LONG-TERM OUTCOMES DATA

As others were reporting technical feasibility at short-term outcomes, the original pioneers were publishing updates (**Table 3**).[37–39]

- Gerber and colleagues[38] presented longer follow-up on 60 of their original 61 patients.
  - ○ The local recurrence was 11.7%, but this was not statistically different from the skin-sparing and non–skin-sparing cohorts.[38]

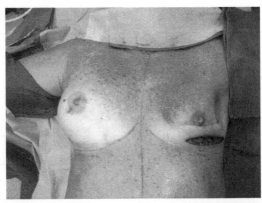

**Fig. 9.** Use of an inframammary incision to perform the nipple-sparing mastectomy and the axillary sentinel lymph node biopsy.

**Table 3**
**Long-term outcomes of nipple-sparing mastectomy**

|  | Petit | Gerber | John Wayne Cancer Center | Moffitt Cancer Center |
|---|---|---|---|---|
| Number of patients | 2000 | 60 | 99 | 111 |
| Follow-up (mo) | 53.2 | 101 | NR | 22 |
| Nipple base with atypia (%) | NR | NR | 14 | 2.1 |
| Partial necrosis (%) | 6.5 | NR | NR | 5.6 |
| Full necrosis (%) | 3.9 | NR | 6 | 0.6 |
| Depigmentation (%) | 31 | NR | NR | 1.2 |
| Sensation present (%) | 36 | NR | NR | NR |
| Local recurrence (%) | 3.9 | 11.7 | 14 | 2.7 |
| Distant metastases (%) | 8 | NR | NR | 0.5 |
| Overall survival (%) | 97.3 | NR | NR | 97 |

*Abbreviation:* NR, not reported.

- Petit and colleagues[39] reported on 1001 patients having subcutaneous mastectomies with ELIOT; the local recurrence rate at 20 months was 1.4%.

In an oral presentation at the San Antonio Breast Cancer Symposium in December, 2010, Petit stated that 37% of their mastectomies are nipple sparing.[40] Their current eligibility criteria for nipple-sparing mastectomy includes all clinical stage T1 and T2 invasive breast cancers but excludes history of previous breast radiation.

- Immediate complications include infection (2.1%) and complications requiring removal of tissue expander/implant (4.2%).
- In these investigators' hands, transverse rectus abdominus myocutaneous reconstruction offers the best cosmetic outcome, and when the reconstruction is a tissue expander/implant, most (75%) have implant alone reconstruction (1-step procedure).
- Complications specific to tissue expander reconstruction were tilting (radiodystrophy) of the nipple toward the axilla and delayed capsular contracture, which occurred in 16.5% of patients.

A few months later, at the 16th Annual Multidisciplinary Symposium on Breast Diseases in Amelia Island Florida (February, 2011), Veronesi[41] reiterated his associate's presentation in San Antonio and included some further updates (see **Table 3**):

- The local recurrence rate was 3.9%, with 12 of 39 local recurrences involving the preserved nipple (11 noninvasive and 1 invasive cancer). Seventy-five patients had a nipple base with cancer (25 invasive and 50 noninvasive cancers) found on final pathology. These nipples were observed in situ and none developed a local recurrence, most likely because of the intraoperative radiation.

Aside from Petit and Gerber, another group to report 5-year data is the John Wayne Cancer Center (see **Table 3**).[42]

- Six percent of patients had the nipple sacrificed for vascular insufficiency. As a result, these investigators have modified their technique to incorporate a delay procedure. A delay procedure entails making an inferior circumareolar incision to obtain a nipple base biopsy and detaching the entire nipple-areola disk from the breast mound. Two weeks later, after skin collateralization has occurred to the nipple and pathologic assessment of the base of the nipple is free of tumor, the nipple-sparing mastectomy is performed. This modified technique, in these investigators' hands, has decreased vascular compromise to the nipple and thus nipple loss.

- Early in their series, patients with a positive nipple base for cancer intraoperatively had a 14% local recurrence rate. By identifying these patients beforehand, they were declared ineligible for nipple-sparing mastectomy.

The Moffitt Cancer Center has been performing nipple-sparing mastectomies over the last several years for genetic carriers and in select women with breast cancer (**Fig. 10**, Video 1). We developed stringent eligibility criteria based on oncologic factors and technical/cosmetic constraints (**Box 1**).

- A total of 187 nipple-sparing mastectomies performed on 111 patients (108 women, 3 men). Their median age was 48.5 years (range 18–82 years) and their median body mass index (BMI, calculated as weight in kilograms divided by the square of height in meters) was 23 (range 17–34).
- Most (68%) had bilateral nipple-sparing mastectomies, with 80% of patients having nipple sparing for an invasive cancer.
- Most women (>80%) experienced some amount of epidermolysis to the nipple tip at 5 to 10 days postoperatively; the area healed without sequelae or intervention.
- Immediate postoperative (<30 days) period included (see **Table 3**):
  - Infection requiring removal of a tissue expander (1.2%)
  - Skin flap necrosis (6.8%)
  - Malposition or leakage of the tissue expander (3.7%)

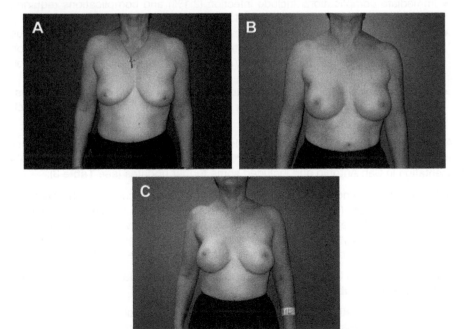

**Fig. 10.** Preoperative (*A*), 6-month postoperative (*B*), and 2-year postoperative (*C*) photographs of bilateral nipple-sparing mastectomy with tissue expander/silicone implant reconstruction.

> **Box 1**
> **Inclusion and exclusion criteria for nipple-sparing mastectomy**
>
> *Inclusion*
>
> 1. Histologically proven diagnosis of breast: unifocal invasive ductal, invasive lobular, or a sarcoma
> 2. The invasive tumor size is 3 cm or smaller based on preoperative breast imaging
> 3. The tumor margin is greater than 2 cm from the areolar edge based on radially and 2 cm from the posterior margin of the nipple-areola base based on preoperative breast imaging
> 4. Clinically, the patient is lymph node negative and has a sentinel lymph node biopsy at the time of the mastectomy on the cancer side (not required on a prophylactic mastectomy)
> 5. Patients who have a prophylactic mastectomy (unilateral or bilateral) for risk reduction are eligible for a nipple-sparing mastectomy of the breast without cancer
> 6. Female, 18 years or older
>
> *Exclusion*
>
> 1. Patients older than 85 years at the time of surgery
> 2. Extensive ductal carcinoma in situ (>3 cm area)
> 3. Previous history of breast cancer (invasive or noninvasive) with radiation
> 4. Previous history of irradiation to the breast area (ie, mantle radiation for lymphoma)
> 5. The invasive cancer is larger than 3 cm, is multicentric, is within 2 cm from the areolar margin, or is within 2 cm from the posterior aspect of the nipple-areolar base
> 6. Clinically suspicious axillary lymph nodes on palpation or by fine-needle aspiration
> 7. History of smoking within 6 weeks of intended surgery
> 8. Obesity (defined as a BMI >30)
> 9. Not a candidate for immediate breast reconstruction
> 10. Candidate for nipple-areola skin-sparing mastectomy (because the location of the nipple is below the inframammary fold with the patient sitting, breast size is >700 g, or there are significant contour abnormalities of the nipple-areola complex itself)

- Delayed complications:
  - Asymmetry of the nipples (8%)
  - Infection requiring intravenous antibiotics (5.6%), irrigation of the surgical site (4.2%), or removal of tissue expander/implant/acellular dermal matrix (12.9%); median time to these delayed infections was 7 months (range 1–51 months)
- Assessment of oncologic safety is limited by short mean follow-up of only 22 months (range: <1–57 months), with 93% of intended nipple-sparing mastectomies maintaining their nipples; 4 of 187 nipples (2.1%) were sacrificed for atypia or cancer at the nipple base on pathology

## LESSONS LEARNED

- Nipple-sparing mastectomy is an oncologically safe procedure for women who have or are at high risk for breast cancer. Knowing that the local recurrence rates for skin-sparing mastectomy are comparable with no–skin-sparing mastectomy, logic predicts that the addition of leaving the nipple in situ should have minimal risk of increased local recurrence.

- Stolier and colleagues[43] reported that only 25% of nipples possess a terminal duct lobular unit, which is the progenitor of all breast cancers. More importantly, the terminal duct lobular unit is always found at the base of the nipple, not within the nipple proper.
- This information has led to a change in surgical technique, away from coring out the nipple proper to frozen sections at the base of the nipple alone. Coring of the nipple has been associated with a higher rate of vascular compromise to the nipple. Avoidance of this maneuver has decreased the nipple loss rate (partial and full) as well as the amount of epidermolysis.
- Additional lessons include selecting the appropriate incision, the nipple-sparing mastectomy technique used, and the effects of several patient factors (heavy smoking, diabetes, and large and very ptotic breasts).[44]
- BMI greater than 25 kg/m$^2$ is also associated with an increased risk for complications, including flap necrosis and wound dehiscence; this risk increases as BMI increases.[45] An excised breast mass of greater than 750 g is associated with an overall increase in complications (especially wound dehiscence), and a sternal notch to nipple distance of greater than 25 cm is associated with a general increase in complications.[45]

## LESSONS TO BE LEARNED: IMPACT ON BODY IMAGE AND QUALITY OF LIFE

In addition, to monitor how all of this affects the woman herself, we and others have launched prospective clinical trials evaluating body image, quality of life, and skin/nipple sensation before surgery and after surgery of women having skin-sparing versus nipple-sparing mastectomy to ascertain what impact the nipple itself has on these components. All women enrolled must meet the eligibility criteria outlined in **Box 1**, regardless of which cohort they are assigned to. Such a study is important, because a dearth of literature exists regarding patient satisfaction and sensation of the preserved nipple (**Table 4**).

- In 1 report by Yueh and colleagues,[46] two-thirds of patients reported being satisfied with their aesthetic result.[46] Although 75% reported preservation of nipple sensation, this sensation was rated poorly on a scale of 1 to 10, with a mean of only approximately 3.0.
- In a similar study by Djohan and colleagues,[47] patients self-rated their appearance, symmetry, color, position, and texture of the breast mound, with most of

**Table 4**
**Nipple loss rates, sensation, and cosmetic outcome from nipple-sparing mastectomy**

| Author, Year | Number of Cases | Nipple Loss (%) | Sensation (%) | Cosmesis |
|---|---|---|---|---|
| Garwood,[32] 2009 | 170 NSM | 13 | NR | NR |
| Petit,[39] 2009 | 1001 NSM + ELIOT | Full 3.5, partial 5.5 | Partial 15 | Yes |
| Sookhan,[30] 2008 | 18 NSM | Partial 11 | NR | NR |
| Yueh,[46] 2009 | 17 NSM | Partial 17.6, full 11.8 | Partial 75 | Yes |
| Didier, 2009 | 159 NSM | 0 | 15 | Yes; quality of life, body image |

*Abbreviations:* NR, not reported; NSM, nipple-sparing mastectomy.

the results rated as good or excellent.[47] This finding correlated with independent observers' ratings. However, although preserved sensation was acknowledged by most patients, it was reported to be only fair or poor.

- MD Anderson Cancer Center[48] reported their experience with nipple-sparing mastectomy and noted an evaluation of nipple sensation in terms of responsiveness to touch preoperatively and postoperatively at 6 months and 1 year. Although response time to erection slowed at 6 months (remained constant at 1 year), data are limited by having only 11 evaluable breasts at 1 year. Although most women had displacement of the nipple position (75%) and breast mound (57.6%), resulting in an excellent to very good overall appearance of nipple (23.1%) and mound (34.6%), most women were not at all self-conscious about their dress.

## SUMMARY

Similar studies worldwide will help objectively answer the value of nipple-sparing mastectomy to the woman choosing that operation. From a breast/general surgeon and plastic surgeon's standpoint, the preservation of the nipple is the ultimate in aesthetic outcome for a patient having mastectomy. However, it is technically challenging, and long-term oncologic safety is unknown (albeit predicted to be low risk). Showing the importance of preserving a nipple, whether sensate or not, in women will encourage surgeons to remain steadfast in their learning curve and acquisition of evidence-based data documenting local recurrence, distant metastasis, cosmetic outcomes, patient satisfaction (quality of life, body image, nipple sensation) and complications/risks of this procedure.

## SUPPLEMENTARY DATA

Video related to this article can be found online at http://dx.doi.org/10.1016/j.soc.2014.03.013.

## REFERENCES

1. Wagner FB, Martin RG, Bland KI. History of the therapy of breast disease. In: Bland KI, Copeland EM, editors. The breast. Comprehensive management of benign and malignant diseases. 2nd edition. Philadelphia: WB Saunders; 1991. p. 1–18.
2. Olson JS. Bathsheba's breast. Women, cancer, & history. Baltimore (MD), London: John Hopkins University Press; 2002. p. 9–45.
3. Haagensen CD. Carcinoma of the breast. New York: American Cancer Society; 1950.
4. Lacour J, Bucalossi P, Cacers E, et al. Radical mastectomy vs. radical mastectomy plus internal mammary dissection. Five-year results of an international cooperative study. Cancer 1976;37(1):206–14.
5. Patey DH, Dyson WH. The prognosis of carcinoma of the breast in relation to the type of operation performed. Br J Cancer 1948;2(1):7–13.
6. Freeman BS. Subcutaneous mastectomy for benign breast lesions with immediate or delayed prosthetic replacement. Plast Reconstr Surg Transplant Bull 1962; 30:676–82.
7. Freeman BS. Complications of subcutaneous mastectomy with prosthetic replacement, immediate or delayed. South Med J 1967;60:1277–80.

8. Cucin RL, Guthrie RH Jr, Luterman A, et al. Transplantation of the cryopreserved nipple-areolar complex. Ann Plast Surg 1980;4:391–5.
9. Rose JH Jr. Carcinoma in a transplanted nipple. Arch Surg 1980;115:1131–2.
10. Allison AB, Howorth MG Jr. Carcinoma in a nipple preserved by heterotopic auto-implantation. N Engl J Med 1978;298(20):1132.
11. Wellisch DK, Schain WS, Noone RB, et al. The psychological contribution of nipple addition in breast reconstruction. Plast Reconstr Surg 1987;80:699–704.
12. Toth BA, Lappert P. Modified skin incisions for mastectomy: the need for plastic surgical input in preoperative planning. Plast Reconstr Surg 1991;87(6): 1048–53.
13. Newman LA, Kuerer HM, Hunt KK, et al. Presentation, treatment, and outcome of local recurrence after skin-sparing mastectomy and immediate breast recon-struction. Ann Surg Oncol 1998;5(7):620–6.
14. Carlson GW, Bostwick J, Styblo TM, et al. Skin-sparing mastectomy: oncologic and reconstructive considerations. Ann Surg 1997;225:570–8.
15. Fersis N, Hoenig A, Relakis K, et al. Skin-sparing mastectomy and immediate breast reconstruction: incidence of recurrence in patients with invasive breast cancer. Breast 2004;13(6):488–93.
16. Greenway RM, Schlossberg L, Dooley WC. Fifteen-year series of skin-sparing mastectomy for stage 0 to 2 breast cancer. Am J Surg 2005;190(6):918–22.
17. Kroll SS, Khoo A, Singletary SE, et al. Local recurrence risk after skin-sparing and conventional mastectomy: a 6-year follow-up. Plast Reconstr Surg 1999;104: 421–5.
18. Kroll SS, Schusterman MA, Tadjalli HE, et al. Risk of recurrence after treatment of early breast cancer with skin-sparing mastectomy. Ann Surg Oncol 1997;4: 193–7.
19. Barton FE, English JM, Kingsley WB, et al. Glandular excision in total glandular mastectomy and modified radical mastectomy: a comparison. Plast Reconstr Surg 1991;88(3):389–92 [discussion: 393–4].
20. Laronga C, Kemp B, Johnston D, et al. The incidence of occult nipple-areola complex involvement in breast cancer patients receiving a skin-sparing mastec-tomy. Ann Surg Oncol 1999;6(6):609–13.
21. Simmons RM, Brennan M, Christos P, et al. Analysis of nipple/areolar involvement with mastectomy: can the areola be preserved? Ann Surg Oncol 2002;9:165–8.
22. Lagios MD, Gates EA, Westdahl PR, et al. A guide to the frequency of nipple involvement in breast cancer. A study of 149 consecutive mastectomies using a serial subgross and correlated radiographic technique. Am J Surg 1979; 138(1):135–42.
23. Smith J, Payne WS, Carney JA. Involvement of the nipple and areola in carcinoma of the breast. Surg Gynecol Obstet 1976;1443(4):546–8.
24. Laronga C, Robb GL, Singletary SE. Feasibility of skin-sparing mastectomy with preservation of the nipple-areola complex. Breast Dis Year Bk Q 1998;19(2): 125–7.
25. Petit JY, Veronesi U, Orecchia R, et al. Nipple-sparing mastectomy in association with intra-operative radiotherapy (ELIOT): a new type of mastectomy for breast cancer treatment. Breast Cancer Res Treat 2006;96:47–51.
26. Gerber B, Krause A, Reimer T, et al. Skin-sparing mastectomy with conservation of the nipple-areola complex and autologous reconstruction is an oncologically safe procedure. Ann Surg 2003;238:120–7.
27. Crowe JP Jr, Kim JA, Yetman R, et al. Nipple-sparing mastectomy technique and results of 54 procedures. Arch Surg 2004;139:148–50.

28. Hartmann LC, Schaid DJ, Woods JE, et al. Efficacy of bilateral prophylactic mastectomy in women with a family history of breast cancer. N Engl J Med 1999;340: 77–84.
29. Rebbeck TR, Friebel T, Lynch HT, et al. Bilateral prophylactic mastectomy reduces breast cancer risk in BRCA1 and BRCA2 mutation carriers: The Prose Study Group. J Clin Oncol 2004;22(6):1055–62.
30. Sookhan N, Boughey JC, Walsh MF, et al. Nipple-sparing mastectomy–initial experience at a tertiary center. Am J Surg 2008;196(4):575–7.
31. Voltura AM, Tsangaris TN, Rosson GD, et al. Nipple-sparing mastectomy: critical assessment of 51 procedures and implications for selection criteria. Ann Surg Oncol 2008;15:3396–401.
32. Garwood ER, Moor D, Ewing C, et al. Total skin-sparing mastectomy: complications and local recurrences in 2 cohorts of patients. Ann Surg 2009;249(1): 26–32.
33. Spear S, Hannan C, Wiley S, et al. Nipple sparing mastectomy. Plast Reconstr Surg 2009;123:1665–73.
34. Garcia-Etienne CA, Borgen PI. Update on the indications for nipple-sparing mastectomy. J Support Oncol 2006;4(5):225–30.
35. de Alcantara FP, Capko D, Barry JM, et al. Nipple-sparing mastectomy for breast cancer and risk-reducing surgery: The Memorial Sloan-Kettering Cancer Center experience. Ann Surg Oncol 2011;18(11):3117–22.
36. Kiluk JV, Santillan AA, Kaur P, et al. Feasibility of sentinel lymph node biopsy through an inframammary incision for a nipple sparing mastectomy. Ann Surg Oncol 2009;15(12):3402–6.
37. Benediktsson KP, Perbeck L. Survival in breast cancer after nipple-sparing subcutaneous mastectomy and immediate reconstruction with implants: a prospective trial with 13 years median follow-up in 216 patients. Eur J Surg Oncol 2008;34:143–8.
38. Gerber B, Krause A, Dieterich M, et al. The oncological safety of skin-sparing mastectomy with conservation of the nipple-areola complex and autologous reconstruction: an extended follow-up study. Ann Surg 2009;249(3):461–8.
39. Petit JY, Veronesi U, Orecchia R, et al. Nipple sparing mastectomy with nipple areola intraoperative radiotherapy: one thousand and one cases of a five years experience at the European Institute Of Milan (EIO). Breast Cancer Res Treat 2009;117:333–8.
40. Petit JY. Nipple sparing mastectomy. Presented at the 33rd Annual San Antonio Breast Cancer Symposium. San Antonio, February 10–13, 2011.
41. Veronesi U. Progress in breast cancer management. Presented at the 16th Annual Multidisciplinary Symposium on Breast Disease. Amelia Island, February 11, 2011.
42. Jensen JA, Orringer JS, Giuliano AE. Nipple-sparing mastectomy in 99 patients with a mean follow-up of 5 years. Ann Surg Oncol 2011;18(6):1665–70.
43. Stolier AJ, Sullivan SK, Dellacroce FJ. Technical considerations in nipple-sparing mastectomy: 82 consecutive cases without necrosis. Ann Surg Oncol 2008;15: 1341–7.
44. Salgarello M, Visconti G, Barone-Adesi L. Nipple-sparing mastectomy with immediate implant reconstruction: cosmetic outcomes and technical refinements. Plast Reconstr Surg 2010;126(5):1460–71.
45. Davies K, Allan L, Roblin P, et al. Factors affecting post-operative complications following skin sparing mastectomy with immediate breast reconstruction. Breast 2011;20(1):21–5.

46. Yueh JH, Houlihan MJ, Slavin SA, et al. Nipple sparing mastectomy: evaluation of patient satisfaction, aesthetic results, and sensation. Ann Plast Surg 2009;62: 586–90.
47. Djohan R, Gage E, Gatherwright J, et al. Patient satisfaction following nipple-sparing mastectomy and immediate breast reconstruction: an 8-year outcome study. Plast Reconstr Surg 2010;125:818–29.
48. Wagner JL, Fearmonti R, Hunt KK, et al. Prospective evaluation of the nipple-areola complex sparing mastectomy for risk reduction and for early-stage breast cancer. Ann Surg Oncol 2012;19(4):1137–44.

# Basal-Like and Triple-Negative Breast Cancers

## Searching for Positives Among Many Negatives

Prasanna Alluri, MD, PhD[a], Lisa A. Newman, MD, MPH[b],*

KEYWORDS

• Triple-negative breast cancer • Breast cancer subtypes • Basal breast cancer

KEY POINTS

- Triple-negative breast cancers (TNBC) are defined as invasive breast cancers that fail to express the estrogen receptor, the progesterone receptor, and the HER2/*neu* marker.
- TNBC and the basal breast cancer subtype (defined by genetic profile) share similarities but are not synonymous.
- The TNBC category includes a spectrum of histopathologically and genetically diverse range of tumors.
- TNBC tend to be more challenging to treat because they are more likely to be of a basal subtype, and because they cannot be manipulated with either endocrine therapy or targeted anti-HER2/*neu* treatments.

## INTRODUCTION

Triple-negative breast cancers (TNBC) are a heterogeneous group of tumors defined by negative immunohistochemical staining for estrogen receptor (ER) and progesterone receptor (PR), and lack of human epidermal growth factor receptor 2 (HER2/*neu*) overexpression.[1] TNBC is often used as a surrogate for identifying the aggressive basal breast cancer subtype, and although the 2 patterns share many similarities, they are not biologically synonymous. The basal subtype is defined by a distinct gene-expression signature characterized by strong expression of basal markers such as cytokeratins 5, 6, and 17, and also encompasses a diverse group of tumors.[2] Both basal-like breast cancers and TNBC are associated with poor clinical outcomes and show disproportionately higher prevalence in women of African descent.[3] Intense investigations are currently under way to study the underlying molecular pathways that

Dr Alluri was partly supported by the National Institutes of Health (T32 CA009672).
[a] Department of Radiation Oncology, University of Michigan, Ann Arbor, MI, USA; [b] Breast Care Center, University of Michigan Comprehensive Cancer Center, 1500 East Medical Center Drive, Ann Arbor, MI 48167, USA
* Corresponding author.
*E-mail address:* lanewman@umich.edu

Surg Oncol Clin N Am 23 (2014) 567–577
http://dx.doi.org/10.1016/j.soc.2014.03.003
1055-3207/14/$ – see front matter © 2014 Elsevier Inc. All rights reserved.

drive the growth and dissemination of these tumors and to develop effective targeted therapies against them.

In one of the earliest illustrations of the utility of gene-expression analyses in unmasking the heterogeneity of a disease process, Sorlie and colleagues[4] used cDNA microarrays to classify breast carcinomas into 5 subtypes that correlated highly significantly with clinical outcomes, including overall survival and recurrence-free survival. These subtypes, in addition to a normal breast-like group, included luminal A and luminal B tumors that encompassed the ER-positive cancers, the ERBB2+ subtype characterized by high expression of ERBB2 and a basal-like subtype that shows high expression of basal markers. Luminal A tumors are the most commonly diagnosed subtype among all breast cancers (40%) and, fortunately, also carry the best prognosis. Luminal B tumors are less common (20%) and differ from the luminal A subtype in having relatively lower expression of ER (while still being ER-positive) and higher expression of proliferation-related genes. The ERBB2+ subtype comprises approximately 15% of breast cancers, and shows high expression of ERBB2 cluster and proliferation-related genes. Finally, the basal subtype constitutes 15% to 20% of breast cancers and is characterized by expression of basal epithelial markers such as keratin 5 and 17, laminin, and fatty acid binding protein 7, and low expression of luminal genes.

Because performing gene-expression analysis on clinical samples is resource and time intensive, simpler immunohistochemical methods were developed to determine the ER, PR, and ERBB2 expression status to categorize tumors into various subtypes that guide treatment decisions. Such subtyping not only provides prognostic information, but also allows tailoring of the therapy to target the specific oncogenic drivers such as estrogen signaling and ERBB2 pathways that drive the growth and dissemination of the tumors. It is this immunohistochemical classification based on ER, PR, and ERBB2 expression status that led to the introduction of the term triple-negative to refer to cancers that are negative for all 3 of these markers.[1] The term also underscores the lack of effective targeted therapies for triple-negative disease that have otherwise revolutionized the treatment of breast cancer.

## CLINICAL AND HISTOPATHOLOGIC FEATURES

It must be borne in mind that although the terms triple-negative and basal-like breast cancer are used interchangeably, they are not synonymous. A variety of prognostically diverse histopathologic patterns are more likely to be triple-negative, further underscoring the heterogeneity of this breast cancer subset. For example, the prognostically favorable medullary and secretory tumors, in addition to the biologically aggressive metaplastic breast cancers, are associated with increased frequency of triple negativity.

In a study aimed at determining the concordance rate between TNBC and the basal breast cancer subtype, Bertucci and colleagues[5] reported that 71% of TNBC were found to be basal-like while 77% of basal-like cancers were triple-negative in nature. Furthermore, because TNBC is a diagnosis of exclusion defined by the lack of expression of certain markers rather than by the presence of any unifying features, it remains a heterogeneous disease entity that presents a formidable challenge to developing effective treatments.[3] Similarly, the basal type has been reported to encompass a diverse array of tumors.

Breast cancers of both basal-like and triple-negative types are associated with aggressive pathologic features and poor clinical outcomes. In a study of 1601 women diagnosed with breast cancer between January 1987 and December 1997 at the

Women's College Hospital in Toronto, Dent and colleagues[6] noted that patients diagnosed with triple-negative disease had younger mean age at diagnosis (53.0 vs 57.7 years) and were more likely to have grade III (66% vs 28%) and larger tumors (mean tumor size of 3.0 vs 2.1 cm) when compared with patients diagnosed with non-TNBC. Furthermore, unlike other breast cancers, TNBC did not show a clear association between tumor size and positive lymph node status. For instance, the risk of lymph node positivity was 19.3%, 39.3%, and 59.5% for tumors less than 1 cm, 1 to 2 cm, and 2 to 5 cm in size, respectively, for non-TNBC. Lymph node positivity for similarly sized triple-negative tumors was 55.6%, 55.6%, and 48.9%, respectively.[6] On the other hand, data also support the prognostic advantage of screening and early detection of TNBC. A study from Memorial Sloan-Kettering Cancer Center reported on nearly 200 cases of node-negative, subcentimenter TNBC. More than two-thirds were screen-detected, and 5-year overall survival rates were excellent (>90%) regardless of whether adjuvant chemotherapy was delivered.[7]

Compared with other breast cancer patterns, TNBC are more likely to be occult on mammography and ultrasonography imaging (36% vs 36%). In a study of 95 interval cancers (ie, breast cancers that develop between screening intervals) diagnosed between 1996 and 2001 as part of a population-based Norwegian Breast Cancer Screening Program, Collett and colleagues[8] noted that patients with interval cancers were more likely to be younger and have ER-negative tumors, basal epithelial phenotype, and dense breasts in comparison with patients with size-matched screen-detected tumors.

Dent and colleagues[6] also noted that patients with TNBC had a shorter median time to death (4.2 vs 6 years), higher propensity for distant recurrence (33.9% vs 20.4%), and shorter mean time to local (2.8 vs 4.2 years) and distant recurrences (2.6 vs 5.0 years) compared with those with other breast cancers. Intriguingly, all deaths in the triple-negative group occurred within 10 years of diagnosis, whereas deaths attributable to other breast cancers continued to accrue up to 18 years after diagnosis. Furthermore, patients with TNBC had higher rates of recurrence in the first 4 years after diagnosis, but this risk declined rapidly after 5 years, and no distant recurrences occurred after 8 years of follow-up. These differences in the patterns of recurrence suggest that the biology of TNBC is likely distinct from other breast cancers. This indication is further corroborated by the observation that the distant sites in TNBC with propensity for recurrence were different from those of other breast cancers.[3] Bone (40%) and liver (30%) are the most common sites of first distant recurrence in non-TNBC, whereas recurrence at these sites is less common in triple-negative disease (10% and 20%, respectively). Instead, distant recurrence in lung (40%) and brain (30%) is more common in TNBC.

## EPIDEMIOLOGY AND RISK FACTORS

Of interest, more than 75% of BRCA1 mutation-carrying patients with breast cancer were found to have triple-negative and/or basal-like phenotype.[9] On the other hand, in patients with a TNBC phenotype, the prevalence of BRCA1 mutations has been found to range from 6.5% to 34.4%.[10] The close correlation between TNBC and BRCA1 mutation-carrier status has led to revised, updated recommendations for genetic counseling and testing among TNBC patients. Patients younger than 50 years diagnosed with TNBC are now routinely recommended to undergo genetic counseling and BRCA mutation testing regardless of whether they have a family history of breast/ovarian cancer, and some centers refer TNBC patients for genetic counseling at any age.[11–13]

Other risk factors for triple-negative and/or basal-like breast cancers include higher body mass index and waist-to-hip circumference ratio, higher parity, and lower duration of breastfeeding.[14,15] It has become clear that reproductive risk factors that historically have been associated with increasing risk for breast cancer (nulliparity; later age at first childbirth) are primarily responsible for higher population-level burden of ER-positive breast cancer. By contrast, multiparity appears to increase the risk for TNBC.[14,16]

The epidemiology of TNBC has attracted significant attention following the observation that racial background may be an independent risk factor for this disease. Initial evidence for such a relationship came from population-based case-control studies such as the Carolina Breast Cancer Study, which showed that basal-like breast cancers were more prevalent among premenopausal African American women.[17] In a subsequent study, Kurian and colleagues[18] determined the lifetime risk of TNBC across various racial/ethnic groups based on data from breast cancers diagnosed in California from 2006 to 2007, and noted that it was highest among African American women (1.98%) and lowest among Asian women (0.77%). Hispanic women (1.04%) and white women (1.25%) had intermediate risk in this study.

In a recent study, the authors carried out a large population-based study on the incidence rates of breast cancer among white, Hispanic, and African American women by analyzing the California Cancer Registry data from 1988 to 2006.[19] The analysis encompassed a total of 375,761 cases of invasive breast cancer, and demonstrated that whereas White Americans had the highest lifetime incidence of breast cancer among the 3 study groups, African American women had the highest incidence of triple-negative disease across all age categories. Incidence rates of stage III and stage IV disease were highest for African American women. For women younger than 44 years, population-based incidence rates of breast cancer were also highest for African American women. Because the risk of TNBC is particularly prominent for African American women younger than 50 years, the study argues that mammographic screening to aid in the early detection of this biologically aggressive disease is particularly relevant among younger African American women. This concept therefore argues against widespread adoption of the 2009 United States Preventive Services Task Force recommendation to delay initiation of screening mammography until the age of 50 years.[20]

The strikingly higher prevalence of triple-negative disease among African American women along with a disproportionately high mortality rate prompted speculation that African ancestry may be an independent risk factor for TNBC. For instance, African Americans account for 8% of all estimated new cases of breast cancer in the United States, but account for 13% of all estimated deaths related to breast cancer. Although in part this is likely related to socioeconomic factors and reduced access to care, the authors hypothesized that African ancestry may contribute to certain unique risk factors that affect breast cancer–specific mortality. In initial work, the authors reviewed the English-language literature on breast cancer published between 1988 and 2004 in the Gold Coast region of Africa (where most of the colonial slave trade occurred).[21] Women from sub-Saharan Africa were found to have a lower incidence of breast cancer, but the average age at diagnosis was around 10 years lower in comparison with patients with breast cancer from Western nations. The African patients also had more advanced disease and a higher mortality rate.

In a subsequent study, the authors examined the prevalence of triple-negative breast disease among white American (n = 1008) and African American women (n = 581) diagnosed with invasive breast cancer between January 1, 2001 and December 31, 2007 at the Henry Ford Health System in Detroit, Michigan, and compared it with prevalence in a study population comprising African women (n = 75) with invasive breast cancer diagnosed or treated at the Komfo Anokye Teaching Hospital, Ghana between January 1, 2007 and December, 31 2008.[22] A dramatically higher proportion of triple-negative disease was observed among the African cohort (82%) than in the African American (26%) or white American (16%) women. The mean age at the time of diagnosis was 48.0 years for Ghanaian women, 60.7 years for African American women, and 62.4 years for white American women. The mean size of primary breast tumor was 3.2 cm, 2.3 cm, and 1.95 cm for Ghanaian, African American, and white American women, respectively. Although the study cohort from Ghana was from a single institution with a relatively small sample size and, thus, subject to selection bias, such a high proportion of triple-negative disease was nevertheless striking. At present, larger multi-institutional studies are under way in Ghana to validate these findings.

Nevertheless, other studies have reported a high proportion of ER-negative and triple-negative disease among African women. For instance, Huo and colleagues[23] looked at the distribution of various molecular subtypes of breast cancer among 507 patients diagnosed with breast cancer in multiple geographic locations in Nigeria and Senegal between 1996 and 2007. The investigators noted that hormone-receptor–negative cancer was predominant and the proportions of ER-positive, PR-positive, and HER2-positive tumors were 24%, 20%, and 17%, respectively. Furthermore, most patients presented with large (4.4 cm) and high-grade tumors (83%), and positive lymph nodes (72%). The mean age at presentation was 44.8 years. Burson and colleagues[24] reviewed the medical records of all patients with breast cancer receiving treatment at Ocean Road Cancer Institute in Tanzania between July 2007 and June 2009, and found that most of the patients had stage III and IV disease and that more than 49% of patients were ER-negative and PR-negative.

To further investigate the molecular basis for the biological aggressiveness of breast cancer in African women, the authors evaluated the expression of aldehyde dehydrogenase 1 (ALDH1) in breast tissue obtained from 173 Ghanaian women receiving treatment at Komfo Anokye Teaching Hospital, Ghana between 2006 and 2010. Among the women with invasive breast cancer, 56.3% had triple-negative disease and 75.7% had ER-negative breast cancer.[25] Interestingly the triple-negative subtype had statistically significantly higher expression of ALDH1 expression when compared with non–triple-negative subtypes. High ALDH1 expression has previously been associated with aggressive features such as high histologic grade, high mitotic rate, and ER/PR negativity.[26]

The strong association between African ancestry and TNBC led investigations to look for inheritable risk factors that account for such a high prevalence in this group. In one such study aimed at searching for risk alleles that differed significantly in frequency between African American and European American women and that contribute to specific breast cancer phenotypes that do not express ER and PR, Fejeman and colleagues[27] performed whole-genome admixture scanning and typing of approximately 1500 ancestry-informative markers after pooling 6 population-based studies of 1484 African American women with invasive breast cancer. The association between breast cancer predisposition loci and disease phenotypes was investigated, whereby significant ancestral differences between ER-positive PR-positive and ER-negative PR-negative breast cancers were found. After controlling for other confounders, patients with ER-positive PR-positive breast cancers and localized tumors were found to have higher European ancestry. Although no specific loci that contribute to differences in the observed risk were identified, more advanced approaches with better resolution, such as whole-genome sequencing technologies, may shed light on the genetic basis of racial differences in prevalence of TNBC. Similarly, Palmer and colleagues[28] found genetically defined African ancestry to be associated with the risk for TNBC in a nested case-control breast cancer study from the Black Women's Health Study.

## TARGETED THERAPIES

The advent of highly effective targeted therapies against ER-positive and HER2-positive breast cancers has dramatically improved clinical outcomes in breast cancer. However, targeted therapies for TNBC remain elusive, and chemotherapy remains the only systemic treatment option at present. No appreciable improvements in survival have been achieved for this patient population over the last few decades. This section reviews recent advances in the development of targeted therapies for TNBC.

### Poly(ADP-Ribose) Polymerase Inhibition

Studies of carriers of germline BRCA1 mutations have shown that these patients predominately have a basal-like and triple-negative phenotype.[9] Furthermore, although most basal-like breast cancers do not carry BRCA1 mutations, a high degree of BRCA1 dysfunction with lower levels of BRCA1 mRNA expression was reported in this group in comparison with matched controls.[29] The specific susceptibility of BRCA-deficient tumors to poly(ADP-ribose) polymerase (PARP) inhibitors has generated interest in evaluating the efficacy of PARP inhibitors in basal-like breast cancer and TNBC. The safety and efficacy of PARP inhibition with oral dosing of olaparib as a single agent has previously been demonstrated in a phase 2 multicenter clinical trial comprising patients with advanced breast cancer with BRCA1 or BRCA2 mutations.[30] The term synthetic lethality is often used to describe the specific susceptibility of BRCA-deficient tumors to PARP inhibition.[31] PARP is an important mediator of genomic stability and is important for repair of DNA single-strand breaks (SSBs) by base excision repair.[32] However, normal cells can withstand PARP inhibition by upregulating homologous recombination (HR), which serves as an alternative error-free DNA repair pathway. Thus, unrepaired SSBs as a result of PARP inhibition collapse replication forks into double-strand breaks (DSBs), which are repaired by BRCA-mediated HR. However, PARP inhibition on a background of deficient HR results in synthetic lethality secondary to accumulation of DNA SSBs and DSBs. Consistent with this hypothesis, in preclinical studies TNBC cells were found to be more sensitive than non-TNBC cells to PARP inhibition, both as a single agent and in combination with gemcitabine and cisplatin.[33] This initial promise promoted clinical evaluation of PARP inhibitors in TNBC. In an open-label phase 2 clinical trial, iniparib, a small-molecule PARP inhibitor, was evaluated in combination with gemcitabine and carboplatin in metastatic TNBC.[34] The combination regimen was found to improve the overall response from 32% to 52%, and prolonged median progression-free survival from 3.6 to 5.9 months and median overall survival from 7.7 to 12.3 months. A follow-up phase 3 clinical trial, however, did not demonstrate any improvement in overall survival. Furthermore, there is controversy surrounding the mechanism of action of iniparib, and the target of this drug remains to be identified. At present, there are multiple clinical trials under way evaluating the clinical efficacy of olaparib in combination with chemotherapy, although a phase 2 study of olaparib as monotherapy in heavily pretreated metastatic TNBC did not show any response.[35]

### Epidermal Growth Factor Receptor Inhibition

The epidermal growth factor receptor (EGFR) is a transmembrane receptor tyrosine kinase that has been shown to be highly expressed in basal-like tumors. For instance,

Nielsen and colleagues[36] used breast carcinoma tissue microarrays from 930 patients, and noted that EGFR expression was observed in 54% of basal-like tumors (vs 11% of non–basal-like tumors) and was a predictor of poor survival independent of nodal status and tumor size. Similarly, EGFR expression was found to be high in basal-like cell lines but low in luminal cell lines. Furthermore, basal-like breast cancer cell lines were found to be more sensitive than luminal cell lines to EGFR inhibition. These findings suggested that EGFR could serve as a targeted therapy for treatment of basal-like breast cancers. In a randomized phase 2 clinical trial, Carey and colleagues[37] evaluated cetuximab, an anti-EGFR monoclonal antibody, as a single agent and in combination with carboplatin in metastatic TNBC. Unfortunately, the response rate in this study was only 6% to cetuximab and 17% for the cetuximab and carboplatin combination. The time to progression and overall survival were short, at 2.1 months and 10.4 months, respectively. Among 16 patients who had tumor biopsies before and 1 week after therapy, activation of the EGFR pathway was noted in 13 patients. However, therapy-induced inhibition of the EGFR pathway was detected in only 5 patients. Given the known efficacy of cetuximab on EGFR, it is likely that constitutive/non–ligand-dependent pathways of EGFR activation may exist in TNBC. Therefore, downstream mediators of the EGFR pathway may be necessary to derive therapeutic benefit. In BALI-1, a randomized phase 2 clinical trial, Baselga and colleagues[38] compared cisplatin with cisplatin and cetuximab for the treatment of metastatic TNBC. Although the overall response rate was improved with the addition of cetuximab (20% vs 10% for cisplatin alone), there was no statistically significant improvement in overall survival. At present, several small-molecule inhibitors of EGFR are in various stages of preclinical and clinical development.[35]

### Angiogenesis Inhibitors

TNBCs are highly vascular, and studies have shown higher levels of expression of vascular endothelial growth factor (VEGF) in TNBC in comparison with non-TNBC.[39] This finding prompted clinical evaluation of VEGF inhibitors in this subgroup of cancers. In a meta-analysis of patients with TNBC from 3 randomized phase 3 trials (E2100, AVADO, and RIBBON-1) of bevacizumab, a monoclonal VEGF antibody, in combination with standard chemotherapeutic agents versus chemotherapy alone as first-line therapy for metastatic breast cancer, O'Shaughnessy and colleagues[40] reported that the addition of bevacizumab improved objective response rate (42% vs 23%) and median progression-free survival (8.1 months vs 5.4 months), but with no statistically significant improvement in overall survival. Brufsky and colleagues[41] reported on a subgroup analysis of the TNBC patient subset of the RIBBON-2 trial, which evaluated the efficacy of bevacizumab in combination with chemotherapy versus chemotherapy alone as second-line therapy for metastatic breast cancer. The investigators reported an improvement in progression-free survival with the combination regimen compared with chemotherapy alone (6.0 vs 2.7 months), with a trend toward improvement in overall survival. However, 2 large randomized clinical trials evaluating the efficacy of bevacizumab in combination with chemotherapy in the neoadjuvant setting produced contrasting results. A large phase 3 clinical trial (BEATRICE Study) evaluating bevacizumab in combination with chemotherapy in the adjuvant setting for TNBC patients is currently under way. However, the recent withdrawal of approval of bevacizumab for the treatment of advanced breast cancer, owing to concerns of significant toxicity, cast a shadow on the safety of this agent in TNBC patients.

In addition to the agents already discussed, several novel targeted therapies for TNBC are at various stages of development, including inhibitors for various pathways/targets such as the PI3K/AKT/mTOR pathway, Hedgehog signaling pathway, Notch signaling pathway, apoptotic pathways, HSP90, JAK2, and androgen receptor.[35,42]

The failure of various targeted therapies to show significant efficacy in clinical trials despite strong preclinical data underscores the challenges that lie ahead for improving clinical outcomes in TNBC. The heterogeneity within the triple-negative and basal-like tumors certainly serves as a major impediment to developing therapies that are efficacious for the entire group. In a genomic landscape study of 104 cases of primary TNBC, Shah and colleagues[43] noted that these cancers exhibited a very broad spectrum of genomic evolution and varied widely in their clonal frequencies. In a study aimed at further subtyping TNBC and identifying "driver" signaling pathways that could be pharmacologically targeted, Lehmann and colleagues[44] analyzed gene-expression profiles of 587 TNBC cases from 21 breast cancer data sets, and used cluster analysis to identify 6 unique TNBC subtypes: basal-like 1 and 2 (BL1 and BL2), immunomodulatory (IM), mesenchymal (M), mesenchymal stem-like (MSL), and luminal androgen receptor (LAR) subtypes. Each of these TNBC subtypes were then matched up with TNBC cell-line models that were representative based on gene-expression analysis. The efficacy of various chemotherapeutic agents and selective inhibitors that target the driver signaling pathways was then evaluated for each subtype. BL1 and BL2 subtypes were characterized by higher expression of cell-cycle and DNA damage response genes, and representative cell lines showed preferential response to cisplatin. M and MSL subtype cell models responded to PI3K/mTOR and abl/src inhibitors, and showed enrichment for genes involved in epithelial-mesenchymal transition and growth-factor pathways. The IM subtype, as the name suggested, showed upregulation of immune signaling pathways. The LAR subtype was characterized by androgen receptor (AR) signaling and decreased relapse-free survival, and representative cell lines were sensitive to the AR antagonist bicalutamide.

The general utility of this approach has been validated in other studies. Speers and colleagues[45] identified distinct kinase expression signatures based on gene-expression microarray analysis, and subtyped ER-negative breast cancers into 4 clusters: cell-cycle regulatory cluster, S6 kinase regulatory cluster, immunomodulatory kinase-expressing cluster, and mitogen-activated protein kinase pathway cluster. In patient survival analyses, these clusters conferred differential survival, with the S6 kinase pathway cluster showing the least favorable prognosis and the immunomodulatory kinase-expressing cluster showing the most favorable prognosis. The investigators went on to identify a panel of breast cancer cell lines with matching kinase expression profile for each of the clusters, and performed kinase knockdown studies to show that many of the overexpressed kinases were necessary for the growth of ER-negative breast cancer cell lines but not ER-positive cell lines.

In a related but slightly different approach, Kothari and colleagues[46] analyzed the transcriptome data from a compendium of 482 cancer and benign samples, including breast cancer, generated by RNA sequencing, to identify "individual sample-specific outlier kinases." An outlier was defined as a kinase with the highest level of absolute expression in a sample compared with the rest of kinome and the highest level of differential expression when compared with the median level of expression of that particular kinase across the compendium. This approach ensures that kinases that are highly overexpressed in only a subset of samples are prioritized and not lost in the noise when their expression is averaged across the whole compendium. The investigators hypothesized that the extremely high level of expression of the outliers is due to their clonal selection, and imparts dependence on the growth of the tumor. Consistent with this hypothesis, they identified several sample-specific outlier kinases, including in TNBC clinical samples and cell lines. Targeting of the outlier kinases with available inhibitors was shown to result in growth inhibition in both cell lines and xenograft models. Clinical evaluation of such highly personalized treatment approaches for TNBC remains a goal for the future.

## SUMMARY

Despite tremendous advances in targeted therapy for breast cancer that have revolutionized clinical care, effective treatment of triple-negative and basal-like breast cancers remains a major challenge. At present, chemotherapy remains the only systemic treatment option for these disease subtypes. Undoubtedly, clinical evaluation of novel targeted therapeutic agents will remain a priority. The failure of some of these agents such as PARP inhibitors and EGFR inhibitors to show efficacy in advanced stages of clinical trials, despite their early promise in preclinical studies, casts doubt on whether a magic bullet for triple-negative disease will ever be a reality. Nevertheless, development of reliable biomarkers that predict susceptibility to these agents in subsets of patients with triple-negative and basal-like breast cancers may allow the design of more effective clinical trials in the future. Furthermore, highly personalized treatment approaches such as kinase outlier profile analyses, which attempt to identify putative oncogenic targets that are essential for the growth of these tumors at an individual patient level, may be necessary to treat this highly aggressive and biologically heterogeneous group of diseases. Although the clinical effectiveness of these approaches remains to be determined, the success of such approaches could herald a new era in the arena of personalized medicine and precision therapy. Until then, the search for positives among many negatives of triple-negative and basal-like breast cancers continues.

## REFERENCES

1. Brenton JD, Carey LA, Ahmed AA, et al. Molecular classification and molecular forecasting of breast cancer: ready for clinical application? J Clin Oncol 2005; 23(29):7350–60.
2. Perou CM, Sorlie T, Eisen MB, et al. Molecular portraits of human breast tumours. Nature 2000;406(6797):747–52.
3. Foulkes WD, Smith IE, Reis-Filho JS. Triple-negative breast cancer. N Engl J Med 2010;363(20):1938–48.
4. Sorlie T, Perou CM, Tibshirani R, et al. Gene expression patterns of breast carcinomas distinguish tumor subclasses with. Proc Natl Acad Sci U S A 2001;98(19): 10869–74.
5. Bertucci F, Finetti P, Cervera N, et al. How basal are triple-negative breast cancers? Int J Cancer 2008;123(1):236–40.
6. Dent R, Trudeau M, Pritchard KI, et al. Triple-negative breast cancer: clinical features and patterns of recurrence. Clin Cancer Res 2007;13(15 Pt 1):4429–34.
7. Ho AY, Gupta G, King TA, et al. Favorable prognosis in patients with T1a/T1bN0 triple-negative breast cancers treated with multimodality therapy. Cancer 2012; 118(20):4944–52.
8. Collett K, Stefansson IM, Eide J, et al. A basal epithelial phenotype is more frequent in interval breast cancers compared with screen detected tumors. Cancer Epidemiol Biomarkers Prev 2005;14(5):1108–12.
9. Foulkes WD, Stefansson IM, Chappuis PO, et al. Germline BRCA1 mutations and a basal epithelial phenotype in breast cancer. J Natl Cancer Inst 2003;95(19): 1482–5.

10. Hartman AR, Kaldate RR, Sailer LM, et al. Prevalence of BRCA mutations in an unselected population of triple-negative breast cancer. Cancer 2012;118(11): 2787–95.
11. Hutchinson L. Screening: BRCA testing in women younger than 50 with triple-negative breast cancer is cost effective. Nat Rev Clin Oncol 2010;7(11):611.
12. Andres R, Pajares I, Balmana J, et al. Association of BRCA1 germline mutations in young onset triple-negative breast cancer (TNBC). Clin Transl Oncol 2014;16(3): 280–4.
13. Rummel S, Varner E, Shriver CD, et al. Evaluation of BRCA1 mutations in an unselected patient population with triple-negative breast cancer. Breast Cancer Res Treat 2013;137(1):119–25.
14. Millikan RC, Newman B, Tse CK, et al. Epidemiology of basal-like breast cancer. Breast Cancer Res Treat 2008;109(1):123–39.
15. Yang XR, Sherman ME, Rimm DL, et al. Differences in risk factors for breast cancer molecular subtypes in a population-based study. Cancer Epidemiol Biomarkers Prev 2007;16(3):439–43.
16. Phipps AI, Chlebowski RT, Prentice R, et al. Reproductive history and oral contraceptive use in relation to risk of triple-negative breast cancer. J Natl Cancer Inst 2011;103(6):470–7.
17. Carey LA, Perou CM, Livasy CA, et al. Race, breast cancer subtypes, and survival in the Carolina Breast Cancer Study. JAMA 2006;295(21):2492–502.
18. Kurian AW, Fish K, Shema SJ, et al. Lifetime risks of specific breast cancer subtypes among women in four racial/ethnic groups. Breast Cancer Res 2010;12(6):R99.
19. Amirikia KC, Mills P, Bush J, et al. Higher population-based incidence rates of triple-negative breast cancer among young African-American women: implications for breast cancer screening recommendations. Cancer 2011;117(12): 2747–53.
20. Nelson HD, Tyne K, Naik A, et al. Screening for breast cancer: an update for the U.S. Preventive Services Task Force. Ann Intern Med 2009;151(10):727–37 W237–42.
21. Fregene A, Newman LA. Breast cancer in sub-Saharan Africa: how does it relate to breast cancer in African-American women? Cancer 2005;103(8):1540–50.
22. Stark A, Kleer CG, Martin I, et al. African ancestry and higher prevalence of triple-negative breast cancer: findings from an international study. Cancer 2010; 116(21):4926–32.
23. Huo D, Ikpatt F, Khramtsov A, et al. Population differences in breast cancer: survey in indigenous African women. J Clin Oncol 2009;27(27):4515–21.
24. Burson AM, Soliman AS, Ngoma TA, et al. Clinical and epidemiologic profile of breast cancer in Tanzania. Breast Dis 2010;31(1):33–41.
25. Schwartz T, Stark A, Pang J, et al. Expression of aldehyde dehydrogenase 1 as a marker of mammary stem cells in benign and malignant breast lesions of Ghanaian women. Cancer 2013;119(3):488–94.
26. Resetkova E, Reis-Filho JS, Jain RK, et al. Prognostic impact of ALDH1 in breast cancer: a story of stem cells and tumor microenvironment. Breast Cancer Res Treat 2010;123(1):97–108.
27. Fejerman L, Haiman CA, Reich D, et al. An admixture scan in 1,484 African American women with breast cancer. Cancer Epidemiol Biomarkers Prev 2009;18(11): 3110–7.
28. Palmer JR, Ruiz-Narvaez EA, Rotimi CN, et al. Genetic susceptibility loci for subtypes of breast cancer in an African American population. Cancer Epidemiol Biomarkers Prev 2013;22(1):127–34.

29. Turner NC, Reis-Filho JS, Russell AM, et al. BRCA1 dysfunction in sporadic basal-like breast cancer. Oncogene 2007;26(14):2126–32.
30. Tutt A, Robson M, Garber JE, et al. Oral poly(ADP-ribose) polymerase inhibitor olaparib in patients with BRCA1 or BRCA2 mutations and advanced breast cancer: a proof-of-concept trial. Lancet 2010;376(9737):235–44.
31. Hiller DJ, Chu QD. Current Status of Poly(ADP-ribose) polymerase inhibitors as novel therapeutic agents for triple-negative breast cancer. Int J Breast Cancer 2012;2012:829315.
32. Dantzer F, de La Rubia G, Menissier-De Murcia J, et al. Base excision repair is impaired in mammalian cells lacking Poly(ADP-ribose). Biochemistry 2000; 39(25):7559–69.
33. Hastak K, Alli E, Ford JM. Synergistic chemosensitivity of triple-negative breast cancer cell lines to poly(ADP-Ribose) polymerase inhibition, gemcitabine, and cisplatin. Cancer Res 2010;70(20):7970–80.
34. O'Shaughnessy J, Osborne C, Pippen JE, et al. Iniparib plus chemotherapy in metastatic triple-negative breast cancer. N Engl J Med 2011;364(3):205–14.
35. Crown J, O'Shaughnessy J, Gullo G. Emerging targeted therapies in triple-negative breast cancer. Ann Oncol 2012;23(Suppl 6):vi56–65.
36. Nielsen TO, Hsu FD, Jensen K, et al. Immunohistochemical and clinical characterization of the basal-like subtype of. Clin Cancer Res 2004;10(16):5367–74.
37. Carey LA, Rugo HS, Marcom PK, et al. TBCRC 001: randomized phase II study of cetuximab in combination with carboplatin in stage IV triple-negative breast cancer. J Clin Oncol 2012;30(21):2615–23.
38. Baselga J, Gómez P, Greil R, et al. Randomized phase II study of the anti-epidermal growth factor receptor monoclonal antibody cetuximab with cisplatin versus cisplatin alone in patients with metastatic triple-negative breast cancer. J Clin Oncol 2013;31(20):2586–92.
39. Linderholm BK, Hellborg H, Johansson U, et al. Significantly higher levels of vascular endothelial growth factor (VEGF) and shorter survival times for patients with primary operable triple-negative breast cancer. Ann Oncol 2009;20(10): 1639–46.
40. O'Shaughnessy J, Romieu G, Diéras V, et al. Meta-analysis of patients with triple-negative breast cancer (TNBC) from three randomized trials of first-line bevacizumab (BV) and chemotherapy treatment for metastatic breast cancer (MBC). Cancer Res 2010;70(Suppl 24). [Abstract P6-12-03].
41. Brufsky A, Valero V, Tiangco B, et al. Second-line bevacizumab-containing therapy in patients with triple-negative breast cancer: subgroup analysis of the RIBBON-2 trial. Breast Cancer Res Treat 2012;133(3):1067–75.
42. O'Toole SA, Beith JM, Millar EK, et al. Therapeutic targets in triple negative breast cancer. J Clin Pathol 2013;66(6):530–42.
43. Shah SP, Roth A, Goya R, et al. The clonal and mutational evolution spectrum of primary triple-negative breast cancers. Nature 2012;486(7403):395–9.
44. Lehmann BD, Bauer JA, Chen X, et al. Identification of human triple-negative breast cancer subtypes and preclinical models for selection of targeted therapies. J Clin Invest 2011;121(7):2750–67.
45. Speers C, Tsimelzon A, Sexton K, et al. Identification of novel kinase targets for the treatment of estrogen. Clin Cancer Res 2009;15(20):6327–40.
46. Kothari V, Wei I, Shankar S, et al. Outlier kinase expression by RNA sequencing as targets for precision therapy. Cancer Discov 2013;3(3):280–93.

# Breast Cancer Disparities
## High-Risk Breast Cancer and African Ancestry

Lisa A. Newman, MD, MPH

## KEYWORDS

- African American • African ancestry • Breast cancer disparities
- Triple-negative breast cancer • Breast cancer subtypes

## KEY POINTS

- Population-based lifetime breast cancer incidence rates are lower for African American women than for white/Caucasian American women.
- Breast cancer mortality rates are higher in African American women than in white/Caucasian American women, and this difference is partially explained by socioeconomic disparities resulting in delayed diagnoses and suboptimal treatment in the African American community.
- Women with African ancestry (African American and Africans) are more likely to be diagnosed with early onset/premenopausal and triple-negative breast cancer (TNBC) than women with Caucasian/European background.
- Male breast cancer is more frequent in populations with African ancestry.
- Genotyping for ancestry informative markers may inform the discussion of how African ancestry may be related to hereditary susceptibility for triple-negative, early onset, and male breast cancer.

## INTRODUCTION

Differences in breast cancer burden (represented by incidence and mortality rates) between white/Caucasian Americans and African Americans have been recognized and documented in the United States during the past several decades. These race/ethnicity-related differences are summarized as follows:

1. Population-based incidence rates for breast cancer are lower in African American women than in white/Caucasian American women.
2. The stage distribution for breast cancer is more advanced in African American women than in white/Caucasian American women.

The author has nothing to disclose.
Breast Care Center, University of Michigan Comprehensive Cancer Center, 1500 East Medical Center Drive, Ann Arbor, MI 48167, USA
*E-mail address:* lanewman@umich.edu

3. African American women have a younger age distribution for breast cancer at time of diagnosis than white/Caucasian American women.
4. Compared with white/Caucasian American women, African Americans are more likely to be diagnosed with breast cancers that are negative for the estrogen receptor (ER), progesterone receptor (PR), and HER2/*neu* marker.
5. Male breast cancer is more common in African Americans than in white/Caucasian Americans.

Contemporary studies of variation in breast cancer subtypes associated with racial/ethnic identity conclusively demonstrate that individuals with African ancestry (African Americans and sub-Saharan Africans) are more likely to be diagnosed with biologically aggressive patterns of disease, but it is clear that inequities in the socioeconomic structure of the United States also play a significant role in explaining these breast cancer differences, just as they account for increased morbidity and mortality burden among African Americans diagnosed with colorectal cancer, lung cancer, and other nonmalignant medical problems such as diabetes or hypertension. Socioeconomic disadvantages such as poverty and absent/inadequate health care coverage are two to three times higher for the African American community, and these issues clearly account for many of the breast cancer disparities listed earlier, by acting as barriers to effective and optimal access to the health care system. The end results are delays in breast cancer diagnosis, less-efficient delivery of multidisciplinary treatment, and ultimately higher mortality rates.

## DISENTANGLING SOCIOECONOMIC RESOURCES FROM RACIAL-ETHNIC IDENTITY IN EXPLAINING BREAST CANCER DISPARITIES

Many investigators have sought to disentangle the confounding effects of socioeconomic disadvantage and race/ethnic identity on cancer survival with interesting and provocative results. In 2004, Ward and colleagues[1] documented that poverty is an adverse oncologic prognostic feature in their landmark study reporting on 5-year survival rates after any cancer diagnosis, stratified by income level. They demonstrated that poverty was associated with worse survival regardless of racial-ethnic identity. As far back as 1994,[2] the National Cancer Institute tried to address this question within the context of breast cancer, with the Black-White Cancer Survival Study, a case-control analysis of 612 African American and 518 white/Caucasian American patients with breast. This comprehensive epidemiologic study used personal interviews and medical record information to account for sociodemographic factors and clinicopathologic cancer features in explaining breast cancer outcomes. Mortality rates were more than twice as high for the African American patients with breast, and approximately 75% of this survival disparity was explained by the various socioeconomic and clinical features studied, leaving 25% of the disparity unexplained and therefore possibly related to some poorly defined, primary race/ethnicity-related factor. Moreover, when the survival data of Ward and colleagues are analyzed from the perspective of outcome stratified by racial/ethnic identity within specific income strata for female cancers (and therefore data largely driven by outcomes from breast cancer), one continues to see incremental decreases in survival for African American patients compared with white American patients. Delving further into adjustments for socioeconomic status in comparisons of outcome between African American and white American patients, Newman and colleagues[3] conducted a meta-analysis of all studies in the medical literature in which a Cox proportional hazard survival analysis had been performed, accounting for racial ethnic identity and some measure of socioeconomic advantage. This pooled analysis yielded a robust sample, more than 13,000 African

American patients with breast cancer whose survival was compared with more than 75,000 white American patients, and African American identity was associated with a statistically significant nearly 30% higher mortality rate (mortality hazard, 1.27; 95% confidence rate, 1.18–1.38).

Results from prospective clinical trials in cancer management provide another strategy for disentangling the effects of poverty and racial/ethnic identity on breast cancer survival, because tumor type, treatment, and follow-up are all standardized and regimented through the clinical trials mechanism. The Southwest Oncology Group[4] conducted this type of analysis and reported outcomes in nearly 20,000 patients with cancer participating in 35 prospective randomized clinical trials between 1974 and 2001. These investigators found that equal treatments indeed did result in equal outcomes (regardless of racial ethnic identity) except for patients treated for hormonally driven cancers. African Americans participating in clinical trials for breast, prostate, and ovarian cancers had statistically significant survival disadvantages compared with participants of other racial/ethnic identities.

## EPIDEMIOLOGY AND RISK FACTORS FOR BREAST CANCER ASSOCIATED WITH AFRICAN ANCESTRY

Several of the features describing the breast cancer burden of African American women cannot easily be ascribed to socioeconomic factors. For example, the age-specific patterns of breast cancer incidence do not lend themselves to a sociodemographic explanation. Approximately 20% of white/Caucasian American patients are diagnosed at younger than 50 years, compared with nearly one-third of African American cases. Although the population-based lifetime risk of breast cancer is lower for African American patients than for white/Caucasian American patients, for women younger than age 45 years, the incidence rates are higher among the African Americans. Similarly, the increased risk of male breast cancer, as well as the increased risk of being diagnosed with adverse primary tumor features, such as high-grade histology, hormone-receptor negative, and triple-negative disease, suggests that some primary race/ethnicity-associated factors also contribute to the reported survival differences.

Reproductive history has been proposed as an explanation for ethnicity-associated variations in age distribution.[5] Multiple pregnancies result in diminished lifetime exposure of the breasts to estrogen, yielding a lower breast cancer incidence among multiparous women than in nulliparous women; however, there is a brief increase in breast cancer risk that occurs in the early postpartum period. Because early childbearing is more common among African American women, it is biologically plausible that a dual effect of parity on breast cancer risk might be observed at a population level, with multiple pregnancies at young ages causing an increased risk of premenopausal disease but a lower lifetime incidence. This theory was supported in an analysis of breast cancer risk in the Black Woman's Health Study,[6] a prospective study of self-reported health and lifestyle issues among African American women subscribers to the magazine *Essence*. More than 50,000 women completed a follow-up questionnaire, representing more than 214,000 person-years of follow-up between 1995 and 1999, and evaluation of breast cancer events revealed that multiparity was associated with an increased incidence rate ratio (IRR) among women younger than 45 years (IRR, 2.4; 95% confidence interval, 1.1–5.1) but was protective against breast cancer among women aged 45 years and older (IRR, 0.5; 95% confidence interval, 0.3–0.9).

In contrast, investigators from the Women's Contraceptive and Reproductive Experience (CARE) study found no differences in effect of parity on age-related breast cancer risk.[7] The Women's CARE study was a population-based, multicenter, case-control study of more than 3000 African American women and nearly 6000 white American women (approximately 50% of both subsets with a history of breast cancer), and this study was specifically designed to analyze the impact of endogenous and exogenous hormonal factors on breast cancer risk in a large, biracial/ethnic dataset. Ursin and colleagues[7] reported that parity was associated with similar degrees of breast cancer risk reduction among younger (age 35–49 years) versus older (age 50–64 years) women in both African American and white American subsets. Risk reduction proportions were 13% and 10% for younger and older white Americans, respectively, compared with 10% and 6% risk reductions for younger and older African Americans.

The increased risk of hormone-receptor-negative disease among African American women and its impact on breast cancer burden is apparent from time trends in population-based incidence and mortality rates. As shown in **Fig. 1**, breast cancer incidence rates have fluctuated since the Surveillance, Epidemiology, and End Results data became available in the early 1970s, but the incidence curves for both population subsets always changed in parallel, with incidence rates being lower for the African Americans. Population-based mortality rates, however, demonstrate a different pattern. Mortality rates for African American and white/Caucasian Americans were actually equivalent until the early 1980s, at which point the curves separate, but the mortality disparity is primarily caused by decreasing mortality rates in white/Caucasian American women but largely unchanged mortality rates in African Americans. This pattern is probably explained by advances in systemic therapy for breast cancer, coupled with differences in the race/ethnicity-specific molecular epidemiology of the disease. In the late 1970s, tamoxifen became available as endocrine therapy for breast cancer, but this treatment disproportionately benefited white/Caucasian American patients, in which case frequency of hormone-receptor-positive disease is

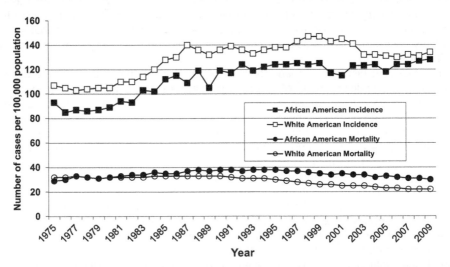

**Fig. 1.** Population-based breast cancer incidence and mortality rates in African American and white American women, from the Surveillance, Epidemiology, and End Results program.[66] Note that disparities in mortality curves do not become apparent until mid-1980s, following availability and adoption of tamoxifen as systemic therapy for breast cancer. (*Data from* Surveillance, Epidemiology, and End Results program. Cancer fast stats 2014. 2014. Available at: http://seer.cancer.gov/faststats/selections.php? Accessed February 26, 2014.)

approximately 2-fold higher than that of African American patients. As shown by Anderson and colleagues,[8] risk of ER-negative breast cancer is higher for African Americans on a population basis, and this pattern persists regardless of age at diagnosis, as well as after stratifying for cases diagnosed as early stage/resectable breast cancer, locally advanced breast cancer, and inflammatory breast cancer. It is likely that outcome disparities have worsened as progress in endocrine therapy for breast cancer has advanced. The armamentarium of endocrine therapies for hormone-receptor-positive disease has expanded to include a variety of aromatase inhibitors for postmenopausal patients, and commercially available genetic profiling analyses (eg, Oncotype Dx Recurrence Score testing) can be performed as a more refined way of identifying ER-positive/node-negative patients with breast cancer who can benefit from adjuvant chemotherapy and endocrine therapy.

In 2007, Carey and colleagues[9] pursued race/ethnicity-related variation further with their landmark report from the Carolina Breast Cancer Study, demonstrating 2-fold higher frequency of tumors that are negative for ER, PR, and HER2/*neu* (TNBC) in premenopausal African American patients with breast cancer when compared with others. Others have confirmed this finding using both single-institution tumor registry data and population-based statistics. As with prior studies of ER-negative disease, the increased risk of TNBC is observed among African American women regardless of age at diagnosis and regardless of stage at diagnosis.

## BREAST CANCER IN AFRICAN AMERICAN WOMEN: IMPLICATIONS FOR SCREENING MAMMOGRAPHY RECOMMENDATIONS

The race/ethnicity-associated differences in population-based incidence of TNBC are also relevant to the controversial discussion of breast cancer surveillance and the age at which American women should initiate screening mammography. In November 2009,[10] the US Preventive Services Task Force (USPSTF) published an updated reevaluation of the historic prospective randomized clinical trials conducted 20 to 30 years ago, comparing mammography screening to usual medical care in the absence of screening. The outcomes data from these 7 trials were pooled together and analyzed by a statistical consortium,[11] forming the evidence basis for the USPSTF's updated recommendations. The statistical experts formulated 2 separate perspectives for interpreting the mammography trials data. The efficiency model studied the number of women that would need to be invited for screening to save 1 life from breast cancer; these age-based numbers were 377 for women aged 60 years and older, 1339 for women aged 50 to 59 years, and 1904 for women aged 40 to 49 years. The longevity model studied the numbers of years of life saved with various mammography screening intervals and demonstrated that more years of life are saved when mammographic screening is initiated at age 40 years. The USPSTF chose to select the efficiency model as being the preferred model for making screening recommendations to American women, and they furthermore opted to choose age 50 years as being the most appropriate age at which to initiate screening, based on their interpretation of the data as suggesting that needing to invite nearly 2000 women to screen to save 1 life is excessive but that needing to invite 1300 women to save 1 life is acceptable. The statistical experts specifically commented in their article that by virtue of their respective study populations, the mammography screening trials almost exclusively reflected the impact of mammography on white/Caucasian women from North America and Europe. These data therefore could not necessarily be generalized to the setting of population subsets such as African American women, in which case the age distribution and disease biology of breast cancer differs. In contrast, the

USPSTF article fails to comment on existing disparities in breast cancer burden associated with racial/ethnic identity and the potential influence of delayed mammographic screening on African American women, whereby incidence rates are higher for the younger-aged women and risk of TNBC is disproportionately higher in the younger women as well. As shown by Amirikia and colleagues[12] in a study from the California Cancer Reglstry, population-based incidence rates of TNBC for African American women in the 40- to 49-year age range is comparable to those of white/Caucasian American women in the 60- to 69-year age range; these data are summarized in **Fig. 2**.

## BREAST CANCER RISK ASSESSMENT AND CHEMOPREVENTION IN AFRICAN AMERICAN WOMEN

Breast cancer chemoprevention studies reveal a unique barrier to ethnic diversity in clinical trial participation, related to the limited understanding of breast cancer risk factor expression in African American women. The National Surgical Adjuvant Breast Project (NSABP) P-01[13] trial randomized more than 13,000 high-risk women to receive chemoprevention with tamoxifen for 5 years versus a placebo, and this study proved the effectiveness of tamoxifen in reducing breast cancer incidence by approximately one-half. Chemoprevention to reduce breast cancer incidence is one potential strategy for decreasing breast cancer mortality among African Americans. Chemoprevention with tamoxifen might be expected to be particularly effective for African American women, because of the fewer adverse effects experienced by premenopausal women using tamoxifen and because of the increased risk for early-onset breast cancer among African American women. On the other hand, tamoxifen is associated with increased risk of thromboembolic phenomena, and it prevents only ER-positive breast cancer.[14] Because morbidity from venous thromboembolism is higher for African

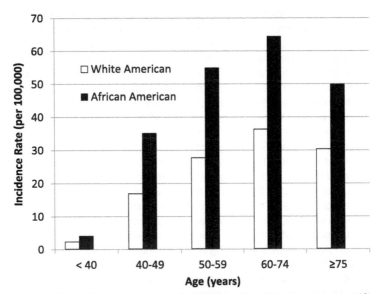

**Fig. 2.** Population-based incidence rates of triple-negative breast cancer stratified by age range at diagnosis, from California Cancer Registry. (*From* Amirikia KC, Mills P, Bush J, et al. Higher population-based incidence rates of triple-negative breast cancer among young African-American women: implications for breast cancer screening recommendations. Cancer 2011;117(12):2747–53; with permission.)

American women and because risk of ER-negative breast cancer is increased among African American women, it is unclear whether the benefits of chemoprevention would outweigh the risks for this population subset. Data from the NSABP P-01 trial should have been able to address these issues, but African Americans accounted for only 1.7% of the study participants. In response to this low accrual, the NSABP developed aggressive outreach strategies for its follow-up chemoprevention trial, the Study of Raloxifene and Tamoxifen. Closer scrutiny of the eligibility criteria for these trials is also warranted, so that any inherent biases against African American participation can be identified. Most chemoprevention trial participants are identified as being high-risk based on their Gail model[15] 5-year breast cancer risk estimate. This statistical tool quantifies a woman's risk of developing breast cancer by studying her age, reproductive history, breast biopsy history, and family cancer history. In its original formulation, the model was developed by studying these risk factors in white American women, and it was modified for the chemoprevention trials so that it would yield ethnicity/race-specific risk estimates. The model accounts for risk of developing breast cancer; it does not account for risk of dying from breast cancer. Furthermore, the modification of the model to calculate risk in African American women was based on small sample sizes, and its performance for African American women is therefore uncertain. As shown by Newman and colleagues,[16,17] the Gail model seems to generate inappropriately low risk estimates for African American women (and especially young African American women). Data from the CARE case-control study has therefore been used to modify the National Cancer Institute's Web-based model for calculating individualized breast cancer risk in African American women, and the modified model has been validated in the postmenopausal participants of the Women's Health Initiative.[18] This updated model, however, requires validation in a cohort of premenopausal women. Boggs and colleagues[19] have studied the model in African American women from the Black Women's Health Study and demonstrated persistent underestimation of breast cancer risk.

## BRCA GENETIC TESTING, HEREDITARY SUSCEPTIBILITY, AND AFRICAN ANCESTRY

Women carrying a mutation in the BRCA1 breast cancer susceptibility gene are more likely to be diagnosed with ER-negative, high-grade tumors that are detected at young ages.[20–22] As discussed earlier, these features are prominent among African American patients with breast cancer,[23] and these parallels motivate questions regarding the extent of hereditary risk in African American women. Studies of hereditary cancer risk among African American women, however, have been limited,[24–27] although some BRCA1 and BRCA2 founder mutations and other unique (but not necessarily deleterious) genotype patterns have been identified.[28–31] It is unclear whether a single high-penetrance, major breast cancer susceptibility mutation will be identified that explains the breast cancer patterns of African American women, as these types of genetic abnormalities are rare. Hurley's research group[32,33] identified a BRCA1 gene founder mutation unique to African American women based on genetic testing in a series of patients from Florida, predominantly with Bahamian Caribbean/African ancestral background. It is furthermore plausible that low- and moderate-risk genetic variants that collectively contribute to the breast cancer burden of selected populations subsets exist.[34,35]

Questions regarding possible germline mutations associated with African ancestry that increase breast cancer susceptibility motivate interest in studying the breast cancer burden of women sharing ancestry with African American women. As discussed by Fregene and Newman,[36] contemporary generations of African American and sub-Saharan African women are likely to have some shared ancestry as a consequence of the colonial-era slave trade posts. These sites were clustered along the southwestern coast of Africa, within present-day Ghana, Nigeria, Senegal, and Gambia. Comparisons of breast cancer in these various populations of women are therefore warranted.

Large-scale, population-based databases that document the cancer burden of Africa are lacking because of limited financial support for the health care and research systems. The World Health Organization estimates that the Americas account for 10% of the global burden of disease and have 37% of the world's health workers spending more than 50% of the world's health financing, whereas Africa has 24% of the global disease burden but possesses only 3% of health workers using less than 1% of world health expenditure.[37] These limited resources leave little for investment into cancer and tumor registries in Africa. However, data available on the epidemiology of breast cancer in Africa reveal some provocative similarities to breast cancer in African American women, thereby strengthening the case for conducting genetic research investigating cancer susceptibility in women with African ancestry.

**Fig. 3** demonstrates breast cancer incidence and mortality data for women from African countries compared with other parts of the world, based on the Globocan program.[38] In general, women of Africa face a low risk of being diagnosed with breast cancer. Although the breast cancer mortality rates are similarly low in comparison to Western nations, the ratio of mortality to incidence tends to be higher. The lifestyle and reproductive history of African women contribute to an overall protective risk factor profile. Childbearing is initiated at younger ages, full-time pregnancies are multiple, postpartum lactation is frequently extended, and menarche may be delayed.[36,39,40] Diminished health care access and lack of breast cancer screening programs result in delayed diagnoses, advanced-stage disease at diagnosis, and higher mortality

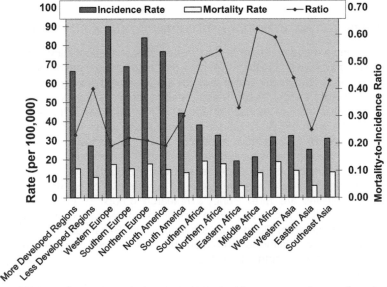

**Fig. 3.** International variation in breast cancer incidence, mortality, and mortality-to-incidence ratios. (*Data from* Jemal A, Bray F, Center MM, et al. Global cancer statistics. CA Cancer J Clin 2011;61(2):69–90; and Globocan 2008. International Agency for Research on Cancer. Available at: http://globocan.iarc.fr/. Accessed March 31, 2011.)

rates.[36,41] However, studies correlating risk factors with breast cancer incidence and tumor features with disease outcome have been inconsistent in ruling out the possibility that African women may have some inherent predisposition for developing biologically more aggressive breast tumors.[41–49]

**Fig. 4** summarizes patterns of breast cancer incidence and outcome for African American, white American, and native sub-Saharan African women. Frequencies of larger tumors, high-grade cancer, ER-negative cancer, and early-onset disease are highest for African women, intermediate for African American women, and lowest for white American women. One particularly impressive clinicopathologic analysis was conducted by Ikpatt and colleagues[47] on 148 Nigerian patients with breast cancer, and the following features were reported: 67% of cases were premenopausal, mean age was 44 years, mean tumor size was 4.2 cm, 78% of cases were grade 2 or 3, only 23% were ER-positive, and Her2/*neu* overexpression was observed in 19%.

It is therefore worthy of speculation that some genotypic variants, perhaps related to estrogen metabolism and/or the ER pathway and associated with African ancestry, might exert some oncogenic effects on mammary tissue that result in lower lifetime risk for endocrine-sensitive breast cancer while increasing the risk for endocrine-resistant, early-onset disease. These patterns might be most apparent in native sub-Saharan African populations, but 4 centuries of genetic admixture might result in an intermediate expression of this pattern of disease among African Americans. Fejerman and colleagues[50] performed admixture scans in nearly 1500 African American patients with breast cancer and confirmed that the extent of African ancestry was associated with risk of hormone-receptor-negative disease, but no specific ancestral marker predicting susceptibility for disease was identified. Several genotyping analyses from the Black Women's Health Study have identified single-nucleotide polymorphisms and patterns associated with African ancestry that are also correlated with risk of TNBC.[51–53]

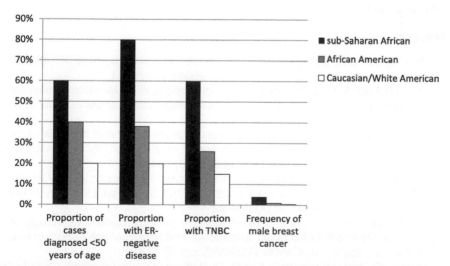

**Fig. 4.** Estimates of breast cancer frequency patterns in African American, Caucasian/white Americans, and African populations. (*Data from* Newman LA. Breast cancer in African-American women. Oncologist 2005;10(1):1–14; and Fregene A, Newman LA. Breast cancer in sub-Saharan Africa: how does it relate to breast cancer in African-American women? Cancer 2005;103(8):1540–50.)

Breast cancer studies from the University of Michigan–Ghana breast cancer partnership have also identified novel patterns of molecular marker expression associated with mammary stem cells in sub-Saharan African populations. Specifically, the mammary stem cell marker ALDH1 was found to be elevated in Ghanaian benign and malignant breast specimens,[54] and the marker EZH2 was also found to have unique patterns in Ghanaian breast tissue compared with white/Caucasian patients with breast cancer.[55]

Advances in gene expression studies are now demonstrating that TNBC is a heterogeneous breast cancer subset, characterized by distinct subsets featuring tumor progression through specific pathways. The Vanderbilt University[56,57] has identified at least 6 different TNBC subtypes: 2 basallike, 1 immunomodulatory, 1 mesenchymal, 1 mesenchymal stem cell-like, and 1 luminal androgen receptor. These subtypes are associated with differential response to neoadjuvant chemotherapy,[58,59] and via androgen receptor expression in the luminal androgen receptor subtype, may serve as a foundation for novel approaches in predicting risk of recurrence as well as in targeted therapy for TNBC with antiandrogen therapy such as bicalutamide.[60–64] Preliminary data suggest novel patterns of androgen receptor expression in Ghanaian women,[65] and additional research is necessary in the study of TNBC subtypes among women with African ancestry.

## SUMMARY

The study of breast cancer disparities related to racial-ethnic identity in the United States has opened the door to unique insights regarding breast cancer subtypes. African American women face higher risk of breast cancer mortality not only because of socioeconomic disadvantages but also because of their increased risk for being diagnosed with biologically aggressive patterns of disease, such as tumors that are negative for the hormone receptors and the HER2/neu marker. Studies of the breast cancer burden in Africa and in African Americans are likely to advance the understanding of the pathogenesis of TNBC and hereditary susceptibility for breast cancer related to African ancestry.

## REFERENCES

1. Ward E, Jemal A, Cokkinides V, et al. Cancer disparities by race/ethnicity and socioeconomic status. CA Cancer J Clin 2004;54(2):78–93.
2. Eley JW, Hill HA, Chen VW, et al. Racial differences in survival from breast cancer. Results of the National Cancer Institute Black/White Cancer Survival Study. JAMA 1994;272(12):947–54.
3. Newman LA, Griffith KA, Jatoi I, et al. Meta-analysis of survival in African American and white American patients with breast cancer: ethnicity compared with socioeconomic status. J Clin Oncol 2006;24(9):1342–9.
4. Albain KS, Unger JM, Crowley JJ, et al. Racial disparities in cancer survival among randomized clinical trials patients of the Southwest Oncology Group. J Natl Cancer Inst 2009;101(14):984–92.
5. Pathak DR, Osuch JR, He J. Breast carcinoma etiology: current knowledge and new insights into the effects of reproductive and hormonal risk factors in black and white populations. Cancer 2000;88(Suppl 5):1230–8.
6. Palmer JR, Wise LA, Horton NJ, et al. Dual effect of parity on breast cancer risk in African-American women. J Natl Cancer Inst 2003;95(6):478–83.
7. Ursin G, Bernstein L, Wang Y, et al. Reproductive factors and risk of breast carcinoma in a study of white and African-American women. Cancer 2004;101(2):353–62.

8. Anderson WF, Chatterjee N, Ershler WB, et al. Estrogen receptor breast cancer phenotypes in the Surveillance, Epidemiology, and End Results database. Breast Cancer Res Treat 2002;76(1):27–36.

9. Carey LA, Perou CM, Livasy CA, et al. Race, breast cancer subtypes, and survival in the Carolina Breast Cancer Study. JAMA 2006;295(21):2492–502.

10. Nelson HD, Tyne K, Naik A, et al. Screening for breast cancer: an update for the U.S. Preventive Services Task Force. Ann Intern Med 2009;151(10):727–37, W237–42.

11. Mandelblatt JS, Cronin KA, Bailey S, et al. Effects of mammography screening under different screening schedules: model estimates of potential benefits and harms. Ann Intern Med 2009;151(10):738–47.

12. Amirikia KC, Mills P, Bush J, et al. Higher population-based incidence rates of triple-negative breast cancer among young African-American women: implications for breast cancer screening recommendations. Cancer 2011;117(12):2747–53.

13. Fisher B, Costantino JP, Wickerham DL, et al. Tamoxifen for prevention of breast cancer: report of the National Surgical Adjuvant Breast and Bowel Project P-1 Study. J Natl Cancer Inst 1998;90(18):1371–88.

14. Gail M, Costantino J, Bryant J, et al. Weighing the risks and benefits of tamoxifen treatment for preventing breast cancer. J Natl Cancer Inst 1999;91:1829–46.

15. Gail MH, Brinton LA, Byar DP, et al. Projecting individualized probabilities of developing breast cancer for white females who are being examined annually. J Natl Cancer Inst 1989;81(24):1879–86.

16. Newman LA, Rockhill B, Bondy ML, et al. Validation of the Gail Breast Cancer risk assessment model in African American women based on a multi-center case-control study of 3,283 African American and 5,974 white American women. Paper presented at: American Society of Clinical Oncology, 38th Annual Meeting. Orlando, May 19, 2002.

17. Newman LA, Gail MH, Selvan M, et al. Proposed revision of the Gail breast cancer risk assessment model for African American women. Paper presented at: American Society of Clinical Oncology, 39th Annual Meeting. Chicago, June 2003.

18. Gail MH, Costantino JP, Pee D, et al. Projecting individualized absolute invasive breast cancer risk in African American women. J Natl Cancer Inst 2007;99(23): 1782–92.

19. Boggs DA, Rosenberg L, Pencina MJ, et al. Validation of a breast cancer risk prediction model developed for black women. J Natl Cancer Inst 2013;105(5):361–7.

20. Robson ME, Boyd J, Borgen PI, et al. Hereditary breast cancer. Curr Probl Surg 2001;38(6):387–480.

21. Newman LA, Kuerer HM, Hunt KK, et al. Educational review: role of the surgeon in hereditary breast cancer. Ann Surg Oncol 2001;8(4):368–78.

22. Thull DL, Vogel VG. Recognition and management of hereditary breast cancer syndromes. Oncologist 2004;9(1):13–24.

23. Newman LA. Breast cancer in African-American women. Oncologist 2005;10(1): 1–14.

24. Hall M, Olopade OI. Confronting genetic testing disparities: knowledge is power. JAMA 2005;293(14):1783–5.

25. Thompson HS, Valdimarsdottir HB, Duteau-Buck C, et al. Psychosocial predictors of BRCA counseling and testing decisions among urban African-American women. Cancer Epidemiol Biomarkers Prev 2002;11(12):1579–85.

26. Lee R, Beattie M, Crawford B, et al. Recruitment, genetic counseling, and BRCA testing for underserved women at a public hospital. Genet Test 2005;9(4):306–12.

27. Nanda R, Schumm LP, Cummings S, et al. Genetic testing in an ethnically diverse cohort of high-risk women: a comparative analysis of BRCA1 and BRCA2 mutations in American families of European and African ancestry. JAMA 2005;294(15):1925–33.
28. Olopade O, Fackenthal J, Dunston G, et al. Breast cancer genetics in African Americans. Cancer 2002;97(Suppl 1):236–45.
29. Gao Q, Neuhausen S, Cummings S, et al. Recurrent germ-line BRCA1 mutations in extended African American families with early-onset breast cancer. Am J Hum Genet 1997;60(5):1233–6.
30. Gao Q, Tomlinson G, Das S, et al. Prevalence of BRCA1 and BRCA2 mutations among clinic-based African American families with breast cancer. Hum Genet 2000;107(2):186–91.
31. Matthews A, Cummings S, Thompson S, et al. Genetic testing of African Americans for susceptibility to inherited cancers: use of focus groups to determine factors contributing to participation. J Psychosoc Oncol 2000;18:1–19.
32. Donenberg T, Lunn J, Curling D, et al. A high prevalence of BRCA1 mutations among breast cancer patients from the Bahamas. Breast Cancer Res Treat 2011;125(2):591–6.
33. Akbari MR, Donenberg T, Lunn J, et al. The spectrum of BRCA1 and BRCA2 mutations in breast cancer patients in the Bahamas. Clin Genet 2014;85(1):64–7.
34. Antoniou AC, Pharoah PD, McMullan G, et al. Evidence for further breast cancer susceptibility genes in addition to BRCA1 and BRCA2 in a population-based study. Genet Epidemiol 2001;21(1):1–18.
35. Gilliland FD. Ethnic differences in cancer incidence: a marker for inherited susceptibility? Environ Health Perspect 1997;105(Suppl 4):897–900.
36. Fregene A, Newman LA. Breast cancer in sub-Saharan Africa: how does it relate to breast cancer in African-American women? Cancer 2005;103(8):1540–50.
37. The World Health Report 2006-Working together for health. 2006. Available at: http://www.who.int/whr/2006/en/index.html. Accessed April 11, 2006.
38. Ferlay J, Bray F, Pisani P, et al. Globocan 2002: cancer incidence, mortality and prevalence worldwide. IARC CancerBase No. 5 version 2.0. Lyon (France): IARCPress; 2004.
39. Anyanwu SN. Breast cancer in eastern Nigeria: a ten year review. West Afr J Med 2000;19(2):120–5.
40. Muguti GI. Experience with breast cancer in Zimbabwe. J R Coll Surg Edinb 1993;38(2):75–8.
41. Hassan I, Onukak EE, Mabogunje OA. Breast cancer in Zaria, Nigeria. J R Coll Surg Edinb 1992;37(3):159–61.
42. Adebamowo CA, Adekunle OO. Case-controlled study of the epidemiological risk factors for breast cancer in Nigeria. Br J Surg 1999;86(5):665–8.
43. Adebamowo CA, Ogundiran TO, Adenipekun AA, et al. Obesity and height in urban Nigerian women with breast cancer. Ann Epidemiol 2003;13(6):455–61.
44. Ademuyiwa FO, Neuhausen S, Adebamowo CA, et al. Early onset breast cancer in black women of African ancestry: Genetic or environmental influence? Abstract No. 3225. Paper presented at: American Association for Cancer Research. Anaheim, April 16–20, 2005.
45. Amir H, Makwaya CK, Aziz MR, et al. Breast cancer and risk factors in an African population: a case referent study. East Afr Med J 1998;75(5):268–70.
46. Ijuin H, Douchi T, Oki T, et al. The contribution of menopause to changes in body-fat distribution. J Obstet Gynaecol Res 1999;25(5):367–72.

47. Ikpatt O, Xu J, Kramtsov A, et al. Hormone receptor negative and basal-like sub-types are overrepresented in invasive breast carcinoma from women of African ancestry. American Association for Cancer Research; 2005. Abstract No. 2550.

48. Ikpatt OF, Kuopio T, Collan Y. Proliferation in African breast cancer: biology and prognostication in Nigerian breast cancer material. Mod Pathol 2002;15(8):783–9.

49. Ikpatt OF, Kuopio T, Ndoma-Egba R, et al. Breast cancer in Nigeria and Finland: epidemiological, clinical and histological comparison. Anticancer Res 2002; 22(5):3005–12.

50. Fejerman L, Haiman CA, Reich D, et al. An admixture scan in 1,484 African American women with breast cancer. Cancer Epidemiol Biomarkers Prev 2009;18(11):3110–7.

51. Ruiz-Narvaez EA, Rosenberg L, Yao S, et al. Fine-mapping of the 6q25 locus identifies a novel SNP associated with breast cancer risk in African-American women. Carcinogenesis 2013;34(2):287–91.

52. Rosenberg L, Boggs DA, Bethea TN, et al. A prospective study of smoking and breast cancer risk among African-American women. Cancer Causes Control 2013;24(12):2207–15.

53. Palmer JR, Ruiz-Narvaez EA, Rotimi CN, et al. Genetic susceptibility loci for sub-types of breast cancer in an African American population. Cancer Epidemiol Biomarkers Prev 2013;22(1):127–34.

54. Schwartz T, Stark A, Pang J, et al. Expression of aldehyde dehydrogenase 1 as a marker of mammary stem cells in benign and malignant breast lesions of Ghanaian women. Cancer 2013;119(3):488–94.

55. Pang J, Toy KA, Griffith KA, et al. Invasive breast carcinomas in Ghana: high frequency of high grade, basal-like histology and high EZH2 expression. Breast Cancer Res Treat 2012;135(1):59–66.

56. Lehmann BD, Bauer JA, Chen X, et al. Identification of human triple-negative breast cancer subtypes and preclinical models for selection of targeted therapies. J Clin Invest 2011;121(7):2750–67.

57. Chen X, Li J, Gray WH, et al. TNBC type: a subtyping tool for triple-negative breast cancer. Canc Informat 2012;11:147–56.

58. Yu KD, Zhu R, Zhan M, et al. Identification of prognosis-relevant subgroups in patients with chemoresistant triple-negative breast cancer. Clin Cancer Res 2013;19(10):2723–33.

59. Masuda H, Baggerly KA, Wang Y, et al. Differential response to neoadjuvant chemotherapy among 7 triple-negative breast cancer molecular subtypes. Clin Cancer Res 2013;19(19):5533–40.

60. McGhan LJ, McCullough AE, Protheroe CA, et al. Androgen receptor-positive triple negative breast cancer: a unique breast cancer subtype. Ann Surg Oncol 2014;21(2):361–7.

61. Thike AA, Yong-Zheng Chong L, Cheok PY, et al. Loss of androgen receptor expression predicts early recurrence in triple-negative and basal-like breast cancer. Mod Pathol 2014;27(3):352–60.

62. Shah PD, Gucalp A, Traina TA. The role of the androgen receptor in triple-negative breast cancer. Womens Health (Lond Engl) 2013;9(4):351–60.

63. Mrklic I, Pogorelic Z, Capkun V, et al. Expression of androgen receptors in triple negative breast carcinomas. Acta Histochem 2013;115(4):344–8.

64. McNamara KM, Yoda T, Takagi K, et al. Androgen receptor in triple negative breast cancer. J Steroid Biochem Mol Biol 2013;133:66–76.

65. Proctor E, Jiagge E, Kleer C, et al. Androgen receptor expression in Ghanaian breast cancer cases: novel correlation with ALDH1 in triple-negative tumors.

Paper presented at: Society of Surgical Oncology Annual Cancer Symposium. Phoenix, March 12–15, 2014.

66. Surveillance, Epidemiology, and End Results program. Cancer fast stats 2014. Available at: http://seer.cancer.gov/faststats/selections.php? Accessed February 26, 2014.

# Nonsurgical Ablation of Breast Cancer

## Future Options for Small Breast Tumors

Michael S. Sabel, MD

### KEYWORDS

- Breast cancer • In situ ablation • Cryoablation • Radiofrequency ablation
- High-intensity focused ultrasonography

### KEY POINTS

- Nonsurgical ablation has several potential advantages over lumpectomy for the treatment of early stage breast cancer.
- A variety of technologies are available for nonsurgical ablation, each with its own advantages and disadvantages.
- Ablate and resect trials have shown the ability of nonsurgical techniques such as cryoablation, radiofrequency ablation, and high-intensity focused ultrasonography to completely ablate breast tumors.
- There are limited data from ablation alone trials, and many questions remain to be answered before nonsurgical ablation can be considered a viable alternative to lumpectomy.

## INTRODUCTION

The surgical management of breast cancer has seen a radical evolution over the past several decades, characterized by equal or improved outcomes, with significantly less morbidity. Eradication of the primary tumor has progressed from radical mastectomy (and extended radical mastectomy), through modified radical mastectomy, to lumpectomy. Management of the regional nodes has transformed from routine axillary lymph node dissection (ALND) to sentinel lymph node (SLN) biopsy and ALND for all SLN-positive patients, and ALND for only a few SLN-positive patients. These changes have been facilitated by a multitude of factors, including improvements in technology and screening, better quality and more widely used adjuvant therapies, and countless patients participating in multi-institutional prospective, randomized trials.

Disclosure: The author is on an advisory board for IceCure.

Department of Surgery, University of Michigan, 3304 Cancer Center, 1500 East Medical Center Drive, Ann Arbor, MI 48109, USA

E-mail address: msabel@umich.edu

The next, seemingly inevitable, step in the evolution of breast cancer therapy would be the replacement of lumpectomy, at least for a select group of patients, with nonsurgical methods for destroying the tumor. Although most of these techniques use thermal energy to destroy the tumor, newer technologies use nonthermal technologies. The potential advantages to nonsurgical breast cancer ablation are multiple, including lower cost of care and simplifying treatment, increased patient comfort, and greatly improved cosmetic outcomes. Various techniques have been used for the in situ ablation of other tumor types, including cancers of the liver, bone, kidney, prostate, and skin. Given recent advances in breast imaging, and our ability to target nonpalpable lesions, it seems logical that breast cancer would be an ideal clinical target. However, many of the technologies for nonsurgical breast cancer ablation have been around for decades, and lumpectomy still remains the absolute standard of care for the treatment of early stage breast cancer. In this article, the clinical experience with a variety of technologies being studied in breast cancer treatment and some of the obstacles to their clinical implementation are reviewed.

## CLINICAL OUTCOMES
### Interstitial Laser Therapy

#### Mechanism
Interstitial laser therapy (ILT) involves the placement of a laser fiber with a diffusing tip through a trocar into a breast cancer. Laser light is then delivered directly to the target lesion, and the resultant thermal effect results from the interaction between the laser photons and the molecules of the tissue. Absorption of the laser light results in transformation of laser energy to heat, which increases the tissue temperature and creates a zone of thermal ablation. One advantage to ILT is that the optical fibers are magnetic resonance (MR)-compatible, allowing for MR imaging (MRI)-guided ILT.

#### Clinical experience
There are a few clinical trials examining ILT in the treatment of breast cancer. Akimov and colleagues[1] treated 35 patients, 7 of whom had no further treatment. Among the 28 patients who had surgery after ILT, the investigators described the common histologic findings but did not quantify the number of patients with complete ablation. Among the 7 patients treated by ILT only, 5 achieved local tumor control. There were also some complications, including skin burns and 1 case in which there was gaseous rupture of the tumor, resulting in pain and subcutaneous emphysema. Dowlatshahi and colleagues[2] treated 56 patients with ILT without MRI guidance before surgery and then examined the excised tissue. All patients had tumors with the greatest diameter no larger than 23 mm. Thirty percent of the patients had residual disease, although 2 women who underwent ILT but did not go through with the subsequent surgery had no evidence of recurrence for 2 years. Haraldsdottir and colleagues[3] performed ILT before surgery in 24 patients, but showed complete ablation in only 3 patients with smaller tumors. The inefficacy was mainly caused by the ability to visualize the tumor and judge the extent of laser damage with ultrasonography. Harms[4] used MRI-guided ILT in a population of women with larger tumors. Although the MRI allowed for better contrast and improved resolution, only 3 women achieved complete destruction, all with tumors smaller than 3 cm.

#### Challenges moving forward
Although ILT has several advantages, including the ability to use MR-guidance and minimal pain, allowing it to be performed under local anesthesia in an outpatient setting, early experience has not shown a reliable ablation of tumors. However,

a multicenter ablate and resect trial of ILT for patients with tumors smaller than 2 cm is currently recruiting participants (ClinicalTrials.gov: NCT01478438).

## RADIOFREQUENCY ABLATION
### Mechanism

Radiofrequency ablation (RFA) involves the placement of an electrode into a tumor. A high-frequency alternating current flowing through the electrode causes ionic agitation, which in turn leads to friction heat and thermal damage, depending on the resultant temperature. Heating to 50°C to 55°C causes irreversible cellular damage in a few minutes, whereas heating between 60°C and 100°C causes instantaneous tissue coagulation. Different types of electrodes are used, including expandable multifilaments and internally cooled and perfusion electrodes.[5] These electrodes determine the size of the area that can be ablated. RFA is typically performed in the operating room (OR) with sedation or general anesthesia.

### Clinical Experience

Early on, RFA was the most widely investigated ablation technique for breast cancer. This technique started in 1999, when Jeffrey and colleagues[6] reported the use of RFA in 5 women with locally advanced breast cancer, showing the potential of RFA for lesions smaller than 3 cm. Subsequently, several investigators reported the results of studies in which patients underwent tumor ablation followed by surgical resection 1 to 4 weeks later. One difficulty with RFA is that histologically, it can sometimes be difficult to assess the success of RFA on hematoxylin-eosin staining, because there are often normal-appearing cells within the area of coagulation. Many investigators therefore perform reduced nicotinamide adenine dinucleotide staining for viability after RFA.

In these early ablate and resect studies, the success rates (rate of complete ablation of the tumor) ranged from 76% to 100% (**Table 1**).[19] The technique was relatively well tolerated, although complications included burns of the skin, local swelling and pain, and thermal damage to the chest muscle and pneumothorax.[16] Based on these results, a handful of investigators have explored the possibility of RFA alone, either

| Table 1 | | | | |
| :--- | :--- | :--- | :--- | :--- |
| **Studies of RFA followed by surgical excision** | | | | |
| Reference | Location | N | Tumor Size (cm) | Complete Ablation (%) |
| Jeffrey et al,[6] 1999 | Stanford, CA | 5 | 4–7 | 80 |
| Izzo et al,[7] 2001 | Naples, Italy | 26 | 0.7–3.0 | 96 |
| Burak et al,[8] 2003 | Columbus, OH | 10 | 0.8–1.6 | 90 |
| Hayashi et al,[9] 2003 | Victoria, BC, Canada | 10 | 0.5–2.6 | 86 |
| Fornage et al,[10] 2004 | Houston, TX | 21 | 0.6–2.0 | 95 |
| Noguchi et al,[11] 2006 | Ishikawa, Japan | 17 | 0.5–2.0 | 100 |
| Earashi et al,[12] 2007 | Yatsuo, Japan | 24 | 0.5–2.4 | 100 |
| Medina-Franco et al,[13] 2008 | Mexico City, Mexico | 25 | 0.9–3.8 | 76 |
| Manenti et al,[14] 2009 | Rome, Italy | 34 | 1.65–1.96 | 97 |
| Imoto et al,[15] 2009 | Tokyo, Japan | 30 | 0.9–2.4 | 92 |
| Wiksell et al,[16] 2010 | Stockholm, Sweden | 31 | 0.7–1.8 | 84 |
| Ohtani et al,[17] 2011 | Hiroshima, Japan | 41 | 0.5–1.8 | 87.8 |
| Kreb et al,[18] 2013 | Hertogenbosch, Netherlands | 20 | 0.4–1.5 | 85 |

with or without radiation therapy. This technique initially started with some small trials in elderly patients who were not believed to be good surgical candidates. Susini and colleagues[20] performed RFA on 3 elderly, unresectable patients and after 18 months of follow-up reported no evidence of local recurrence by either MRI or core needle biopsy. In a similar approach, Marcy and colleagues[21] had no local recurrences in 3 elderly women treated with hormonal therapy, RFA, and radiation.

Several larger series examined RFA as an alternative to lumpectomy. Oura and colleagues[22] treated 52 patients with tumors 2 cm or smaller as confirmed by mammogram, ultrasonography, and MRI. Under general anesthesia, patients had RFA of the primary tumor and SLN biopsy. To rule out residual disease, fine-needle aspiration was performed 1 month after the operation and MRI was performed 1 to 3 months later. No patients had residual disease, and after 15 months of follow-up there were no recurrences. In a similar trial, Yamamoto and colleagues[23] treated 30 tumors less than 2 cm in 29 patients. Again, this treatment was performed in the OR with SLN biopsy, and after treatment, MRI and Mammotome vacuum-assisted breast biopsy (Mammotome, Cincinnati, OH, USA) were used to ensure no residual disease. Twenty-seven of 29 patients who had posttreatment biopsies showed no viable cells. The 2 patients with viable cells refused additional surgery and went on to whole breast radiotherapy with a boost. With a median follow-up of 17 months, there were no recurrences.

### Challenges Moving Forward

As with other hyperthermic ablative techniques, there have been reports of skin burn or burns to the underlying chest wall, and so a subset of tumors, even if they are within the appropriate size limits, would not be good candidates for RFA secondary to proximity to the skin or pectoralis muscle. The 2 most significant challenges facing the use of RFA for the percutaneous ablation of breast cancer are the skills required to perform breast RFA and the difficulty monitoring the ablation with current imaging modalities. To perform RFA, the needle electrode is inserted percutaneously through the tissues until the tip abuts the lesion. The prongs are then deployed. Real-time sonographic monitoring is needed to verify that the prongs are deployed in a symmetric fashion around the lesion, which is more challenging in the breast than other areas in which RFA is used. To ensure successful RFA, the device needs to be at the geometric center, which requires accurate three-dimensional mental images of the location of the tips of the deployed prongs and the anticipated shape and size of the ablation volume.[24] Thus, the level of skill required to perform breast RFA makes it less desirable than other modalities.

Compared with some other techniques, there are no specific sonographic changes during the procedure that can assure the physician that the lesion is reliably ablated.[24] Instead, as the procedure progresses, the visibility of the lesion decreases and by the end can be completely obscured. It is therefore more difficult to be assured that the entire lesion has been adequately treated. Given these challenges, several investigators have shifted away from using RFA as an alternative to lumpectomy and instead are examining its use in combination with excision, either lumpectomy or percutaneous excision.[25–27]

### CRYOABLATION
#### Mechanism

Cryoablation is performed by placing a cryoprobe at the center of a tumor. A cryoprobe is a high-pressure, closed-loop gas expansion system, in which the metal probe is insulated, except for the tip. The cryoprobe is rapidly cooled by means of the Joule-Thomson effect (rapid expansion of a gas results in a change in the temperature of the gas), removing heat from the tissue contacting the probe. For ablation of smaller tumors, a single probe is typically placed under ultrasound guidance through the center of a tumor. For larger tumors, multiple probes can be placed to generate cytotoxic isotherms.[28-30]

Although cryoablation refers to the freezing of tissues, cell damage is induced by a variety of mechanisms during both the freezing and thawing process, as well as indirect damage to the microcirculation. The method by which the cells die is related to the lowest temperature reached, the amount of time at subzero temperatures, and the number of freeze-thaw cycles (allowing the frozen tissue to thaw before freezing again).[31,32] Close to the cryoprobe, the freezing rates are high enough to induce freezing of the intracellular fluid, or intracellular ice formation.[29,33] This is a lethal event associated with irreversible membrane damage. Further from the probe, freezing rates are slower. Here, the extracellular fluid freezes, but the intracellular fluid has better protection by the lipid membrane. This situation leads to osmotic forces that shift pure water out of the cell, or cellular dehydration. When the tissue is thawed, the intracellular compartment is hypertonic, and as the ice melts, fluid rushes into the damaged membranes, and the cells burst.[34,35] In addition, large ice crystals may form during recrystallization in the warming period, and these create direct shearing forces, which further disrupt the tissues. When the freezing is repeated, the damaged tissue conducts the cold more efficiently, increasing the area of necrosis beyond the first cycle. Cells not killed by direct cryoinjury may also suffer apoptotic dell death secondary to cryoinduced destruction of the microvasculature and postthaw platelet aggregation and vascular stasis.[36]

## Clinical Experience

Initial experience with cryoablation for breast cancer centered on palliation of locally advanced disease.[37-39] An initial preclinical and clinical study of in situ cryoablation[40] led to several small series of cryoablation followed by surgical resection (**Table 2**). Pfleiderer and colleagues[41] treated 16 tumors of any size in 15 patients under ultrasound guidance. The investigators reported that for the 5 tumors smaller than 16 mm, there was no residual invasive cancer after cryoablation, whereas for the 11 tumors greater than 23 mm, ablation was incomplete. Following on this work, these investigators reported a series of 29 patients, limited to tumors 15 mm or smaller, and reported 100% ablation of the visualized tumor.[47,48] Similar findings were reported in 3 additional series of ultrasound-guided cryoablation. Niu and colleagues[43]

**Table 2**
**Studies of cryoablation followed by surgical excision**

| Reference | Location | N | Tumor Size (cm) | Complete Ablation (%) |
|---|---|---|---|---|
| Pfleiderer et al,[41] 2002 | Jena, Germany | 16 | 0.9–4.0 | 31 |
| Sabel et al,[42] 2004 | Multicenter, United States | 27 | 0.6–2.0 | 78 |
| Pfleiderer et al,[78] 2005 | Jena, Germany | 29 | 0.5–1.5 | 100 |
| Niu et al,[43] 2007 | Guangzhou, China | 27 | 0.8–2.5 | 85.2 |
| Morin et al,[44] 2007 | Quebec City, Canada | 25 | 1.2–6.0 | 52 |
| Pusztaszeri et al,[45] 2007 | Geneva, Switzerland | 11 | 0.5–2.6 | 20 |
| Manenti et al,[46] 2011 | Rome, Italy | 15 | 0.4–1.2 | 93 |

reported on 27 patients who underwent successful ultrasound-guided cryoablation, followed by surgery 8 to 35 days later. No invasive cancer was seen in 85.2% of the patients, and as with the study by Pfleiderer and colleagues, this was 100% when restricted to the patients with tumors less than 15 mm. Sabel and colleagues[42] reported on 27 patients treated as part of a multicenter trial, followed by surgery 7 to 30 days later. Complete ablation was seen in 21 (78%), with a success rate of 100% for all tumors smaller than 1.0 cm, and for tumors smaller than 1.5 cm if lobular carcinomas and those patients with an extensive intraductal component on their initial core biopsy were excluded. Manenti and colleagues,[46] limiting cryoablation to lesions 4 to 12 mm in size, had complete ablation in 14 of 15 (93%) patients, with the 1 patient having residual disease secondary to a technical failure. Morin and colleagues[44] treated 25 women, 4 weeks before their scheduled mastectomy. Using MRI guidance rather than ultrasound, these investigators attempted to treat larger tumors (only 2 were <2.0 cm). Complete ablation was achieved in only 13 of 25 women, but this study did show the ability of MRI (combined with scintomammography) to predict the histopathologic results, with an accuracy of 96%.

Two studies have looked at cryoablation alone, without surgical excision. Littrup and colleagues[30] treated 22 lesions in 11 patients who refused surgery. Using ultrasound and computed tomography guidance to place multiple cryoprobes (average of 3), 100% procedural success (defined as 1 cm visible ice around all tumor margins) was obtained, and with a mean follow-up of 18 months, there were no local recurrences. Fukuma and colleagues[49] have presented (but not published) results of 2 clinical trials of cryoablation alone for small breast cancer. In the first study, 38 patients with luminal A invasive ductal carcinoma or ductal carcinoma in situ (DCIS), less than 10 mm in size, were treated. With a median follow-up of 43 months, there were no local recurrences. In the second study, 20 similar patients were treated. MRI and core biopsy failed to detect residual disease after treatment.

### Challenges Moving Forward

Early on, breast cancer cryoablation was slow in building momentum, because the equipment needed (often requiring large tanks of gas) made it less desirable than, for example RFA, which requires only a table top device. However, with the increasing use of cryoablation in the treatment of several other malignancies, its US Food and Drug Administration (FDA)-approved use in the treatment of fibroadenomas of the breast, and design improvements that made the equipment more portable and user friendly, momentum has grown. Cryoablation seems to be the most popular ablative technique being investigated, as shown by the recently completed multicenter national trial of cryoablation by the American College of Surgeons Oncology Group (ACOSOG Z1072).

Before cryoablation becomes a viable alternative to lumpectomy, there are still several questions that need to be addressed. Outside the work by Littrup and colleagues,[30] most of the experience with cryoablation has been with a single cryoprobe, limiting treatment to small, well-visualized tumors. Further investigation is needed to determine if this is truly the optimal method for cryoablation. Although ultrasonography and MRI can be used to monitor the procedure, whether MRI can be used to select appropriate patients and accurately predict whether patients have had a complete ablation, or have residual disease after cryoablation (thus requiring excision), is unknown. This question is being examined in the Z1072 trial, and the results of this trial are anxiously awaited. However, the Z1072 trial examined the use of MRI within a few weeks of cryoablation. Inflammatory changes, which can be confused for residual enhancing tumor, can be seen up to 3 months after cryoablation. Further study of

MRI, and other breast imaging modalities, may be necessary to determine the appropriate before and after cryoimaging.

Although there is some experience with cryoablation without excision, there are still several unknowns about what happens to the cryolesion after treatment. After cryoablation of fibroadenoma, the lesion initially gets larger, and can take several months before it completely resorbs. This situation may not only be of psychological concern to patients who have breast cancer, but it is not clear how this might affect the delivery of radiation, and how radiation might affect the resorption of the lesion. In a case report by Littrup,[50] 1 patient did have radiation therapy 3 months after cryoablation (delayed to allow healing) and did report resorption of the mass to have stalled during radiation, although it resolved. Although cryoablation and radiation have been used in combination in the treatment of prostate cancer, there are unanswered questions about the timing and complications of radiation therapy to the breast after cryoablation, the impact on surveillance imaging, and the ability to detect recurrence.

## HIGH-INTENSITY FOCUSED ULTRASONOGRAPHY
### Mechanism

Ultrasound ablation is a truly noninvasive ablation technique, because it does not require the minimally invasive placement of a catheter or probe at the tumor site. Ultrasound beams are generated by an ultrasound transducer and propagate through tissue as a high-frequency pressure wave. When an ultrasound beam is focused at a specific point at a certain distance from the source, the acoustic energy is converted to heat, leading to tissue coagulation.[51] Using frequencies in the range of 0.5 to 4 MHz, it is possible to increase the temperature at the focal point during a single sonication to between 60°C and 95°C.[52]

A single ultrasound beam ablates only a small volume of tissue (approximately the size of a rice grain), so the skin and surrounding tissue show minimal temperature changes. However, the entire volume of the tumor (and margins) needs to be covered by overlapping multiple beams. This necessity increases the duration of the procedure compared with some of the other ablative techniques. This precise targeted procedure can be accomplished by using ultrasound guidance, or more commonly MRI guidance.

### Clinical Experience

There have been several studies examining the efficacy of high-intensity focused ultrasonography (HIFU) at ablating breast cancer. As with other forms of ablation, the initial studies consisted of HIFU followed by resection. Initial results were variable (**Table 3**). Zippel and Papa[55] achieved complete ablation in only 2 of 10 patients undergoing MR-guided focused ultrasonography 1 week before surgery. Gianfelice and colleagues[53,57,58] also reported the difficulty with residual cancer either outside the

**Table 3**
**Studies of focused ultrasonography followed by surgical excision**

| Reference | Location | N | Tumor Size (cm) | Complete Ablation (%) |
|-----------|----------|---|-----------------|----------------------|
| Gianfelice et al,[53] 2003 | Montreal, Canada | 17 | <3.5 | 24 |
| Wu et al,[54] 2003 | Chongqing, China | 23 | 2.0–4.7 | 100 |
| Zippel & Papa,[55] 2005 | Tel Hashomer, Israel | 10 | <3.0 | 20 |
| Furusawa et al,[56] 2006 | Miyazaki, Japan | 30 | 0.5–2.5 | 53.5 |
| Khiat et al,[57] 2006 | Montreal, Canada | 26 | 0.1–11.2 | 27 |

targeted area or at the periphery. Furusawa and colleagues[56] achieved complete ablation in 53.5% of 25 breast cancers undergoing treatment with a 5-mm margin. Wu and colleagues,[54] using a target that included 1.5 to 2.0 cm margin of normal tissue, achieved 100% ablation in 23 patients. In addition to showing the need to ablate a wide margin around the visualized tumor, these studies also showed the ability of MRI to assess residual disease after ablation, allowing selection of patients to proceed with radiation versus surgery or repeat ablation.

These studies subsequently led to trials of HIFU without surgical resection. In a study of patients who either refused surgery or were poor surgical candidates, Gianfelice and colleagues[59] ablated the tumor with MR-guided focused ultrasonography as an adjunct to their systemic therapy. Using both MRI and percutaneous biopsy to determine the presence of residual tumor, 10 of 24 patients underwent a second treatment. Overall, 19 of 24 patients (79%) achieved negative core biopsies. Wu and colleagues[60] reported long-term data from a trial in which 22 patients underwent ultrasound-guided HIFU, followed by chemotherapy, radiation therapy, and hormonal therapy. The 5-year recurrence-free survival rate was 89%, with the cosmetic result judged to be good to excellent by 94% of patients. Furisawa and colleagues[61] also reported 21 patients who underwent MRI-guided HIFU without surgical resection. With a mean follow-up of 14 months, 1 of 21 patients had a local recurrence.

### Challenges Moving Forward

Although the fact that HIFU is noninvasive (compared with cryoablation or RFA, which are minimally invasive) is in some ways advantageous, it is also challenging, in that there is a risk that if the target lesion moves during treatment, complete ablation might not be achieved. The biggest challenge facing the clinical implementation of HIFU for the treatment of breast cancer is the heterogeneity of the results, with histopathologic analysis showing complete tumor necrosis in 20% to 100% of patients treated. Ultrasound-guided HIFU is the only technique reporting 100% tumor necrosis, although MRI would be expected to be the most reliable imaging modality to delineate the tumor margins and guide the ablation. It may be that the difference is the significantly larger margins treated by this group than those using MRI-guided HIFU. However, treating large margins increases the size of the treatment zone considerably, which in the case of HIFU substantially increases treatment time, which is already a concern for this technology. It also decreases the population of eligible patients, excluding patients with larger tumors and tumors closer to the skin.

### MICROWAVE THERMOTHERAPY
#### Mechanism

Another truly noninvasive approach to breast cancer ablation is microwave ablation therapy. As with HIFU, no probe needs to be placed percutaneously. Instead, the breast is compressed between 2 microwave phased array waveguide applicators. Microwaves produce dielectric heat through the rapid agitation of water molecules within the tissue and the cells, leading to thermoinduced coagulation necrosis. It takes advantage of the fact that tissues with high water content, such as breast cancer cells, are preferentially heated compared with cells with less water content, such as adipose or connective tissue or the nonmalignant breast parenchyma.

#### Clinical Experience

There is minimal experience using microwave ablation, with most experience coming from a single group.[62–65] In their initial pilot study, Gardner and colleagues[62] performed focused microwave ablation before mastectomy and showed some tumor necrosis or apoptosis, but no complete ablation and several complications, including skin burn and flap necrosis. In a follow-up dose-escalation study,[65] the results were mildly improved, with a higher rate of necrosis (68%) and 2 of 25 women having complete ablation. Complications improved slightly as well.

### Challenges Moving Forward

Although the principle of microwave ablation is intriguing, the results have not supported its consideration as a potential alternative to lumpectomy.

## NOVEL TECHNOLOGIES

Although several modalities are being examined for breast cancer ablation, newer technologies continue to be developed. Irreversible electroporation (IRE) involves inserting needle electrodes in or around a tumor and then delivering short-length, high-voltage electric pulses.[66] Depending on the change in potential, the electroporation pulse can either reversibly open the cell membranes, allowing the cell to survive, or irreversibly open the cell membrane, resulting in cell death.[67] The former has been used to increase permeability to allow the introduction of small drugs or macromolecules to a targeted area,[68] whereas the latter can be used for percutaneous ablation of tumors.[69] The safety of IRE in humans was shown in a series of 30 patients with advanced malignancy, although it must be used with electrocardiographically synchronized delivery to minimize the risk of cardiac arrhythmias. The therapy has also been tested in large animals[70] and used (in addition to chemotherapy) for the successful treatment of a sarcoma in a dog.[71] In the only study looking at breast cancer, 5 of 7 mice with MDA-MB231 human mammary tissues implanted in Nu/Nu mice regressed after treatment. Further research is ongoing. However, given the complexity of the modeling, the need for general anesthesia, and the potential risks, the potential of IRE for the percutaneous ablation of early breast cancer is unclear.

An interesting new area of research is the use of nanoparticles to enhance tumor ablation. Because tumor vasculature is more porous than normal blood vessels, nanoparticles can accumulate within the tumor from the blood stream. Combining nanoparticles with antibodies can increase binding, allowing for improved imaging, drug delivery, and potentially, tumor ablation. Using magnetofluorescent gold nanoshells conjugated with monoclonal antibodies to HER2, Dowell and colleagues[72] showed the potential of these nanoshells to generate heat and cause hyperthermic cell death in an in vitro study of breast cancer. Sun and colleagues[73] used superparamagnetic poly(lactic-co-glycolic acid)–iron oxide nanoparticles in combination with HIFU to treat VX2 breast tumors in rabbits. The nanoparticles significantly improved the ability of HIFU to ablate the tumors, presumably by both changing the acoustic microenvironment and by improving the heat transfer rate.

## CONCERNS FOR THE FUTURE

A wide variety of technologies may be used in the ablation of a tumor in vivo. Some are minimally invasive (requiring the percutaneous placement of a probe or catheter[s]), whereas others are truly noninvasive. Some use hyperthermic ablation, some hypothermic, and others use physical destruction without a change in tissue temperature. Although each technology may have its own unique advantages and disadvantages, there are some common obstacles facing clinical implementation.

For many, it seems surprising that in situ ablation has seen a more rapid adoption in other tumor types, such as prostate, kidney, or liver, than it has in breast cancer, especially given the high incidence of breast cancer, the emphasis on cosmesis after treatment, and the sophistication of breast cancer imaging and image-guided interventions. However, although there may be several benefits to in situ ablation, when compared with the gold standard of lumpectomy, the incremental gains are less impressive than when compared with, for example, an alternative to partial nephrectomy or prostatectomy. Given the excellent results seen with breast conservation, with minimal morbidity and good rates of local control, there is little room for error when introducing a novel technology. For this reason, enthusiasm for approaches like ILT and microwave thermotherapy, which have limited data suggesting reliably achievable complete ablation, has understandably diminished.

Beyond the outcomes, lumpectomy is a simple procedure, with low morbidity and, for the most part, good cosmetic results. Therefore, technologies for tumor ablation need to show equal or lower morbidity and dramatically improved cosmesis. Avoidance of complications such as skin burns with hyperthermic modalities is critical, and although improved technique and patient selection have minimized this, it remains a concern. Ease of delivery is also a consideration. An ablative technology that is painful, such that it requires intravenous sedation or general anesthesia, represents a minor step forward compared with a minimally invasive or noninvasive technology, which can be performed with only local anesthetic in a doctor's office. The more complex a technology is, such that it can be performed only by a limited number of practitioners with the needed technical expertise, the less likely it will be adopted. Thus, more complex technologies, such as RFA or multiprobe cryoablation, have a greater hurdle to overcome in justifying their use.

Another obstacle is the steps necessary to show equivalency with breast conservation surgery. Most data are from ablate and resect studies, with strong data for cryoablation, HIFU, and RFA, but there is limited experience with ablation only trials. These data are summarized in **Table 4** and, as shown, have limited follow-up. What data do exist are from small, highly select groups of patients, and in some cases, remain unpublished. Although the completion of the ACOSOG Z1072 trial, a large-scale ablate and resect trial of cryoablation, represents a major step forward, a more concerted effort to design and implement multicenter trials is needed for in situ ablation to become a viable alternative to lumpectomy.

But what level of evidence is necessary for ablation to become a viable alternative? The next step seems obvious: there need to be large multicenter phase 2 trials examining ablation as an alternative to lumpectomy. These trials require adequate numbers and follow-up to ensure local recurrence rates on a par with breast conservation. They also need to carefully examine complication rates, cosmetic outcomes, and long-term impact on breast imaging. These trials understandably require a significant amount of time to accrue and follow, and as with many phase 2 trials, will be likely limited to select patients, with a low overall risk of local recurrence. But what about the next step after that? Is a prospective, randomized trial necessary before nonsurgical ablation becomes an accepted alternative to lumpectomy for select patients?

A model for this strategy comes from the adoption of accelerated partial breast irradiation (APBI) as an alternative to whole breast irradiation (WBI) for breast conservation. Many proponents and critics of nonsurgical ablation argue that a phase 3 randomized trial would be too difficult and costly given the low number of events, the number of patients required, and the difficulty accruing to surgical trials, in which patients have significant difficulty with randomization between 2 vastly different arms. However, it is feasible, and evidence for this theory comes from the joint NSABP (National Surgical Adjuvant Breast and Bowel Project) and RTOG (Radiation Therapy Oncology Group) trial (NSABP B-39/RTOG 0413) comparing APBI with WBI.[74] This

**Table 4**
**Studies of in situ ablation without surgical excision**

| Reference | N | Ablation | Tumor Size | Posttreatment Assessment | Results |
|---|---|---|---|---|---|
| Gianfelice et al,[59] 2003 | 24 | HIFU | 6–25 mm | MRI, core biopsy | 5 (21%) with residual disease |
| Wu et al,[60] 2003 | 22 | HIFU | <5 cm | MRI, single-photon emission computed tomography | 5-year recurrence-free survival of 89% |
| Oura et al,[22] 2007 | 52 | RFA | ≤2 cm | Fine-needle aspiration, MRI | No local recurrences after median follow/up of 15 mo |
| Furusawa et al,[61] 2007 | 21 | HIFU | 5–50 mm | MRI | 1 local recurrence (5%) with a mean follow-up of 14 mo |
| Littrup et al,[30] 2009 | 11 | Multiprobe cryo | Varied | MRI | No local recurrences after median follow-up of 18 mo |
| Yamamoto et al,[23] 2011 | 29 | RFA | ≤2 cm | Mammotome, MRI | No residual disease in 27/29 No local recurrences after median follow-up of 17 mo |
| Fukuma et al,[49] 2012 | 38 | Single-probe cryo | Luminal A or DCIS, ≤1 cm | MRI | No local recurrences after median follow-up of 43 mo |
| Fukuma et al,[49] 2012 | 20 | Single-probe cryo | Luminal A or DCIS, ≤1 cm | MRI, core biopsy | No residual disease |

trial, with local recurrence as the primary outcome, also requires many patients, yet is on target to meet its accrual goals. Nonetheless, in the absence of any prospective, randomized data supporting its use, it has become an option routinely offered to selected patients after breast conservation surgery, and the American Society of Breast Surgeons and American Society of Radiation Oncology have published guidelines for patient selection.[75,76] More recent evidence has suggested a possible increased local recurrence rate with brachytherapy.[77] Proponents of nonsurgical breast cancer ablation need to carefully examine both the positive and negative aspects of how APBI has become a clinical option in breast cancer treatment.

## SUMMARY

Although technologies for the nonsurgical ablation of breast cancer, such as cryoablation or HIFU, show clinical promise in early trials, more data are needed before these can be considered as viable alternatives to lumpectomy. Most current and pending data are from ablate and resect trials, with limited information from ablation alone trials. More information is needed on how nonsurgical ablation might affect subsequent radiation, adjuvant therapy, and breast imaging. Lumpectomy, with minimal complications, good cosmetic outcome, and excellent local control rates, is a daunting gold standard to compare with. The next level of clinical trials needs to be carefully designed so as to not only show equivalency with breast conserving surgery in regards to local control but also validate the potential advantages over lumpectomy to the patient. Care must be taken to discourage early adoption until there is adequate evidence supporting its use.

## REFERENCES

1. Akimov AB, Seregin VE, Rusanov KV, et al. Nd:YAG interstitial laser thermotherapy in the treatment of breast cancer. Lasers Surg Med 1998;22:257–67.
2. Dowlatshahi K, Francescatti DS, Bloom KJ. Laser therapy for small breast cancers. Am J Surg 2002;184:359–63.
3. Haraldsdoittir KH, Ivarsson K, Gootberg S, et al. Interstitial laser thermotherapy (ILT) of breast cancer. Eur J Surg Oncol 2008;34:739–45.
4. Harms SE. Percutaneous ablation of breast lesions by radiologists and surgeons. Breast Dis 2001;13:67–75.
5. Goldberg SN, Grassi CJ, Cardella JF, et al, Society of Interventional Radiology Technology Assessment Committee. Image-guided tumor ablation: standardization of terminology and reporting criteria. J Vasc Interv Radiol 2005;16:765–78.
6. Jeffrey SS, Birdwell RL, Ikeda DM, et al. Radiofrequency ablation of breast cancer. First report of an emerging technology. Arch Surg 1999;134:1064–8.
7. Izzo F, Thomas R, Delrio P, et al. Radiofrequency ablation in patients with primary breast carcinoma: a pilot study in 26 patients. Cancer 2001;92:2036–44.
8. Burak WE Jr, Agnese DM, Povoski SP, et al. Radiofrequency ablation of invasive breast carcinoma followed by delayed surgical excision. Cancer 2003;98:1369–76.
9. Hayashi AH, Silver SF, van der Westhuizen NG, et al. Treatment of invasive breast carcinoma with ultrasound-guided radiofrequency ablation. Am J Surg 2003;185:429–35.
10. Fornage BD, Sneige N, Ross MI, et al. Small (< or = 2-cm) breast cancer treated with US-guided radiofrequency ablation: feasibility study. Radiology 2004;231:215–24.
11. Noguchi M, Earashi M, Fujii H, et al. Radiofrequency ablation of small breast cancer followed by surgical resection. J Surg Oncol 2006;93:120–8.
12. Earashi M, Noguchi M, Motoyoshi A, et al. Radiofrequency ablation therapy for small breast cancer followed by immediate surgical resection or delayed mammotome excision. Breast Cancer 2007;14:39–47.
13. Medina-Franco H, Soto-Germes S, Ulloa-Gomez JL, et al. Radiofrequency ablation of invasive breast carcinomas: a phase II trial. Ann Surg Oncol 2008;15:1689–95.
14. Manenti G, Bolacchi F, Perretta T, et al. Small breast cancers: in vivo percutaneous US-guided radiofrequency ablation with dedicated cool-tip radiofrequency system. Radiology 2009;251:339–46.
15. Imoto S, Wada N, Sakemura N, et al. Feasibility study on radiofrequency ablation followed by partial mastectomy for stage I breast cancer patients. Breast 2009;18:130–4.
16. Wiksell H, Lofgren L, Schassburger KU, et al. Feasibility study on the treatment of small breast carcinoma using percutaneous US-guided preferential radiofrequency ablation (PRFA). Breast 2010;19:219–25.
17. Ohtani S, Kochi M, Ito M, et al. Radiofrequency ablation of early breast cancer followed by delayed surgical resection–a promising alternative to breast-conserving surgery. Breast 2011;20(5):431–6. http://dx.doi.org/10.1016/j.breast.2011.04.007.

18. Kreb DL, Looij BG, Ernst MF, et al. Ultrasound-guided radiofrequency ablation of early breast cancer in a resection specimen: lessons for further research. Breast 2013;22(4):543–7. http://dx.doi.org/10.1016/j.breast.2012.11.004.
19. Zhao Z, Wu F. Minimally-invasive thermal ablation of early-stage breast cancer: a systemic review. Eur J Surg Oncol 2010;36:1149–55.
20. Susini T, Nori J, Olivieri S, et al. Radiofrequency ablation for minimally invasive treatment of breast carcinoma. A pilot study in elderly inoperable patients. Gynecol Oncol 2007;1004:304–10.
21. Marcy PY, Magne N, Castadot P, et al. Ultrasound-guided percutaneous radiofrequency ablation in elderly breast cancer patients: preliminary institutional experience. Br J Radiol 2007;80:267–73.
22. Oura S, Tamaki T, Hirai I, et al. Radiofrequency ablation therapy in patients with breast cancers two centimeters or less in size. Breast Cancer 2007;14:48–54.
23. Yamamoto N, Fujimoto H, Nakamura R, et al. Pilot study of radiofrequency ablation therapy without surgical excision for T1 breast cancer. Breast Cancer 2011; 18:3–9.
24. Fornage BD, Edeiken BS. Percutaneous ablation of breast tumors. In: Sonnenberg E, McMullen W, Solbiati L, editors. Tumor Ablation: Principles and Practice. New York: Springer; 2005. p. 428–39.
25. Klimberg VS, Boneti C, Adkins LL, et al. Feasibility of percutaneous excision followed by ablation followed by local control in breast cancer. Ann Surg Oncol 2011;18:3079–87.
26. Klimberg VS, Kepple J, Shafirstein G, et al. eRFA: excision followed by RFA–a new technique to improve local control in breast cancer. Ann Surg Oncol 2006;13:1422–33.
27. Noguchi M, Motoyoshi A, Earashi M, et al. Long-term outcome of breast cancer patients treated with radiofrequency ablation. Eur J Surg Oncol 2012;38:1036–42.
28. Permpongkosol S, Nicol TL, Khurana H, et al. Thermal maps around two adjacent cryoprobes creating overlapping ablations in porcine liver, lung and kidney. J Vasc Interv Radiol 2007;18:283–7.
29. Rewcastle JC, Sandison GA, Muldrew K, et al. A model for the time dependent three-dimensional thermal distribution within iceballs surrounding multiple cryoprobes. Med Phys 2001;28:1125–37.
30. Littrup PJ, Jallad B, Chandiwala-Mody P, et al. Cryotherapy for breast cancer: a feasibility study without excision. J Vasc Interv Radiol 2009;20:1329–41.
31. Smith DJ, Fahssi WM, Swanlund DJ, et al. A parametric study of freezing injury in AT-1 rat prostate tumor cells. Cryobiology 1999;39:13–28.
32. Rui J, Tatsutani KN, Dahiya R, et al. Effect of thermal variables on human breast cancer in cryosurgery. Breast Cancer Res Treat 1999;53:185–92.
33. Bischof JC, Smith D, Pazhayannur PV, et al. Cryosurgery of dunning AT-1 rat prostate tumor: thermal, biophysical, and viability response at the cellular and tissue level. Cryobiology 1997;34:42–69.
34. Zhang A, Xu LX, Sandison GA, et al. A microscale model for prediction of breast cancer cell damage during cryosurgery. Cryobiology 2003;47:143–54.
35. Gage AA, Baust J. Mechanisms of tissue injury in cryosurgery. Cryobiology 1998;37:171–86.
36. Baust JM, Van B, Baust JG. Cell viability improves following inhibition of cryopreservation-induced apoptosis. In Vitro Cell Dev Biol Anim 2000;36:262–70.
37. Tartour E, Dorval T, Mosseri V, et al. Serum interleukin-6 and C-reactive protein levels correlate with resistance to IL-2 therapy and poor survival in melanoma patients. Br J Cancer 1994;69:911–3.

38. Tanaka S. Cryosurgical treatment of advanced breast cancer. Skin Cancer 1995; 10:9–18.
39. Suzuki Y. Cryosurgical treatment of advanced breast cancer and cryoimmuno-logical responses. Skin Cancer 1995;10:19–26.
40. Staren ED, Sabel MS, Gianakakis LM, et al. Cryosurgery of breast cancer. Arch Surg 1997;132:28–33 [discussion: 34].
41. Pfleiderer SO, Freesmeyer MG, Marx C, et al. Cryotherapy of breast cancer under ultrasound guidance: initial results and limitations. Eur Radiol 2002;12:3009–14.
42. Sabel MS, Kaufman CS, Whitworth P, et al. Cryoablation of early-stage breast cancer: work-in-progress report of a multi-institutional trial. Ann Surg Oncol 2004;11:542–9.
43. Niu LZ, Xu KC, He WB, et al. Efficacy of percutaneous cryoablation for small solitary breast cancer in term pathologic evidence. Technol Cancer Res Treat 2007;6:460–1.
44. Morin J, Traore' A, Dionne G, et al. Magnetic resonance-guided percutaneous cryosurgery of breast carcinoma: technique and early clinical results. Can J Surg 2007;47:347–51.
45. Pusztaszeri M, Vlastos G, Kinkel K, et al. Histopathological study of breast cancer and normal breast tissue after magnetic resonance-guided cryotherapy ablation. Cryobiology 2007;55(1):44–51.
46. Manenti G, Perretta T, Gaspari E, et al. Percutaneous local ablation of unifocal subclinical breast cancer: clinical experience and preliminary results of cryo-therapy. Eur Radiol 2011;21:2344–53.
47. Berwick M, Armstrong BK, Ben-Porat L, et al. Sun exposure and mortality from melanoma. J Natl Cancer Inst 2005;97:195–9.
48. Holick MF. Vitamin D deficiency. N Engl J Med 2007;357:266–81.
49. Fukuma E, Nakashima H, Tozaki M. Nonsurgical cryoablation for small breast cancer (oral presentation). In: American Society of Breast Surgeons 13th Annual Meeting, Edition. Phoenix, April 27–May 1, 2012.
50. Littrup P. Breast ablation for breast imagers and interventional radiologists. In: Dupay DE, editor. Image-guided cancer therapy, edition. New York: Springer Science-Business Media; 2013. p. 857–76.
51. Cline HE, Hynynen K, Watkins RD, et al. Focused US system for MR imaging-guided tumor ablation. Radiology 1995;194:731–47.
52. Schmitz AC, Gianfelice D, Daniel BL, et al. Image-guided focused ultrasound ablation of breast cancer: current status, challenges, and future directions. Eur Radiol 2008;18:1431–41.
53. Gianfelice D, Khiat A, Amara M, et al. MRI imaging-guided focused ultrasound surgery of breast cancer: correlation of dynamic contrast-enhanced MRI with histopathologic findings. Breast Cancer Res Treat 2003;12:32–8.
54. Wu F, Wang ZB, Cao YD, et al. A randomized clinical trial of high-intensity focused ultrasound ablation for the treatment of patients with localized breast cancer. Br J Cancer 2003;89:2227–33.
55. Zippel DB, Papa MZ. The use of MR imaging guided focused ultrasound in breast cancer patients; a preliminary phase one study and review. Breast Cancer 2005;12:32–8.
56. Furusawa H, Namba K, Thomsen S, et al. Magnetic resonance-guided focused ultrasound surgery of breast cancer: reliability and effectiveness. J Am Coll Surg 2006;203:54–63.
57. Khiat A, Gianfelice D, Amara M, et al. Influence of post-treatment delay on the evaluation of the response to focused ultrasound surgery by breast cancer by dynamic contrast enhanced MRI. Br J Radiol 2006;79:308–14.

58. Gianfelice D, Khiat A, Amara M, et al. Imaging-guided focused US ablation of breast cancer: histopathologic assessment of effectiveness–initial experience. Radiology 2003;227:849–55.

59. Gianfelice D, Khiat A, Boulanger Y, et al. Feasibility of magnetic resonance imaging-guided focused ultrasound surgery as an adjuvant to tamoxifen therapy in high-risk surgical patients with breast carcinoma. J Vasc Interv Radiol 2003;14:1275–82.

60. Wu F, Wang ZB, Zhu H, et al. Extracorporeal high intensity focused ultrasound treatment for patients with breast cancer. Breast Cancer Res Treat 2005;92:51–60.

61. Furusawa H, Namba K, Nakahara H, et al. The evolving non-surgical ablation of breast cancer: MR guided focused ultrasound (MRgFUS). Breast Cancer 2007; 14:55–8.

62. Gardner RA, Vargas HI, Block JB, et al. Focused microwave phased array thermotherapy for primary breast cancer. Ann Surg Oncol 2002;9:326–32.

63. Fenn AJ, Wolf GL, Fogle RM. An adaptive microwave phased array for targeted heating of deep tumours in intact breast: animal study results. Int J Hyperthermia 1999;15:45–61.

64. Vargas HI, Dooley WC, Garnder RA, et al. Success of sentinel lymph node mapping after breast cancer ablation with focused microwave phased array thermotherapy. Am J Surg 2003;186:330–2.

65. Vargas HI, Dooley WC, Garnder RA, et al. Focused microwave phased array thermotherapy for ablation of early-stage breast cancer: results of thermal dose escalation. Ann Surg Oncol 2004;11:139–46.

66. Weaver JC, Chizmadzhev YA. Theory of electroporation: a review. Bioelectrochem Bioenerg 1996;41:135–60.

67. Neal RE, Singh R, Hatcher HC, et al. Treatment of breast cancer through the application of irreversible electroporation using a novel minimally invasive single needle electrode. Breast Cancer Res Treat 2010;123:295–301.

68. Mir LM. Mechanisms of electrochemotherapy. Adv Drug Deliv Rev 1999;35: 107–18.

69. Al-Sakere B, Andre F, Bernat C, et al. Tumor ablation with irreversible electroporation. PLoS One 2007;2:e1135.

70. Edd JF, Davalos RV. Mathematical modeling of irreversible electroporation for treatment planning. Technol Cancer Res Treat 2007;6:275–86.

71. Neal RE, Rossmeisi JH, Garcia PA, et al. Successful treatment of a large soft tissue sarcoma with irreversible electroporation. J Clin Oncol 2011;29:e372–7.

72. Dowell A, Chen W, Biswal N, et al. Calibrating the imaging and therapy performance of magneto-fluorescent gold nanoshells for breast cancer. In Proc. SPIE 8233, Reports, Markers, Dyes, Nanoparticals and Molecular Probes for Biomedical Applications, Edition. 2012.

73. Sun Y, Zheng Y, Ran H, et al. Superparamagnetic PLGA-iron oxide microcapsules for dual-modality US/MR imaging and high intensity focused US breast cancer ablation. Biomaterials 2012;33:5854–64.

74. Julian TB, Costantino JP, Vicini FA, et al. A randomized phase III study of conventional whole breast irradiation vs partial breast irradiation (PBI) for women with stage 0, 1 or 2 breast cancer. NSABP B-39/RTOG 0413 (Abstract OT2-06-02). Cancer Res 2011;71:618s.

75. American Society of Breast Surgeons. Consensus statement for accelerated partial breast irradiation. Available at: https://www.breastsurgeons.org/statements/PDF_Statements/APBI_statement_revised_100708.pdf. Accessed April 22, 2014.

76. Smith BD, Arthur DW, Buchholz TA, et al. Accelerated partial breast irradiation consensus statement from the American Society for Radiation Oncology (ASTRO). Int J Radiat Oncol Biol Phys 2009;74:987–1001.

77. Smith GL, Xu Y, Buccholz TA, et al. Association between treatment with brachytherapy vs whole-breast irradiation and subsequent mastectomy, complications and survival among older women with invasive breast cancer. JAMA 2012;307: 1827–37.

78. Pfleiderer SO, Marx C, Camara O, et al. Ultrasound-guided, percutaneous cryotherapy of small (<15mm) breast cancers. Invest Radiol 2005;40(7):472–7.

# Surgical Leadership and Standardization of Multidisciplinary Breast Cancer Care

## The Evolution of the National Accreditation Program for Breast Centers

Jessica Bensenhaver, MD[a],*, David P. Winchester, MD[b,c]

KEYWORDS

• Multidisciplinary breast cancer care • Breast cancer • Breast center • NAPBC

KEY POINTS

• Multidisciplinary team approach is the preferred method of cancer care both nationally and internationally.
• Multidisciplinary care has resulted in better outcomes.
• The National Accreditation Program for Breast Centers has helped standardized multidisciplinary breast cancer care.

## HISTORY OF MULTIDISCIPLINARY CARE

The concept of establishing a multidisciplinary approach to cancer care initiated in the early 1990s after observational evidence identified better outcomes among patients treated by specialists for various common cancers.[1] The Calman-Hine report was published in the European system to address discrepancies of cancer care.[2] This report proposed that all patients with cancer should be seen by surgeons who specialized in their type of cancer, who worked with colleagues in multidisciplinary teams.[3] Specifically for breast cancer, the multidisciplinary approach was introduced following report of better local and regional treatment of disease by specialist surgeons,[4] with

---

No Disclosures.
[a] Department of Surgery, University of Michigan Health System, 1500 East Medical Center Drive, Ann Arbor, MI 48109, USA; [b] Cancer Programs, American College of Surgeons, 633 North Saint Clair Street, Chicago, IL 60611-3211, USA; [c] Department of Surgery, NorthShore University HealthSystem, Evanston Hospital, 2650 Ridge Avenue, Evanston, IL 60201, USA
* Corresponding author.
E-mail address: jbensenh@umich.edu

Surg Oncol Clin N Am 23 (2014) 609–616
http://dx.doi.org/10.1016/j.soc.2014.03.005
1055-3207/14/$ – see front matter © 2014 Elsevier Inc. All rights reserved.

a reported 11% to 17% reduction in risk of death among women treated for breast cancer by specialist surgeons[5] and a survival benefit between specialist and nonspecialist breast cancer surgeons.[6]

Today many countries, including the United States, use multidisciplinary teams as the preferred method of delivering cancer care.[7–11] The team is composed of surgeons, clinical and medical oncologists, specialist nurses, radiologists, pathologists, and others who operate along the whole care pathway from diagnosis to follow-up and beyond.[7] Patients are discussed at many points along the treatment pathway, initially at diagnosis, following each treatment, and also at times of recurrence or progression.[12] The key task of the team during a multidisciplinary team meeting, often under the leadership of a surgical oncologist, is to collate and review information about the patient and their disease, discuss it, and make a decision for further investigation and treatment.[13,14]

## STANDARDIZATION OF THE MULTIDISCIPLINARY BREAST CANCER CARE

Since the introduction of multidisciplinary teams in breast cancer care, there have been concerns as to whether improved survival is due to earlier detection, improved treatment, improved organized care, or a combination of each.[15] An international review of 21 studies in 2010, including 5 on breast cancer, cited 3 reasons for inability to identify a causal relationship between multidisciplinary teams and cancer survival, including an imprecise and heterogeneous definition of multidisciplinary care.[16] An intervention study in 2012 aimed to address this dilemma found that multidisciplinary teams for breast cancer were associated with 18% lower breast cancer mortality at 5 years and 11% lower all-cause mortality at 5 years.[15] Although evidence suggests survival advantage due to local and regional treatment by specialist surgeons,[4] surgical specialty alone is unlikely to explain the survival advantage seen with a multidisciplinary team.[15]

Breast care deficiencies, including fragmented evaluation and management, led Silverstein[17] to pioneer the first free-standing breast center in the United States in 1979, the Van Nuys Breast Center. Since Silverstein's center, there has been an exponential increase in the number of breast centers across the United States with the purpose of conducting high-quality, timely multidisciplinary team evaluation and management of both benign and malignant breast disease. These breast centers were focused multidisciplinary facilities of excellence that dealt with the complete range of breast problems; however, there was diversity across the centers and across their stated missions without an established definition of what constitutes a quality program. Recognizing that evidence-based and consensus-developed standards have gained increasing importance and recognition, the US health care system has concentrated on quality measurement and improvement with documentation of adherence to accepted standards of care. Accreditation of facilities and provider reporting are becoming expectations.

The National Consortium of Breast Centers has defined many breast center variations.[18] The European Accreditation of Breast Units was founded in 1986 to establish breast center standards in Europe. No similar body existed in the United States until 2008 when the National Accreditation Program for Breast Centers (NAPBC) was strategically built by the experts that deliver breast disease care to offer credible evidence-based standards for existing breast centers. Getting there started with Silverstein's Van Nuys Breast Center, the prototype model for most breast centers developed in the United States.[17] The evaluation and management offered in these centers have been standardized with the establishment the NAPBC.

**Box 1**
**Breast Center Components recommended by the NAPBC**

1. Imaging
   a. Screening mammography
   b. Diagnostic mammography (additional views beyond screening mammography and workup of a clinical abnormality)
   c. Ultrasound
   d. Breast magnetic resonance imaging (MRI)
2. Needle biopsy
   a. Needle biopsy—palpation-guided
   b. Image guided—stereotactic
   c. Image guided—ultrasound
   d. Image guided—MRI
3. Pathology
   a. Report completeness/College of American Pathologists (CAP) protocols
   b. Radiology-pathology correlation
   c. Prognostic and predictive indicators
   d. Gene studies (if available)
4. Interdisciplinary conference
   a. History and findings
   b. Imaging studies
   c. Pathology
   d. Pretreatment and posttreatment interdisciplinary discussion
5. Patient navigation
   a. Facilitates navigation through system
6. Genetic evaluation and management
   a. Genetic risk assessment
   b. Genetic counseling
   c. Genetic testing
7. Surgical care
   a. Surgical correlation with imaging/concordance
   b. Preoperative planning after biopsy
   c. Breast surgery: lumpectomy or mastectomy
   d. Lymph node surgery: sentinel node/axillary dissection
   e. After initial surgical correlation/treatment planning
8. Plastic surgery consultation/treatment
   a. Tissue expander/implants
   b. Transverse rectus abdominis myocutaneous (TRAM)/latissimus flaps
   c. Deep inferior epigastric perforator (DIEP) flap/free flap (if available)

9. Nursing
   a. Nurses with specialized knowledge and skills in diseases of the breast
10. Medical oncology consultation/treatment
    a. Hormone therapy
    b. Chemotherapy
    c. Biologics
    d. Chemoprevention
11. Radiation oncology consultation/treatment
    a. Whole breast irradiation with or without boost
    b. Regional nodal irradiation
    c. Partial breast irradiation treatment or protocols
    d. Palliative radiation for bone or systemic metastasis
    e. Stereotactic radiation for isolated or limited brain metastasis
12. Data management
    a. Data collection and submission
13. Research
    a. Cooperative trials
    b. Institutional original research (not part of national trials)
    c. Industry sponsored trials
14. Education, support, and rehabilitation
    a. Education along continuum of care (pretreatment, during, after treatment)
    b. Psychosocial support
       i. Individual support
       ii. Family support
       iii. Support groups
    c. Symptom management
    d. Physical therapy (ie, lymphedema risk, shoulder range of motion)
15. Outreach and education
    a. Community at-large education (including low-income/medically underserved)
    b. Patient education
    c. Physician education
16. Quality improvement
    a. Continuous quality improvement through annual studies
17. Survivorship program
    a. Follow-up surveillance
    b. Rehabilitation
    c. Health promotion/risk reduction

*Adapted from* National Accreditation Program for Breast Centers. 2013 NAPBC Breast Cancer standards manual. Chicago: American College of Surgeons; 2013. Available at: http://napbc-breast.org/standards/2013standardsmanual.pdf. Accessed March 5, 2014.

**Box 2**
**Breast Center Standards recommended by the NAPBC**

*Standard 1: Center leadership*

Purpose: To establish the medical director and/or co-directors, or interdisciplinary steering committee as the breast program leadership (BPL) responsible and accountable for breast center activities.

- *Standard 1.1—Level of Responsibility and Accountability:* The organizational structure of the breast center is in accord with the BPL responsibility and accountability for provided breast center services.

- *Standard 1.2—Interdisciplinary Breast Cancer Conference:* The BPL establishes, monitors, and evaluates the interdisciplinary breast cancer conference frequency, multidisciplinary and individual attendance prospective case presentation, and total case presentation annually, including American Joint Committee on Cancer (AJCC) staging and discussion of nationally accepted guidelines.

- *Standard 1.3—Evaluation and Management Guidelines:* The BPL identifies and references evidence-based breast care evaluation and management guidelines.

*Standard 2: Clinical Management*

Purpose: To identify the scope of clinical services needed to provide quality breast care to patients. The managing physician is essential to coordinating a multidisciplinary team approach to patient care.

- *Standard 2.1—Interdisciplinary Patient Management:* After diagnosis of breast cancer, the patient management is conducted by an interdisciplinary team.

- *Standard 2.2—Patient Navigation:* A patient navigation process is in place to guide the patient with a breast abnormality through provided and referred services.

- *Standard 2.3—Breast Conservation:* At least 50% of all eligible patients diagnosed with early-stage breast cancer (stage 0, I, II) are treated with breast-conserving surgery (BCS), and the BCS rate is evaluated annually by the BPL.

- *Standard 2.4—Sentinel Node Biopsy:* Axillary sentinel lymph node biopsy is considered or performed for patients with early-stage breast cancer (clinical stage I, II), and compliance is evaluated annually by the BPL.

- *Standard 2.5—Breast Cancer Surveillance:* A plan is in place for assuring follow-up surveillance of patients with breast cancer.

- *Standard 2.6—Breast Cancer Staging:* The BPL develops a process to monitor physician use of AJCC staging in treatment planning for patients with breast cancer. The process and results of such monitoring are discussed among the BPL and breast center staff, and the findings are documented annually.

- *Standard 2.7—Pathology Reports:* The CAP Committee guidelines are followed for all breast cancers, including estrogen and progesterone receptors, and Her2 status for all invasive breast cancers. Estrogen is recommended for ductal carcinoma in situ (DCIS).

- *Standard 2.8—Diagnostic Imaging:* Screening mammography and diagnostic mammography are performed at Mammography Quality Standards Act (MQSA)-certified facilities and interpreted by MQSA-certified physicians.

- *Standard 2.9—Needle biopsy:* Palpation-guided or image-guided needle biopsy is the initial diagnostic approach rather than open biopsy.

- *Standard 2.10—Ultrasonography:* Diagnostic ultrasound and/or ultrasound-guided needle biopsy are performed by an American College of Radiology (ACR) ultrasound-accreted facility or by and American Society of Breast Surgeons (ASBS) Breast Ultrasound-certified surgeon.

- *Standard 2.11—Stereotactic Core Needle Biopsy:* Biopsy is performed at an ACR accredited facility, or by surgeons under the standards and requirements developed by the ACR and American College of Surgeons and by an ASBS Breast Procedure Program-certified surgeon.

- *Standard 2.12—Radiation Oncology:* Treatment services are provided by or referred to radiation oncologists that are board certified or in the process of board certification; the center either has been accredited by the ACR/American Society for Radiation Oncology Accreditation Program or has a quality assurance program in place, and the breast cancer quality measure endorsed by the National Quality Forum (NQF) for radiation therapy is used.

- *Standard 2.13—Medical Oncology:* Treatment services are provided by or referred to medical oncologists that are board certified or in the process of board certification, and the breast cancer quality measures endorsed by the NQF for medical oncology are used.

- *Standard 2.14—Nursing:* Care is provided by or referred to nurses with specialized knowledge and skills in diseases of the breast. Nursing assessment and interventions are guided by evidence-based standards of practice and symptom management.

- *Standard 2.15—Support and Rehabilitation:* Services are provided by or referred to clinicians with specialized knowledge of diseases of the breast.

- *Standard 2.16—Genetic Evaluation and Management:* Cancer risk assessment, genetic counseling, and genetic testing services are provided or referred.

- *Standard 2.17—*Culturally appropriate educational recourses are available for patients along with a process to provide them. The materials provided are reviewed on an annual basis and adjusted for the patient population.

- *Standard 2.18—Reconstructive Surgery:* All appropriate patients undergoing mastectomy are offered a preoperative referral to a reconstructive/plastic surgeon. Reconstructive surgery is provided by or referred to reconstructive/plastic surgeons that are board certified or in the process of board certification. Compliance is evaluated annually by the BPL.

- *Standard 2.19—Benign Breast Disease:* The evaluation and management follow nationally recognized guidelines.

*Standard 3: Research*

Purpose: To promote advancement in prevention, early diagnosis, and treatment through the provision of clinical trial information and patient accrual to breast cancer–related clinical trials and research protocols.

- *Standard 3.1—Clinical Trial information:* Information about the availability of breast cancer–related clinical trials is provided to patients through a formal mechanism.

- *Standard 3.2—Clinical Trial Accrual:* 2% or more of all eligible patients with breast cancer are accrued to treatment-related breast cancer clinical trials and/or research protocols annually.

*Standard 4: Community Outreach*

Purpose: To ensure that breast cancer education, prevention, and early detection opportunities are provided to the community, patients, and their families.

- *Standard 4.1—Education, Prevention, and Early Detection Programs:* Each year, 2 or more breast cancer education, prevention, and/or early-detection programs are provided on-site or coordinated with other facilities or local agencies targeted to the community and follow-up is provided to patients with positive findings.

*Standard 5: Professional Education*

Purpose: To promote increased knowledge of breast center staff through participation in local, regional, or national educational activities.

- *Standard 5.1—Breast Center Staff Education:* Professionally certified/credentialed members of the breast cancer staff participate in local (in addition to breast cancer conference attendance), state, regional, or national breast-specific educational programs annually.

*Standard 6: Quality Improvement*

Purpose: To ensure that breast services, care, and patient outcomes are continuously evaluated and improved.

- *Standard 6.1—Quality and Outcomes:* Each year the breast program leadership conducts or participates in 2 or more studies that measure quality and/or outcomes and the findings are communicated and discussed with the breast center staff, participants of the interdisciplinary conference, or the cancer committee, where applicable.

- *Standard 6.2—Quality Improvement:* Annual performance rates are reported for each of the measures identified by the NAPBC, and performance is evaluated annually by the BPL.

*Adapted from* National Accreditation Program for Breast Centers. 2013 NAPBC Breast Cancer standards manual. Chicago: American College of Surgeons; 2013. Available at: http://napbc-breast.org/standards/2013standardsmanual.pdf. Accessed March 5, 2014.

## THE NATIONAL ACCREDITATION PROGRAM FOR BREAST CENTERS

The NAPBC Mission Statement states the following: The NAPBC is a consortium of national, professional organizations focused on breast health and dedicated to the improvement of quality care and outcomes of patients with diseases of the breast through evidence-based standards and patient and professional education.

The NAPBC Standards Manual clearly defines the standards of what accredited centers demonstrate. These standards include a multidisciplinary team approach to coordinate the best care and treatment options available. These centers provide access to breast cancer–related information, education, and support. All the subspecialties involved in breast cancer diagnosis and treatment undergo data collection for quality indicators. The centers will have information about clinical trials and new treatment options, and there is ongoing monitoring and improvement of care. Accreditation is only awarded after a successful survey process and thorough full-day site visit. It maintains annual reporting and regular reaccreditation.[19]

NAPBC accreditation for a breast center is accomplished once this high level of standardized care is met by commitment to 17 component services offered (**Box 1**) and 6 categories of standards (**Box 2**) as defined by the NAPBC Standards Manual.[19] The categories include center leadership (3 standards), clinical management (19 standards), research (2 standards), community outreach standards (1 standard), professional education (1 standard), and quality improvement (2 standards).

The NAPBC has accomplished standardization of multidisciplinary breast cancer care. No breast centers are exactly alike with models varying from freestanding to institution-based, from physician-owned to hospital-owned, from imaging-only to comprehensive support programs, from cancer center–affiliated to women's center–affiliated, and all the intervening gradations.[19] Regardless of modeling, having accreditation is a fundamental component for a successful breast center because it clearly defines the center as one that understands and adheres to strict criteria across each discipline that meets or exceeds national expectations.

## REFERENCES

1. Selby P, Gillis C, Haward R. Benefits from specialized cancer care. Lancet 1996; 348:313–8.
2. Expert Advisory Group on Cancer. A policy framework for commissioning cancer services: a report to the chief medical officers of England and Wales. The Calman–Hine Report. London: Department of Health; 1995.

3. Tattersall MH. Multidisciplinary team meetings: where is the value? Lancet 2006; 7:886–8.
4. Kingsmore D, Hole D, Gillis C. Why does specialist treatment of breast cancer improve survival? The role of surgical management. Br J Cancer 2004;90:1920.
5. Kingsmore D, Ssemwogerere A, Hole D, et al. Specialization and breast cancer survival in the screening era. Br J Cancer 2003;88:1708–12.
6. Gillis CR, Hole DJ. Survival outcome of care by specialist surgeons in breast cancer: a study of 3786 patients in the west of Scotland. BMJ 1996;312:145–8.
7. The Department of Health. Manual for cancer services. London: The Department of Health; 2004.
8. McAvoy B. Optimising cancer care in Australia. Melbourne: National cancer control initiative. Aust Fam Physician 2003;32:369–72.
9. American College of Surgeons: Commission on Cancer. Cancer program standards. Chicago: American College of Surgeons; 2004. Revised 2009. Available at: http://facs.org/cancer/coc/cocprogramstandards.pdf.
10. Wright FC, De Vito C, Langer B, et al. Multidisciplinary cancer conferences: a systematic review and development of practice standards. Eur J Cancer 2007;43: 1002–10.
11. Chan WF, Cheung PS, Epstein RJ, et al. Multidisciplinary approach to the management of breast cancer in Hong Kong. World J Surg 2007;30:2095–100.
12. Lamb BW, Taylor C, Lamb JN, et al. Facilitators and barriers to teamworking and patient centeredness in Multidisciplinary Cancer Teams: Findings of a National study. Ann Surg Oncol 2013;20:1408–16.
13. Fleissig A, Jenkins V, Catt S, et al. Multidisciplinary teams in cancer care: are they effective in the UK? Lancet Oncol 2006;7:935–43.
14. Lamb BW, Brown KF, Nagpal K, et al. Quality of care management decisions by multidisciplinary cancer teams: a systematic review. Ann Surg Oncol 2011;18: 2116–25.
15. Kesson EM, Allardice GM, George DW, et al. Effects of multidisciplinary team working on breast cancer survival: retrospective, comparative, interventional cohort study of 13722 women. BMJ 2012;344:2718–26.
16. Hong NJ, Wright F, Gagliardi A, et al. Examining the potential relationship between multidisciplinary cancer care and patient survival: an international literature review. J Surg Oncol 2010;102:125–34.
17. Silverstein MJ. The Van Nuys Breast Center: the first free-standing multidisciplinary breast center. Surg Oncol Clin N Am 2000;9(2):159–75.
18. Lee CZ. Comprehensive breast centers: Priorities and pitfalls. Breast J 1999;5(5): 319–24.
19. American College of Surgeons: 2013 NAPBC Breast Cancer Standards Manual. Chicago. Available at: http://napbc-breast.org/standards/2013standardsmanual. pdf. Accessed March 5, 2014.

# Index

*Note:* Page numbers of article titles are in **boldface** type.

Surg Oncol Clin N Am 23 (2014) 617–627
http://dx.doi.org/10.1016/S1055-3207(14)00041-6
1055-3207/14/$ – see front matter © 2014 Elsevier Inc. All rights reserved.

surgonc.theclinics.com

# Moving?

## Make sure your subscription moves with you!

To notify us of your new address, find your **Clinics Account Number** (located on your mailing label above your name), and contact customer service at:

**Email: journalscustomerservice-usa@elsevier.com**

**800-654-2452** (subscribers in the U.S. & Canada)
**314-447-8871** (subscribers outside of the U.S. & Canada)

**Fax number: 314-447-8029**

**Elsevier Health Sciences Division**
**Subscription Customer Service**
**3251 Riverport Lane**
**Maryland Heights, MO 63043**

ELSEVIER

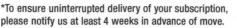

Printed and bound by CPI Group (UK) Ltd, Croydon, CR0 4YY

03/10/2024

01040491-0004